From the Gita to the Grail

Exploring Yoga Stories and Western Myths

Bernie Clark

Blue River Press
Indianapolis

www.brpressbooks.com

From the Gita to the Grail © 2014 Bernie Clark
ISBN: 9781935628316
Library of Congress Control Number: 2013950236

Cover designed by Heather Phillips
Packaged by Wish Publishing

Printed in the United States of America
10 9 8 7 6 5 4 3 2 1

Distributed in the United States by
Cardinal Publishers Group
www.cardinalpub.com

For Sam, Cillian and Toby

May you dream mythic dreams
May they fire your imagination
May you visit new and old realms –
Deep and profound
May you be whole

Table of Contents

Preface

You can hear the music even in the stairwell as you climb the three floors to the studio that sits just above the everyday world of downtown Manhattan. The beat is strange and foreign and you cannot quite catch the words, but you think they are chanting Sita and Rama, Govinda and Radha—unfamiliar names. Upon opening the door to the studio, other senses awaken; while your eyes are dazzled by the bright colors, wafting incense tells you that you are not in Kansas anymore—you have taken a step beyond your ordinary world, a cause to pause at the threshold. Your friend takes your arm and gently urges you in. Behind the receptionist, who is dressed in a brightly colored printed top with the image of a man with an elephant's head, you see a big wooden sign that says something like "30"—it is hand-carved in looping swirls. On the counter is a statue of some fellow with four arms and two legs, one of which is raised, the other perched on an unidentifiable creature. A snake loops his hips like a belt, his hair is wild and wavy, and a ring of fire surrounds the whole scene. Your friend sees where you are looking and names the images: on the wall is the symbol Om, the primordial sound of the universe, and the statue is the Hindu deity Shiva, dancing. Your mind and your senses are overwhelmed: What have you gotten yourself into? Welcome to your first yoga class!

The studio is weird, and you feel a bit uneasy. A video is playing on a screen mounted in a corner of the room, showing a man flowing through his practice, moving like a Cirque du Soleil acrobat, perfectly sculpted and consciously serene in his movements. You can't move like that—never in a million years! Looking at the other students, you notice that they are mostly women, and mostly very fit-looking, flexible, young women. Your resolve begins to waver; you know you don't belong here. You told your friend that you *can't* do yoga and that you are too inflexible. She simply responded by saying that was like being too dirty to take a shower. Then she reminded you why you needed to come: Your life is way too stressful; you have put on more weight than you'd like; and you are easily tired. Even just climbing the three flights of stairs to reach the studio winded you. You need to do something to get back some control over what's been happening to you—and now you find yourself in this very strange land.

This is a book about stories and myths for people who love stories and who love to understand what the stories mean down deep inside. It is a book for yogis of the West who frequently encounter all kinds of images taken from the East, but to whom those images seem quaint or meaningless. The Eastern stories are fun, although on first contact they have no power to stir us. After all, we were raised on different stories: stories of Romeo and Juliet, Lancelot and Guinevere, and even Tristan and Isolde—Western stories. We know little or nothing of Rama and Sita, or Krishna and Radha. We have at least heard about Yahweh, Allah and Jesus, but Brahma, Vishnu and Shiva are cartoon creatures to us. We know about the great flood, the Garden of Eden, *the* Virgin Birth, but nothing about great floods that come in grand cycles, about heavens and hells that come and go, about the multitude of virgin births—Eastern ideas that sound very strange to our ears. We know about the rights of man and the individual pursuit of liberty and happiness, but we know little of the might of society, of dharma and duty, and of proper forms of marriage. This book is designed to shine a light on the source of all these stirring stories from the East and West and to illuminate their meanings, so that we can consciously choose which stories to buy into, which stories to take to heart and, once these stories are integrated within, allow them to guide us along our passage through life.

Hopefully even Westerners who have not taken a single yoga class will find value in understanding the source and meanings of the stories stored within these pages. We all have our stories, our dreams and our deep inner landscapes from which our actions and reactions to life arise. By shining the light of conscious awareness onto the deep within, we can begin to evaluate whether our reactions to life are serving us skillfully and, if not, begin to adopt new strategies and cultivate new habitual patterns. It all begins with the stories within: Change the stories or understand them in a new light and we can change what happens on the surface of our personalities. This book is about gaining a choice as to how we see and live our lives.

For over a decade I have been offering workshops to aspiring yoga teachers on the history and philosophy of yoga, explaining the rich variety of thought found in the Eastern teachings, showing how it has evolved and changed over time, and contrasting these ideas and ideals with the default patterns found in our Western culture. Greatly influenced by the teaching of Carl Jung and Joseph Campbell, among many others, I've chosen to contrast East and West through the stories that illustrate the way life is lived in distinct cultures, past and present, near and far. This book has arisen from my workshops; it is a distillation of many hours of talks, slideshows and music. My fondest hope is that this book, like the workshops it came from, will cause readers to wonder and look with renewed interest and new eyes at the stories through which they live their lives.

A Note on Mythology

Myths are stories, and good stories are entertaining, but not all entertaining stories are mythic. Defining exactly what myths are and why we have them is not easy and is subject to great debates. One academic definition is that myths are "traditional stories a society tells itself that encode or represent the worldview, beliefs, principles and often fears of that society."[1]

Some scholars believe myths serve aetiological purposes, which means they explain the causes of the world we find ourselves in. These myths explain why the world is the way it is. Other scholars believe the purpose of a myth is to provide a justification for the way that particular society behaves or to justify the existence and authority of certain social institutions. Naturally, myths also deal with the existence and behavior of gods and mystical powers beyond the normal day-to-day world of ordinary experience.

For the last two centuries, modern thinkers have tried to explain how myths originated and developed. Some, like the ancient Greek mythographer Euhemerus (~300 B.C.E), posit that myths are simply misremembered history, but these views rob myths of their wonder and ability to move people.[2] Others, like the 19th century's Max Müller (1823–1900), think that all myths are allegorical: They are purely symbolic and have no historical truth in them at all. Müller felt that not only were myths allegorical, but they all represented the single fact that the sun rose each morning and chased away the darkness of the night. His theory did not last very long. To Müller, myths were a "disease of language"—mistakes in understanding the original intent of the story that accumulated over time.[3]

To Andrew Lang (1844-1912) myths were primitive forms of science: attempts to explain the way thing are, but without the benefit of the modern scientific method.[4] To Sir James Frazer (1854-1941), author of the immense work written around the turn of the 20th century called *The Golden Bough*, myths were created to explain and guide rituals.[5] Frazer has been assailed by claims of selective editing and of taking myths out of their native contexts and arranging the snippets in ways that support his theory.[6] Many mythologists felt that we cannot take one pattern in a culture's story over here and assume it means the same thing to a similar pattern found in a different culture's story over there. The context is missing when we do that.

Bronislaw Malinowski (1884-1942), marooned on the island of Trobriand during World War I, observed that myths are fundamentally functional–that is, they helped societies to function.[7] Myths explain why the social order is the right order for the people.

As we can see, there is no unanimity about what myths are and why they exist. They can serve all the above functions and sometimes none of them. Joseph Campbell (1904-1987), the great popularizer of myths in the 20th century, often said there were four main functions of myths: the mystical function, the cosmological function, the social function and the psychological function.[8] Within this framework Campbell assigned much of the aetiological reasons for myths, such as the ideas of Lang, to the cosmological function and the ideas of people like Malinowski and Frazer to the sociological function. Campbell also borrowed freely from the newest theories in depth psychology, especially the work of Carl Jung (1875–1961), in describing the psychological and mystical functions of myths.

Campbell was not treated kindly by many mythologists, who accused him, as they did Frazer earlier, of being selective in his stories and of extracting certain aspects of a culture's mythology, stripping away the cultural context, and then presenting the naked theme as a proof of his own reasoning.[9] One considerable accusation leveled at Campbell is that he did not demonstrate the validity of his position and that "assertion is not evidence."[10] In other words, his idea that all myths are inflections of a monomyth that crosses all cultures and times is unproven and unprovable; just by saying it is so, does not make it so. However, the popularity of Campbell's work shows that despite the criticisms pointed at him, his teaching touches people: His stories work.

The other critique of Joseph Campbell's work was that his insistence on the existence of a monomyth was unsupportable and simply a projection of his own personal philosophy. He was accused of being a metaphysicist rather than a mythologist.[11] Campbell came upon the idea of a monomyth, more popularly known as "the hero's journey," through the writings of James Joyce. Through his own studies, Campbell noticed how many cultures' myths saw their heroes pass through similar challenges and stages in their respective quests. Campbell wrote his book *The Hero With a Thousand Faces* in 1949, but in the years to follow, he expanded his idea of the monomyth. Borrowing from the ideas of Adolf Bastian (1826–1905) and Carl Jung, Campbell discovered constant motifs, "elementary ideas" in Bastian's words, or "archetypes" in Jung's terminology, reoccurring over and over again in myths quite far apart in time and geography. He came to believe that these common themes were important and that they pointed to a transcendent reality that was poking up through the stories.

The original working title of this book was *Map Making 101*. The intention was to show how stories and myths are simply maps that are used to guide people's lives. A map is never truth: It is a symbolic representation of reality, but it cannot be reality itself. What is important about a map or a myth is not whether it is true or not, but whether it is useful. Joseph Campbell's presentation of mythology to the modern reader has proven to be useful: If it weren't, it would not be popular. I will leave it to the scholars to argue about the validity and accuracy of his work, but the utility of his work cannot be denied.

While this book contains novel ideas and associations, I have made no attempt to prove any of the particular points of view, and I am not qualified to do so. The book is meant to educate and provoke thought, not to cite sources and dates. For those who like sources and dates, endnotes are available. What I hope to do is to share some of the stories I have come across that have proven interesting and useful, especially to the yoga students and teachers I have taught.

Occasionally, the way the stories are explained may cause some distress for readers who happen to believe that the story is factually or historically true and is not a myth. This never happens when describing a myth found in someone else's religion but often happens when one's own religious stories are said to be mythical. For many people their maps provide great comfort and a sense of direction to their lives. If we take away the belief that their stories are true, they may feel left adrift and without purpose. However, virtually all religions have a deeper teaching available: When the stories are no longer taken as literally true, the student is able to delve much more deeply inside a more profound mystery. The Christian mystic experiences a "cloud of unknowing," and the Sufi mystic experiences a dance with the beloved, while the Jewish mystic finds deeper understanding of the mind of God through the teachings of the Kabbalah.

It is not my intent to take away anyone's cherished beliefs but rather to open a door that may help them go deeper in whatever direction their beliefs point them. The start is knowing that there is more to mythic or spiritual stories, and that we can shine a light on what is hidden.

One last point worth making is that I have made no attempt to reproduce the original mythic stories. Written myths are frozen slices of something that was once alive and changing. It is very difficult to understand the impact of a myth on its original audience because we are *not* they. We do not live in their time and culture, and we do not understand what their lives were like. All we can know is that these stories meant something to them; exactly what, we can only surmise. For this reason, I have tried to tell most of these old stories in a modern, folksy vernacular, not in the original, archaic verse. Through this I hope the stories will resonate with today's reader. I am hoping these stories will prove useful to you.

An Introduction to Myths, Maps and Models

This is the truth of truths, this is what the gods and myths are all about, so find them in yourself, take them into yourself, and you will be awakened in your mythology and in your life.
—Joseph Campbell[1]

❧ ❧

A man named Laghu desperately wanted to find Shiva, to see Shiva with his own eyes. He found Thay, a meditation master who promised to teach him how to behold Shiva. After four years of study and practice with Thay, Laghu was still unable to see Shiva. Thay considered Laghu's situation carefully and, after much deliberation, sent him to the mountains to study with Guruji. "In the mountains you will surely find Shiva!"

Laghu lived with Guruji for three years. Life upon the mountain was physically hard, but Laghu did not complain. He did all that Guruji asked and learned his teacher's demanding exercises well, but still, even after three years, he could not see Shiva. Guruji meditated on Laghu's desire and said, "You need to go to the city and study with Kritya. Living with Kritya, you will find Shiva."

Laghu lived and worked with Kritya in the heart of the city, where he saw many desperate souls and broken lives. He tended each person with kindness but still felt distant from everyone, so intent was he upon one thing alone: to behold Shiva. After two years Kritya told Laghu, "You must go on your own to the forest. There you will see Shiva!"

At the entrance to the forest Shiva stood watching Laghu approach. Laghu was filled with equal measures of hope and doubt, excitement and resignation. He stopped before entering the forest and scanned the great, tangled mass of life ahead of him. He turned and looked in Shiva's direction, but just as his eyes were about to fall upon Shiva, Shiva turned around. There on Shiva's back was a tree covered in vines; Laghu's eyes saw only the tree and moved on.

Laghu walked along a path that led him deep into the soul of the forest. In a small meadow, Shiva sat looking directly at Laghu. Laghu paused in the opening and looked straight at Shiva, who quickly turned around. Upon Shiva's back was a large boulder covered in moss, and this was all that Laghu knew. Laghu resumed his travel.

Shiva walked alongside Laghu, following no path. One time Shiva stepped upon a dead branch, snapping it in two. Laghu, upon hearing the sound, turned and looked straight at Shiva, but Shiva had turned again, and there on his back was a deer running through the woods. Laghu focused again upon the path and watched his feet continue walking.

⚐ ⚑

To paraphrase Carl Jung, of what use is an image of Shiva dancing on a dwarf named Avidya to a hockey player in Montreal? Symbols have meaning, and through their meaning they obtain power, but symbols can only wield such power when we can relate to them. If the symbol is unknown or foreign, it can't touch us—it strikes no chord in our unconscious mind. If the symbol is known to us, even if we don't consciously acknowledge it, we can be moved by it.

The story above is a story about Shiva, one of the three big deities of the Hindu trinity of gods. If it were written, however, with the word *Shiva* replaced by the word *God*, the impact of the story would be quite different on Westerners who do not know Shiva. Read it again and hear *God* every time you see *Shiva*, and see if the resonance changes.

* * *

Joseph Campbell was a leading mythologist of the 20th century and arguably the most famous one. He loved to tell stories that he culled from his vast readings of, and visits to, different cultures all over the world. He would hear a story in one culture and discern the latent imagery in their myth and realize that it also occurred in stories from other cultures separated by time and distances. They were the same stories.

Campbell's understanding of why so many cultures shared the same mythic images grew through his investigation of the psychological models being developed in the 20th century. He was deeply steeped in the ideas of the new depth psychology, especially the work of Carl Jung, who created a template of the mind that depicted our unique psychic landscapes. While the terrain of the mind is shaped uniquely by a person's biography, there are certain landmarks and themes shaped by our biology that are constantly appearing in all maps. These Jung called *archetypes*: symbols of psychic energies that are common throughout humanity regardless of background and era. What differs is the way these archetypes are inflected by the individual and by the culture or society he lives within.

Joseph Campbell's fascination was in the way these archetypes manifested themselves in people's stories. His bliss was to follow these maps of the deep psyche and explain them in terms that we, people living in the West in the 21st century, could understand and thus tap into to help us experience our own life more fully.

Both Campbell and Jung shone a light, the light of consciousness, into the dark landscape of our souls. Where Jung worked with the individual intimately and helped her understand her own struggle for completeness, a process that he called *individuation*, Campbell worked with the full breadth of mankind. Both men sought to illuminate that which was hidden within: Campbell through his stories and Jung through his counseling. To understand what these great men were bringing into our conscious awareness requires us to understand the symbols they discovered and the maps they described. That is the purpose of this journey. While this book is directed toward students and teachers of Yoga, and the stories culled and presented illuminate certain yogic philosophies and practices, the importance and value of these stories are not limited only to Western yogis: Everyone growing up in our modern Western culture can benefit from light cast inward.

✳ ✳ ✳

Like Laghu, we walk in dreams, often confused by what we see and helpless to change our own circumstances. Terrific and sometimes terrible powers move around and through us. We are in the land of myths and stories, and we feel as if we are awake, but we are sleepwalking through life. We look at life, but do not see; we hear but do not comprehend. The symbols elude us, their meanings unfathomable. So we do our best; we follow the path that is in front us and hope it will lead us somewhere pleasant.

⚐ ⚑

Walking in your neighborhood one fine morning, you notice a new Indian restaurant on your main street. "When did that open up?" you ask yourself. You peek at the menu in the window: yummm … mango lassis—looks great. You make a mental note to remember the restaurant, and this creates a mental map in your mind.

That afternoon a friend mentions a great new place they ate at last night; coincidentally, it's the same place you came across earlier. Your friend confirms your hunch that it is really good. You add this piece of information to your mental map.

Later that week you dine at the restaurant and are greatly pleased: The food is excellent; the service is good and the ambiance perfect. You update your map and resolve to share what you know with other friends.

＊ ＊

A map is a story, a conceptualization of an experience told in symbolic language that will help the user of the map come to the same experience the creator of the map had. The map is not the experience itself—that is not its purpose. No map is the territory it describes. The intention of the map is to help one navigate the territory.

Normally, we think of maps as being descriptions of geography, but the concept is much broader than that. Maps can be metaphors for anything we experience. A map models reality, but it is not reality itself. This is why a map is simply a story and every story is just a map. The whole point of any map is to be useful, not to be true.

To explain more clearly: Take a map of your city and lay it on the floor; find out exactly where you are right now on this map, and place your finger on that spot. Conceptually you might say, "I am here." If that were literally true, then a huge finger would come out of the sky and squish you into the floor. Of course you don't get squashed, because the map is not the territory. Suppose this particular map showed you the location of all the Starbucks coffee shops in your city. You might think this is a great map, but your friend, who doesn't drink coffee, says he has a better map. His map shows where all the dog parks are. Since you don't have a dog, you think his map is useless.

One day, some genius named Einstein comes along and creates a new map that shows all the Starbucks *and* all the dog parks. This is a great map! This map is more useful to more people than the earlier maps, but still the map is not the territory. For the map to be complete, it would have to show all the trees in each park; it would have to show all the cups in each coffee shop; it would have to show all the yoga studios and all the mats within the studios, all the students, their water bottles, etc. The map, to be completely faithful to reality, would have to contain everything that reality contains. This would turn it into reality, and not a concept of reality.

It is impossible for any map to be complete or completely accurate, but that is not the point of a map. The map is not "truth," but it can be useful. A story is not the truth either, but a good story can be very useful. The degree to which we judge a map to be good is the degree to which we can use it without being deceived or misdirected.

* * *

Jesus said, "I am the way."[2] We can consider His way as a map. The "Dao" in Chinese means "path" or "way": again— Daoism is another map. Maps make us feel comfortable: We sense where we are; we are not lost. It is a comforting illusion, one that we will not surrender easily. People love their maps, their opinions, their beliefs in the way the world is and works—they cling to these concepts fiercely and will fight to maintain the illusion. Since we all need maps, it would be cruel to try to remove someone's without providing a better one in its place. Only when you can see that there is a better way offered will you be ready to switch your conceptual view of the world. Some people are content with their life as it is, and they are not open to new maps, no matter how much better the new map might serve them. That is their choice, and no one can insist that they should adopt a different map. However, when your maps no longer serve you well, then it may well be time for you to seek a better way.

A map is a story, and if you wanted to think of it this way, you could say that these stories *want* to be believed. There is a part of our deep darkness that needs to be expressed, and these stories allow this expression. Anyone who says *our* story is not true is often considered an evil person or an outsider. There is danger in shining the light on another person's map if the other person does not wish to see the light.

Often our stories provide a pretext for actions we would like to take: The facts are not important. The stories found in the book of Genesis are not meant to be factually true; they are meant to be believed. The pretext is more important than the text. This is found often in the art of power and politics: President Lyndon Johnson took the United States into a war in Vietnam under the pretext that the North Vietnamese attacked two boats in international waters on August 4, 1964. The attack was known as the Gulf of Tonkin incident. The Secretary of Defense Robert S. McNamara later admitted that there was no such attack. Wayne Morse was one of only two senators who opposed the Gulf of Tonkin resolution, and his reward for speaking out and showing that the story was not true was to lose his seat in the next election. He was out of Washington for good and never managed to come back. In 2003, George W. Bush also used a story to take his country into a war with Iraq, the pretext being that Saddam Hussein had weapons of mass destruction. The story was proclaimed to be false at the time by many, including the weapons inspectors in Iraq. It was proven to be false after the invasion, but let's not let the facts ruin a good story! Stories do not need to be true to be effective.

Shining the light of conscious awareness into deep, dark places within is not without its risks: resistance can develop. The warning signs include tension, judgments and negative emotions, all of which result in a shutting down of the reason faculty and a rejection of inputs that might lead to illumination. If, as you wander through the stories herein, you notice these effects occurring within you, you may want to pause and linger longer in the place that yields the most discomfort: something interesting may happen.

※ ※

A Zen master sat with her students at the end of their zazen practice. Tea was steeping in a black, metallic teapot set upon a small table in the middle of the room around which the students and master sat. Normally the master would get up and pour each student a cup of tea, but she just sat there looking puzzled at the teapot; the students waited patiently.

For a few moments, there was stillness; then the master asked a question, "What is a teapot?" The students knew they were being tested, so they paused before answering. Was this a kôan? She was always trying to trick them. No one wanted to be the first to respond, but unless they responded, there would be no tea today!

A clever student responded first. He went to the teapot and poured himself a cup of tea and sat down again. He raised the cup in a salute to the teacher and promptly drank his tea. The master simply looked at him with curiosity and repeated her question, "What is a teapot?" She looked at the other students for help.

A new student shrugged and spoke, pointing at the teapot and said, "*That* is a teapot."

"What is?" asked the master.

"That there," replied the student while shaking his finger.

"Ah!" said the master. "A shaking finger is a teapot! Thank you for enlightening me."

"No, no!" said the student. "That is the teapot! What my finger is pointing to is the teapot."

"The table?"

"No, what is on the table!"

Another student got a brilliant idea, took the teapot and placed it in the master's hands. "This is a teapot," she explained.

"Oh, now I see," said the master as she moved the teapot around in her hands. "A teapot is a black object that weights about five pounds and is hot. Now I know what a teapot is; anything that weighs about five pounds, is black and is hot is a teapot."

"Not quite," said the student as she sat back down on her zafu. "The color and weight are irrelevant. It has to have a certain shape in order to be a teapot. It must have a spout, for example, and a handle."

"Ah! Now I understand," said the teacher, and then she paused for a moment. "Curious, though, when I came into the zen-dô this evening I passed a nun watering the flowers. She was using something that had a spout and a handle. I didn't realize at the time, but she was using a teapot to water the flowers!"

"No," replied the student, "that was a watering can. You don't brew tea in a watering can."

"But it had a spout and a handle. Isn't that what makes something a teapot?" asked the master.

"Just because something has a spout and a handle, it is not necessarily a teapot. A handle is a necessary, but not sufficient, condition for a teapot to be."

"Oh, so if this teapot had no handle, if the handle was broken or missing, it would then no longer be a teapot?"

"Hmmm," puzzled the student, "yes–it would still be a teapot; it would just be a broken teapot."

Another student ventured into the discussion, "A teapot is a pot that holds tea."

"I don't understand," replied the master.

"A pot is something that holds water, and tea is a beverage made from brewing leaves in the pot."

"But I was just told that a teapot was something that has a handle and a spout. I know that a watering can also has a handle and a spout, and I presume I could pour water and brew tea in it, too, couldn't I? Then why isn't it a teapot?"

"A watering can is too big to be a teapot."

"Oh, so size is important! Only if an object is this size," said the master as she held up the teapot still in her hands, "can it be a teapot."

"Well, no," admitted the student, "a teapot could be bigger or smaller than that."

"Well then, the size is not what makes this a teapot. The color, the weight, or the shape doesn't make this a teapot. What makes this a teapot? Is it the material? Can a teapot only be made out of metal?"

"No," said the student. "It can be made out of metal like the watering can, but it can also be made of ceramic," and after a little more reflection he added, "and of course, the watering can could also be made of ceramic, so that doesn't help much."

The newest student chimed in again, "A teapot is called a teapot because it is *used* for brewing tea."

"Ah—so the *use* is what is important! So if I took that big pot that Chef is using for boiling rice each night for dinner, boiled some water in it and added some tea leaves, it would be a teapot?"

"Yes! Because then it would be a pot that was being used to brew tea," exclaimed the student triumphantly.

"How grand! Thank you. So tonight when I go to Chef and hold up his big pot and tell him, 'this is a teapot,' he will know I am speaking the truth and will agree?"

"Um, no—he will probably think you are testing him by saying something not true to see his reaction."

"But you have confused me again: A teapot is used for brewing tea, but if I use something else to brew my tea, it is not a teapot? Sorry, I am still lost. What is a teapot?"

The group fell silent as they tried to work through the puzzle. Neither the color nor the shape of an object defines it. Many objects have similar shapes. What the object is made of, its weight and size are not the important things. Its use is not the important thing either, because other things could be used in a similar way and yet not be named the same. What does make a teapot a teapot?

The clever student finally spoke, "there actually is no teapot, but we call this a teapot because we all agree to call this a teapot." Saying this he got up, took the pot from his master's hands, and started to serve everyone a cup of tea.

The master applauded and then held out her cup for some tea, too, which by now had grown quite cold.

જ ફ

First there is a teapot, then there is no teapot, and then there is. What applies to a teapot applies to any thing: a teapot or a mountain—no difference. First we see a mountain, but then we realize that *mountain* is merely a concept, and there really is no mountain. There is no difference between a mountain and a teapot because there are no *things*. But if you try to explain to friends who invited

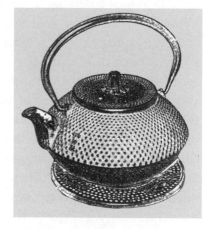

Figure 1: Ceci n'est pas une teapot!

you to go skiing on Grouse Mountain that actually there is no such thing as Grouse Mountain, don't be surprised if you never get invited to go skiing with them again. If there is no Grouse Mountain, then where are they when they are skiing without you?

An artist is one who looks at the conventional world with unconventional eyes. Where you or I may simply see a teapot, the artist sees a flowerpot for her beautiful geraniums. She looks beyond the confinement of the word—beyond the boundaries of the map. Crush an old teapot, and its pieces may be used to make a lovely mosaic. A mouse may see a teapot as home. To an ant trying to cross your table, the teapot is a mountainous obstacle. A mystic sees the teapot like a reflection in a window: the teapot exists, but its name is only a reflection, and the concept is not real. When we say "teapot," we constrain the object to a preconceived notion and use. We no longer worry about who made the teapot, all the people who have used the teapot, or how the teapot will one day meet its end. We don't see the clay it is made from and dust it will return to.

This is true of all words: if we can't really know what a simple teapot really is, how will we ever know what *God* is? What is *truth*? How will I know if I am in *love*? A word is simply a map, which by convention we agree points toward some aspect of reality. If we look up the definition of any word in the biggest dictionary in the world, we will find that word defined by other words. If we then look up those other words in the same dictionary, we will discover that they, too, are defined by yet more words that are also found in the dictionary. Ultimately, like an enormous house of cards, there is no absolute foundation upon which all these words rest. All of our ideas, our concepts, our words, our maps and stories have no reality in and of themselves. But, believe that there actually is no teapot, and you may never be served tea again!

✳ ✳ ✳

It is important to remember the true nature of maps and the true reason for stories. The important thing is the utility, the usefulness, and that they work! This applies whether we call the representation of an experience a story or a map. In science we create maps, too, but they are called theories or models. These stories model the experience of the scientist in such a way that others can recreate the same experience the first scientist had. A scientific model is a hypothesis based upon observations (these observations are called *facts*). This is similar to the way you may have noted the address of the new Indian restaurant you came across in our earlier imagining. The address is a fact noted on your map.

When the scientist collects enough facts, she tries to create a map that relates all the facts together coherently so that others can also reproduce these facts, and, more excitingly, predict new facts that have not yet been observed. If later scientists, by performing new experiments, observe these new facts, then the model is a strong one. If the observations don't agree with the predicted facts, the model is a weak one. A weak map may still be useful, but it is not as good as a strong map, which describes reality better.

Sometimes the maps, or scientific models, are so good at describing reality that the model shows things the scientists can't bring themselves to accept. Albert Einstein [1879-1955], when he worked out his general theory of relativity, saw that his math predicted the universe was either contracting or expanding. Einstein did not believe his own model, because he knew the universe was constant, neither growing nor shrinking (this was the nature of his previous map), and so he ignored what his new map was showing him and missed out on being the first to predict the expanding universe.[3]

Science does not pretend that its theories are "true," in terms of some absolute, unchangeable understanding that will be correct for all time and in all places. Theories are not supposed to be confused with "the truth." Scientists work toward truth, knowing that it can never be obtained. Science itself is a continuous thrust forward to answer questions raised by the incompleteness of existing models. And all scientific models are incomplete and must always be so. Reality is ultimately undefinable and unknowable. This conclusion has become part of the way of science: It has been shown in many ways that we cannot know everything about our universe. Immanuel Kant (1724-1804) spoke of this when he said things exist only so far as we can perceive them, but the ultimate "thingness" (he called it *ding an sich* or the "thing in itself") cannot be experienced. All we can know is what our perceptions reveal, but the reality is far more than what we can perceive or conceptualize.[4]

Werner Heisenberg (1901-1976), who helped develop quantum mechanics in the 1920s, showed that we cannot know everything about a piece of matter. More specifically, he showed that we cannot know both an object's position and its velocity. Let's use the example of an electron: The simple act of observing the electron, which we do by bouncing a photon off it, causes it to change its position. This unknowingly became known as the "Uncertainty Principle," and many scientists, including Albert Einstein, disliked it tremendously: "What do you mean that we can't know the universe!"[5] Heisenberg's model ultimately became accepted as a good representation of truth: Indeed we can't know everything.[6]

Kurt Gödel (1906-1978) was a Czech-born mathematician who postulated a theory of incompleteness. He showed that it is impossible to prove as true all statements in a set of mathematics using the rules of only that set of mathematics. To prove everything in a universe requires us to go outside the bounds of the knowledge that exists in that universe.[7] A simplistic way to understand Gödel's point is to consider the

"Liar's Paradox." Ask someone to tell you whether the following statement is true or not: "This statement is false." There is no adequate answer to the question. If your friend says the statement is true, then the statement is false and thus can't be true, so your friend is wrong. If he says the statement is false, then the statement is true and he again is wrong. (You may want to think about this for a while.)

Where Heisenberg demonstrated that we can never know or experience reality completely, Gödel showed that we can never completely describe reality, either. We can quest toward truth, but that truth is inherently unknowable. All of our conceptualizations are mere menus describing delicious dinners, but a menu is not the dinner: It's not the experience of eating the dinner, nor is it a complete description of what you will experience when you dine.

Since they are only human beings, sometimes our scientists fail the ideals of science, and they become as attached to their stories as any conservative society or theologian might. The big danger for a scientist is confusing his theories for reality and believing that his map is the right one. Notwithstanding such human frailties, there is a big difference between religion's search for truth and science's search. Religions are conservative in nature, and their hierarchies seek to maintain what is. Truth for religious organizations is that which has already been revealed and described in a special book. For science, *facts* may already exist, but *truth* is always out there awaiting discovery.

Scientific models must be falsifiable. This means they could be proven false if certain results were obtained in an experiment. If a theory is not falsifiable, then it is not a very good theory. This does not mean they have to be proven false—if they were proven false, then they are not good theories, either. More important than being proven right, the possibility has to exist that the scientific theories could be proven wrong, but they pass the test, showing they are not wrong. Religious truths are never falsifiable: for example, can you prove that God does not exist? Religious truths are *asserted* to be true but not proven to be true, and they are not capable of being proven to be false. (And you may have to think about that for a while, too.)

* * *

Images and feeling can be described: Ideas can be expressed in words, and sometimes they are rendered in pictures, music or dance. Stories are the same, for if the story is a good one, images and feeling will arise in resonance with the ideas presented in the story. Good stories have power; they have the power to move us. Great stories have even greater power, the power to arrest us. Stories teach us about our surroundings, our family, friends and neighbors, our own life and our role in this life. This is the role of mythic stories.

A radio station host once invited Joseph Campbell to be interviewed on air.[8] Right from the start of the show, the host was on the attack and said that myths were out-and-out lies. Campbell begged to differ and explained that myths were metaphors, but through the back and forth of their debate Campbell came to realize that the host did not understand what a metaphor was.

"A myth is a metaphor. Do you know what a metaphor is? Give me an example of a metaphor," Campbell commanded.

The host stumbled and could not articulate the definition of a metaphor, but when pushed, offered an example. "A metaphor is when you say, 'Johnny runs like a deer.'"

What the host offered was a simile. "That's not a metaphor," responded Campbell. "A metaphor is 'Johnny *is* a deer!'"

"That's a lie!" exclaimed the host.

"That's a metaphor!" replied Campbell.

The show ended on that note.

⋅⊰ ⊱⋅

The host of the above interview was reflecting a common misperception about myths: A myth is a story that is not true. Since the myth is a lie, it cannot be believed; therefore, it has no value. This is a common perception, and yet we crave our stories. We flock to theatres to see great movies, and we rent or download for private viewing dozens of videos every year. Novels in all forms captivate us, whether in old-fashioned hardcover books or on electronic tablets. On a more personal level, we listen intently whenever a friend starts to tell us some gossip about people we know. The blockbuster best sellers and the whispered tattles are the stories that captivate, motivate, and stop us. These stories are far from valueless, and yet they are not true.

What is there about these lies that are so important to us, and how can they be so valuable if they are just lies? Again, the reality is that stories do not have to be true to be compelling; they just have to be useful.

✳ ✳ ✳

If people think their map is reality, they are likely to think that the places outside the map—areas where there are no details or areas where they have never been—are areas of chaos and danger. The ancient cartographers warned of these areas by writing, "Here be dragons." We fill in the blank areas of our maps not with experience, but with fantasies.

If you have a map that continuously leads you to the wrong places, if you get lost every time you try to follow the map, you are going to be frustrated, angry and upset most of the time. Life is not much fun when you try to follow a map that lies to you. You need to have some faith that your map is right, or, if you are wise, you will stop following it. The unwise are those who keep following their old maps, even though they know they will get lost.

Beyond being useful, your map needs to be believable. The power of faith is legendary. While faith may not literally move a mountain, it is faith that takes you to that mountain. Remember, no map is the literal truth, but a good map is functionally true. The same is true of our myths. It is the functionality and the believability of the myth, not its literalness, that makes it powerful.

This was not just true in ancient times; it is equally true today. Take one of the most compelling, unexplained facts of modern medicine—the power of the placebo. The placebo is a story; it is a bit of medicine you are told will work, even though it factually has no healing property whatsoever. It is simply a sugar pill: sweet, innocent and useless—or, at least, it should be useless. A strange thing happens to that little sugar pill when we are told, and we believe, that it is powerful medicine. It works!

Placebos work because we believe they will work. A placebo is a mythic image. When a placebo is dressed up with a really good story, it works even better. If your doctor raves about this great new treatment and cites lots of arcane articles, you are more likely to believe the story, and the placebo is more likely to work. (A study of Danish physicians discovered that 48% had deliberately prescribed placebos for their patients at least 10 times in the last year![9]) The doctor's story is even more convincing when the doctor himself dresses up in a special costume, one that you don't wear (a white lab coat, for example), uses magical devices in a prescribed ritualistic way (taking your blood pressure or using a stethoscope to listen to your heart while chanting the magic mantra of "hmmm"), and exhibits his prowess through a wall full of diplomas and certificates. Who would not believe a doctor like that?

Belief works at the unconscious level. An interesting study showed that even if a patient is told that the pill she is being given is simply a sugar pill and has no medical value, but still it has been shown to help others, it works![10] What is happening here? The unconscious mind hears the story and doesn't care whether it is true or not. The mind behaves "as if" the story were true. Rational logic does not matter: If this helped someone else, even someone I never met, then it can help me. There is a magic here that the great mythic stories tap into: If the story is believable, then the story can work. However, if the story is no longer believable, it stops working.

✳ ✳ ✳

Stories change; times change. Maps are always changing, too, at least good maps are. Old maps are interesting and have some sentimental or artistic value, but they are out of date and no longer useful. For stories to remain useful, they must change with the times, or their power is lost.

ᴈ ᴇ

An ancient seer sitting under a tree in the forest had a revelation. Deep in meditation, understanding awoke. The yogi sat completely still while the vision expanded. He knew what it meant. He felt himself being transformed. For seven days the experience worked its alchemical magic within and upon him until, finally, he was completed. Getting up, he walked purposely back to his village, where he thought to share his understanding with his old friends. Along the way he pondered how best to help them reach the same place he was now: He created a story. The yogi compared his path to the path one would take when following the footprints of a lost cow. His story spoke of lions and bulls, eagles and snakes, dwarves and boars, gods and goddesses.

⅏ ⅌

The story the prophet spun was couched in words of that time and of that place: how else could his friends understand? If the story were told in archaic words and with obtuse imagery, there would be no hope of the story being useful. Ancient stories contain a myriad of images that today strike our senses strangely. The old stories no longer speak to us. We find their metaphors quaint and powerless. How many people today have even seen a wild boar or danced with dwarves? Truth may be eternal, but new maps are required to help us find the way to them.

* * *

Jacques Cartier (1491-1557) is well known to Canadian school children: In 1534 he became the first European to map the Saint Lawrence Seaway and claimed the land, which he named the Canadas, for France. In the early 1600s, Samuel de Champlain (1567-1635) became the first European to map the Great Lakes. The early map made by Cartier was not as good as the later one created by de Champlain; de Champlain had explored further and consequently mapped more places than Cartier. Today, Google Maps has a rendering of Canada that is far better than either explorer's early map. But Google Maps notwithstanding, Cartier's map was useful for what he needed the map to do. Cartier's map was a rendering of his experiences in the New World. The map rendered by de Champlain covered more area than Cartier's, but his map was also simply a rendering of his experiences, different as they were from Cartier's.

The prophets, seers, rishi and ancient yogis were all pioneers. They were *psychonauts*[11] exploring inner realms, and when they returned from their travels they created maps to help others visit the same places. These maps were couched in the language of their time and culture. Later psychonauts used these same maps, just as de Champlain did, but then they went further than their predecessors. These new maps were more useful, but that did not mean the older stories were wrong. Modern explorers of the mystical realms use modern terminology, modern imagery, and we understand them far better than we do the ancient stories. The poets and mystics of today speak to us far more clearly than do the ancient teachers.

Stories and myth, like maps and models, have power when they speak to us in our own language and when they use images that help us relate to the story. The old stories don't touch us anymore because they have not kept up with the changing times. No one in Montreal today would try to navigate the corridors of their city using Jacques Cartier's hand-drawn scribbles. Is it any wonder the stories of the grand old religions move so few of us today in the West?

But what if they could?

* * *

Joseph Campbell observed that mythologies serve four main functions. There is the grand cosmological function that explains the universe, how it came to be and what it is made of. Campbell was not the first to discover myth's aetiological function (as described in the Note on Mythology, which preceded this chapter). The function of the creation myths, whether they are the four-thousand-year-old idea of a three-layer universe, with the heavens above, the waters below and the earth in between, or the modern view of a tremendous explosion, the Big Bang, which set everything in motion, is to create a sense of awe and wonder toward that which is so much vaster than ourselves. We can say the cosmological function puts us in accord with the entire universe, and through that accord we understand our place in it.

The second function of mythology is the sociological function. The myths serving this function put us in accord with our society. These are the myths that tell us how we are supposed to act in society and how to behave in our dealings with other people. These myths are inflected in many ways in various cultures and times; these are the laws of society, both written and unwritten. Societies do not exist to serve people; people exist to serve the society they were born into. How to serve the society is spelled out in the mythologies of that culture.

The third function of mythology is the psychological one of putting oneself in accord with the inevitable arc of aging and the stages of life. No matter where you go, no matter what culture you were born into, we all go through the same stages of birth, dependency, adolescence, adulthood and the challenges of retiring, old age and ultimately departure through the grey door. How we are supposed to deal with these challenges is described and laid out for us in our mythologies. There are fewer variations in these myths from culture to culture and from age to age than in any of the other mythologic functions.

Finally, the mystical function of mythology or religion is to put us in accord with the great mystery that is life itself. Why am I here? What is the purpose of life? What is the purpose of *my* life? Beyond even this, Joseph Campbell felt that the ultimate power of a great mystical myth is to go beyond purpose and meaning to the actual *experience* of life itself. The mystical function is the transcendent function, which helps us look beyond the mere facts of mundane existence to something greater and more profound. It is mystical awareness that is awoken by the awe generated through the cosmological function of mythology; and thus we come full circle.

There is no one myth or story that can evoke all of these functions. Cultures are made up and maintained through a tapestry of stories: Each thread relates us in one particular way to the whole. We can choose to examine each individual mythic strand or step back and enjoy the grand design of the complete tapestry. We can also come to understand and enjoy the tapestries of other cultures and see how they differ and how they are similar to our own.

✳ ✳ ✳

The four functions of mythology help us relate to our environment, our people, our individual life and finally to the mystery of life itself. This was true five thousand years ago and it remains true today. What has changed are the stories that help us come into these concordances. When the old stories no longer work, new stories are required. If the changes are happening too quickly, then the stories can't keep up and we feel lost. We enter what Joseph Campbell calls (citing T.S. Eliot's story) *The Waste Land*, a place where people live inauthentic lives, doing what they are told, believing what they are told, but having no sense of joy. It is a barren place, as barren as the land of King Arthur before the healing quest of the Holy Grail.

It was in early 1900s that Carl Jung looked for the myth by which he was living his life and discovered he did not know.[12] His work with psychotic patients at the Burghölzli Psychiatric Hospital at the University of Zurich introduced him to the depths of the individual psyche. He discovered powerful mythic images and learned how terrible it was to live with these myths when they were raw and exposed. He also discovered that it was equally terrible to not have any myths at all. He set out to find what mythology he was living by.

We all have our own myths: They show up at night in our most profound and disturbing dreams. The dreams you remember most easily are dreams spun out of the mythic energies of your own psychic landscape. Freud noted that dreams are private myths and myths are public dreams. Myths then are the dreams of an entire society, possessing the power to speak to each individual in that society. The myth is a shared dream, but you have your own private myths, as well.

These myths are maps to our inner landscapes. These myths are models of the way we are supposed to behave. We all have our own maps, our own myths by which we live our lives. It cannot be otherwise because we all travel the path of our unique life. The path we have chosen to follow is determined by the map we use, and this choice may be unconsciously selected or consciously. Most people, though, are simply sleepwalking along their unconsciously chosen path. It is a rare individual, like Jung, who asks, "What is the myth I am living by?"

A clue to your map can be found any time you find yourself thinking about the way things or other people, or even yourself, *should* be. The idea of *should* is based upon a map you hold internally; the map defines the way life is *supposed* to be. When life doesn't meet this expectation, a dissonance is created, often manifesting as irritation, frustration, anger or even fear or anxiety. When someone or something is not behaving properly, that is a map talking through you. Can you see your own map? Probably not, because it is shrouded in darkness and hidden from you. It is easier to blame the outside world for not meeting our expectations of it than to go inward and find the flaws in our own map.

To explore a dark territory requires a light, and the light we use to explore the darkness of our deep, inner realms is the light of consciousness. To bring something into conscious awareness requires us to go down into that darkness and turn on the light. Be prepared to be shocked or pleasantly surprised—in either case, what you will find will be unexpected.

✳ ✳ ✳

Remember, we all follow maps, which are the mental models or patterns in our mind. These maps are not normally known to consciousness, but they are there and they are powerful. If we are not happy with the way our life is unfolding, perhaps we are following a map that is not very useful. If we are doing OK in life but wonder how we could do even better, then we can shine a light on the map we are using and see if there are better ones available. And there may be times when our map is perfectly fine, although our path through that map is not well chosen: A better path may be necessary even though we keep using the same map. In any case, we need to know our map!

Once we can see the map in the full light of day, once we can bring it fully into conscious awareness, then we can start to determine whether the map is useful or not. If not, we may decide whether to get a new map or plot a new course within the existing map. Here is some good news: We can always get a new map or take a new path! It is not easy, but it is possible.

Notice, we are not asking whether the map is *right*! And here again is the big point: None of our maps is right! Every map we follow, every story we believe in, whether consciously or unconsciously, is a *representation* of the way things actually are; it is not reality. Our maps are not real in this sense. They are real maps, but the maps aren't reality—no matter how attractive and compelling they feel. The game we play is to act "as if" the maps were real—that is where belief is required.

We do not use just one map, and even one map can lead us to many places. We have a multitude of maps in the bureau drawers of our mind. Throughout our life, from childhood to old age, we are told stories that become our maps. Before we can choose a new map or a new way to live, we need to know what stories we believe now.

The journey in this book is one of shining the light of conscious awareness on some of the maps we are using by sharing many of the stories that created the maps. Knowing this, we can decide whether these maps are useful or not. If not, we can gain some idea of where we might find better maps to follow. We can tell ourselves new stories. Perhaps we can incorporate some stories from the East, but this is only possible if we can relate to the images and ideas in those stories. To do that we have to understand what these stories mean. Understanding the meaning of these foreign myths makes it possible to select or reject them as candidates for updating our current maps.

Knowing that a myth is a map to our deep psychic landscape, we come to the intention of this book: to shine the light of consciousness inwardly and answer these questions.

What myths do I live by?

Are these myths useful?

Do I need to find better myths?

Which new myths would serve me better?

The Cosmological Function

What I want to know is whether God had any choice in the creation of the universe.

—Albert Einstein

Chapter 1: The Creation of All Things

⁂

In the beginning there was the Self. One day, before there were any days, the Self had a thought: It thought "I". And as soon as it thought "I" it became afraid. (As soon as you have the concept of existence, you also have the possibility of nonexistence.) But then the Self reasoned, "Since I am the only one that exists, what is there to be afraid of?" Reassured by this thought, the Self then noticed that it was lonely: "I wish there was someone else to be with!"

So the Self swelled and grew until it became as big as two people, and then it split apart, into a man and a woman. As soon as the man and the woman separated, they immediately clung together, in the nature of male and female, and out of this first union came all of us—the human race began.

After a little while, the female Self thought, "Hey wait a minute, this doesn't seem right. I mean, he is like my brother and I am his sister and we shouldn't be doing this." So the female Self disengaged and ran away. The male Self, being a normal male Self, ran after her. She hid from him by turning herself into a cow, but he found her, became a bull, and went into her. From this union cattle were created. She thought, "Well, this isn't working!" and ran away again. This time she turned herself into a mare. He found her again, became a stallion and bingo! Horses were begotten. She ran again and again. Finally she turned herself into an ant; he still found her and all the ants were created.

After a while the Self looked around, amazed, and thought, "Wow! All this came from me, and I am in all of this!"

⚛ ೞ

One of the four main functions of mythology is the cosmological function. Its purpose is to put us in accord with nature and our surroundings. To revisit, the other functions of myths are the sociological function, putting us in accord with our society; the psychological function, putting us in accord with our human nature and the inevitable stages of life; and the mystical function, which helps us relate to the mystery that is existence itself. The creation myths explain how we came to be, and they explain our relationship to everything else we see. Knowing our place in the universe helps us act properly toward the environment we find ourselves in, but there are many different myths of creation. Depending upon which map we follow, our attitudes and actions toward our environment and other beings may be drastically different.

The creation myth cited above is a very old story. It is from one of the earliest Upanishads, the Brihadaranyaka Upanishad, which was perhaps created around 800 B.C.E., approximately the same time that the earliest biblical creation story was rendered.[1] The Upanishads are a collection of mythic writings from a revolutionary time in India when the much more ancient teachings of the Vedas were being questioned and surpassed.[2]

This particular creation story is a nondualistic myth: All of creation is part of the creator, and the creator is part of all creation. There is no self and other—you are it! You *are* the other. If this was the map you had in your psyche, if your most fundamental belief structures were based upon this idea, how do you think it would affect your attitude toward creation, toward nature and toward your fellow man?

3

Compare this to our creation stories in the West. In the West the Creator is *not* a part of creation, and as His creatures, we are not part of Him. The clockmaker is not the clock. In the West we have what is known as a *dualistic* philosophy. To say in the West, "I am God!" is the highest blasphemy. Jesus was crucified for saying, "I and the Father are one."[3] The 10th-century Sufi mystic Mansur Al Hallaj was also executed for saying he and his beloved were one.[4] In India, if you were to go up to a guy on the street and say, "I am God!" he would simply shrug and say, "So what? I am also God." In the East, nondualistic views of the universe are common but not universal. In the West, with our strictly dualistic view of creation, we believe we are not divine, creation is not divine, and therefore nature is not divine. If this was someone's guiding mythology, the base map operating at his deepest psychic level, how do you think it would affect his actions toward creation, toward nature and toward his fellow man?

The Eastern myths tell us we are divine, we are God, and God is everywhere. Like Laghu, however, as described in the introduction, we walk through the world and miss its divinity. Our task of tasks is to realize our *identity* with God. This is not the task we have set out for ourselves in the West. In the West we are told, through our stories, that we are *not* divine and God is *not* a part of us, so our task of tasks in the West is to come into a *relationship* with the divine. These are two very different imperatives that differentiate Eastern and Western spirituality and philosophy: Are you seeking a relationship with God (Western), or are you trying to identify with God (Eastern)? This basic philosophical understanding of the nature of the universe underlies much of the differences between the stories we will hear, East and West.

* * *

4

A BABYLONIAN STORY

The divide between East and West can be drawn quite nicely through modern Iran: East of Iran (east of Persia or Mesopotamia in earlier eras) we have mostly nondualistic philosophies, those found in India and China. To the west of this line, we find the dualistic philosophies of the Levant and Europe. These dualistic philosophies are revealed in the creation myths that grew in Levantine soils. They evolved to suit changing needs, as myths must do, but it is useful to hear the original stories and try to see what they may have meant to the people of those times and places, and to see how they came to affect the mythos by which we live today.

⊰ ⊱

Before anything was named, there was only water. Within the waters were Tiamat, the Waters of the Ocean and her husband, Apsu, the Waters of the Land. This was a time before the heavens were called *heaven* and before land was called *land*. It was a time of no gods and no names to determine destinies.

The River poured into the Ocean; Apsu's sweet waters joined with the salty waters of Tiamat, and life was created within her. Tiamat's powerful children, upon being named, became gods, but they were still children nonetheless, and they made quite a loud babble of noise that annoyed their mother and father greatly. The Waters of the Land, their father, said to the Ocean, their mother, that they should kill these noisy brats within her to regain some peace and quiet. Tiamat did not agree and warned the gods. In their own self-defense the gods acted first, and the great god Ea killed his grandsire Apsu.

Ea had a son, Marduk, who was given a gift of the winds to play with by his doting grandfather, Anu, the sky god. Marduk's four winds disturbed Tiamat's great body. Annoyed, the gods still residing within the Ocean persuaded her to attack Ea and the others who had killed her husband. She agreed and a cosmic war began, but Marduk won the battle and tore Tiamat's great body in two. From these two halves Marduk created the heavens and the earth. He then created the sun, the moon and the stars and ordered their movements to follow in great cycles his calendar.

When his work was done, Marduk was praised by the gods and was inspired: From the clay of the earth he decided to create a race of savages to be called *man* to free the gods from labor. Ea warned his son that only the shedding of the lifeblood of a god could accomplish this task. Marduk made an easy choice: He sacrificed the second husband of Tiamat, Kingu, the general who opposed him in the great battle, and through Kingu's blood man was brought to life: a life of service to the gods.

⁓ ⁖

This Babylonian myth, the Enuma Elish, composed around 1700 B.C.E. and derived from even earlier Sumerian myths, tells of the sweet waters of the rivers, the Tigris and Euphrates, mingling with the salt and bitter waters of the sea. And it is from this mixing that life is created within the mother, but at this point the land is not yet fertile. The fertile soil must be wrestled out of the desert; a struggle is required, for anything great must come from a great effort. Here we have a mythology that is halfway between the Eastern view of nonduality and the modern Western view of strict duality. All of creation, according to the Enuma Elish, is divine—it is the body of the original goddess mother. Man, however, is a secondary creation; he is semi-divine because he does have the lifeblood of a god flowing through him, but he is also an animal brought forth for one purpose only—to serve the gods.

If you lived four thousand years ago in Mesopotamia and if this was the story you had been hearing since you were a small child, how would you see your purpose in life? Would you have any doubt that you are in service to a higher power, put here only to toil and suffer? Still, you are partly divine; you exist because of the sacrifice of a god who himself was formed from the original waters of the universe—but but it was not a willing sacrifice. Like Kingu you are to submit to the dominance of those more powerful than you: That is your only purpose, your only reason for being.

✳ ✳ ✳

A Buddhist Story

The waters of the universe: This is a common theme in many creation mythologies. For Carl Jung, the ocean represents the deep psychic landscape of our soul. *Psyche* is a Greek word that literally means "life" or "breath," but also "self, spirit" or "soul"; in modern depth psychology (there is the word again—*psyche-ology*!), it refers to the totality of our personality, the conscious and unconscious components of our total self. The deep psyche then refers to the layers of ourselves that we have no conscious awareness of, despite the vastness lurking within.[5] There are mysteries hidden in the deep, mysteries which sometimes push through into conscious awareness; when they do, they always appear in symbolic language. It is only when the deep stirs that things happen. In the time prior to the waters moving, there was no time at all and no universe. The original waters are calm, but then a breath is breathed, as happened in this Buddhist cosmology:

⇜ ⇝

At first there is nothing, a nothingness created by the consuming fires that ended the earlier universe. Time is the only thing that moves. From the highest heaven, a Buddha watches the nothingness without thought, without feeling, without a body, a heart or a mind.

After a great pause, another age begins, the age of arising. The wind begins to move, moved by the consequences of human activity performed in the previous universe. The air of this newborn universe swirls faster, moving in a grand circle, spiraling like a galaxy. The wind moves, molds and condenses water, which forms a smaller disk floating on top of the wind circle.

The water, affected by the swirling wind, hardens, begetting a disk of land that floats on top of it. This disk of earth is the same diameter and circumference as the water disk, but it is thinner. The earth forms on the water like a skin forming on heated milk. It is golden. Upon this golden earth arise seven mountain ranges, several seas and four continents. The outer Iron Mountain range, named Cakravâ

a, contains the oceans, which in turn create islands of the four continents. The southern continent is our home, bounded to the north by the mountains of snow, the Himavat, and to the east and west the continent tapers to a point flanked on each side by the ocean. North of the Himavat is a great lake from which the four great rivers flow.

In the center of the golden earth disk is the wonderful, holy mountain Sumeru, on whose sides many gods live in their four heavens. Below, buried deep within the golden earth are the eight hot hells, the eight cold hells and the innumerable individual hells where, in torment, solitary souls purge themselves of their consequences.

Around the center of the holy mountain, swirling in the wind, floats the circle of stars; above them, the moon; above it, the sun. The 33 gods in another heaven found on the summit of Sumeru look down upon the sun and the moon, but theirs is not the highest of the heavens. Indra rules this summit, and above Indra, higher in the sky above Sumeru, are four other heavens. The lowest of these is the heaven of Yama, the god of death. Above Yama is *Tushita* heaven, where the bodhisattvas await their return to the human lands below.

All we have seen are in the Realm of Desire, where pain and suffering are constant companions to all life. Above this realm are the four superior heavens in the Realm of Form: the lowest of these heavens, the first *Dhyana* realm, is ruled by Brahma who, through his meditation, has gone beyond desire and evil; above him are three more Dhyana heavens, and above them all, which is nowhere at all, is the ultimate Realm of Formlessness, where the Buddhas dwell. There they are beyond space, matter, thought and all suffering and delight, but not beyond the reach of time.

The time of creation gives way to the time of duration: One age follows another, each lasting for 20 kalpas, which is a terribly long time. One kalpa is the time it would take to erode away a rock that is two kilometers high, two kilometers wide and two kilometers long by softly rubbing across it the robe of a celestial woman once every hundred years. In other words, it is a very, very long time.

Six forms of beings work out their lives within this universe, being born, dying, being reborn and re-dying: the gods, humans, animals, ghosts, the hell-bound creatures and the anti-gods, whom men call demons and devils. When no one is reborn in hell anymore and the first human is born in Brahma's heaven, the hells begin to empty. When the hells are empty, they disappear. When the land of living beings is empty and all have been reborn in the Realm of Form, the land, too, disappears. When all the gods in the first Dhyana heaven are reborn in the second Dhyana heaven, then the first Dhyana heaven also disappears.

When the karma of all living beings is extinguished, then seven suns appear, and fire destroys the universe totally, up to and including the first Dhyana heaven. The age of nothingness begins: Burnt up are the wind circle, the water circle, the golden earth, the four continents, the six mountain ranges and wonderful Sumeru. Gone, gone, all gone ... for now. And then they come again.

9

After seven more turnings of the ages, even the second Dhyana heaven dissolves, this time through a great flood. After eight times eight turnings of the wheel of time, the universe is extinguished even to and including the third Dhyana heaven, this time by the wind that begins it all again. Only the fourth Dhyana heaven and the Buddhas remain safe ... for now.

⚛ ⚛

The universe begins with a wind, which moves the waters. It is tempting to say the universe begins with a breath or a voice pronouncing a word, by a sound, but that would be personalizing the energy of creation, making it into a Him. That is the temptation we in the West have given in to. This is not the metaphor of Buddhism; there is no personal god who begins the world nor ends it. All that which happens, happens by the inexorable laws of Nature itself. There is no intention, no judgment and no prime mover willing all to happen; there is no one to pray to asking that things be different.

Like most myths, this story of creation evolved over centuries. Unlike our earlier stories, it is a dry story—actually a bit boring. It is filled with confusing facts, lists, numbers, and has no personality to it. There are no heroes or bad guys. The story evolved during the first thousand years after the time of the Buddha, who was born around 500 B.C.E.[6] The universe comes into existence and goes back into the nothingness from which it will arise again. The animating energy that causes everything to unfold and dissolve is *karma* (a word which comes from the Sanskrit root*kr*, which means "action"); karma can be thought of as simply consequence. Anything that can ever happen comes about only from the consequences of prior happenings, and in turn these current happenings create new consequences from which the future arises. Nothing exists in and of itself; everything is a consequence of something else. This is known in Buddhism as the Theory of Dependent Origination, and we will return to this topic in great detail later on.

The arising of the universe comes about because of the consequences, or the karma, of the previous universe. No god is required: We are not divine, nor are we even divinely created; we are but participants in an ongoing, never-ending cycle of becoming, being, dissolving, waiting and becoming again. All the people, all the animals, all the gods are just agents of the great cycles;[7] and all the worlds, all the heavens and all the hells are stages and props created for this particular telling of the same old tale.

If this mythology was your guiding worldview, how would you see your life? Where would you find the room for optimism, or even pessimism? Through countless incarnations, we progress, regress and progress again, until finally we all make it to heaven; which only means it is time for the whole world to be destroyed again. Nothing lasts; everything changes. You have been here before, done all this before, read this particular sentence before, and will come back and do it all again next time.

❋ ❋ ❋

If this creation myth leaves you wanting, you are not alone. This myth has no answers to the question of where people came from. How did the humans, gods and devils arise in the first place? How did the very first cycle of creation get started? This myth arose after the Buddha's passing, and he was not the one who developed the ontology suggested by it. The Buddha was reticent to talk of such matters. He was a pragmatist and rarely got caught up in such speculations, as this story demonstrates:

᪶ ᪷

One time a monk filled with questions came up to the Buddha. After saluting the Honored One, kissing his feet, and enquiring as to his health, the man laid out his burden. In quick succession he asked, "Please tell me whether the universe is eternal or will it one day end? Or can it be that it is both eternal and not eternal, or neither eternal nor not eternal? Is the universe finite or infinite, or is it both finite and infinite, or is it neither finite nor infinite? And, please tell me, is the self identical to the body or is the body separate from the self? And when a saint dies, does he still exist or not, or is he both existent and nonexistent, or neither existing or not existing?

The Buddha considered the monk carefully. "Did I ever promise to answer such questions?"

"Well, no," admitted the monk.

"Did I ever say that if you follow a spiritual life, these questions would be answered for you?"

"No," repeated the monk.

The Buddha fell silent for another moment and then offered a parable:

❧ ❦

There was once a man who was wounded by an arrow that was dipped in deadly poison. His friends and family quickly brought a doctor to him, but before the physician could tend to his wound, the man stopped him. "Wait! Before you remove the arrow, I must know, who shot me? Why? Was he an enemy or was this an accident? And where did the arrow come from, who made the arrow, from what bird did the feathers of the arrow come, and from what animal was the string of the bow made? I need to understand all this!"

The doctor then replied to the suffering man, "I can try to answer your questions, but in the meantime the poison will kill you; or I can get on with saving your life and end your suffering!"

◄ ►

"In the same way," explained the Buddha, "following a spiritual path does not require you to know whether the universe is eternal or not; whether it is finite or not; whether the self is separate from the body or not; or whether a saint exists after death or not."

"It is of no value to know these things, my dear monk. Instead, invest your time in finding the end to suffering that is afflicting you right now; let go of desire, hatred and your confusion about the causes of suffering."

◄ ►

THE BIBLICAL STORIES OF CREATION

It seems logical to think that if there is a creation, there must be a creator. But does that creator have to be a person or can it simply be a power, an energy by which all things come into being? And whether there is an impersonal power that causes everything to be, or there is a personifiable entity that brought about the creation of the universe, are we supposed to identify with it or merely relate to it? Our myths give us answers, but the answers are very different between East and West and even within the Eastern philosophies. In the West, there is but one philosophy. The mythologies found today in the West are very different than any found in the East: The main mythologies extant today in the West, the myths of Christianity, Judaism and Islam, flow from two (!) biblical creation mythologies:

◄ ►

In the beginning God created the heaven and the earth. The earth was without form, and void; darkness was upon the face of the deep. The breath of God moved upon the face of the waters. God said, "Let there be light" and there was light. God saw the light, that it was good, and He divided the light from the darkness. God called the light

13

Day, and the darkness He called Night. The evening and the morning were the first day.

God said, "Let there be a structure in the midst of the waters, and let it divide the waters from the waters." God made the structure and divided the waters that were under the structure from the waters that were above the structure. God called the arc of the structure Heaven. The evening and the morning were the second day.

God said, "Let the waters under heaven be gathered together unto one place, and let the dry land appear." It was so. God called the dry land Earth and the gathering together of the waters He called Seas. God saw that it was good. Then God said, "Let the earth bring forth grass, plants yielding seed, and trees yielding fruit." It was so. The earth brought forth grass, plants and trees, and God thought that He had done a good job. The evening and the morning were the third day.

God said, "Let there be lights in the structure of heaven to divide the day from the night, and let them be there as signs for the seasons, and for days, and for years. Let them give light upon the earth." It was so. God made two great lights: the greater light to rule the daytime and the lesser light to rule the nighttime. He made the stars also and set them in the structure of heaven to give light upon the earth. God thought that this was pretty good, too. The evening and the morning were the fourth day.

God said, "Let the waters bring forth many swimming creatures and birds that may fly above the earth." God created great whales and every living creature that moved in the seas. God saw that this was also good, so He blessed them, saying, "Be fruitful, and multiply, and fill the seas and sky." The evening and the morning were the fifth day.

God said, "Let the earth bring forth living creatures: cattle and creeping things and beast of the earth." It was so.

God made the beasts of the earth and cattle and everything that creeped upon the earth. God saw that it was good.

God said, "Finally, let us make man in our image, after our likeness, and let them have dominion over the fish of the sea, and over the birds of the air, and over the cattle, and basically over the whole blessed planet." So God created man in His own image, in the image of God created He man: male and female. God blessed them, and God said to them, "Be fruitful, and multiply, and replenish the earth, and subdue it and have dominion over the fish of the sea, and over the birds of the air, and over every living thing that moves upon the earth."

God said, "Behold, I have given you every plant bearing seed and every tree that bears fruits, nuts and seeds; to you it shall be food. And every creature of the land, sea or air will be for your use." It was so. God saw everything that He had made and—behold!—it was very good. The evening and the morning were the sixth day.

Thus the heavens and the earth and all the good stuff in them were finished. On the seventh day, God ended His work and took a break. God blessed the seventh day and sanctified it because in it He had rested from all His labors.

⅋ ⅊

This story is the first of two creation myths found in Genesis, the first book of the Bible. Genesis, which means "the beginning," gives us our word *generate*. This story of generation, which includes the first chapter entirely and three lines of the second chapter, was compiled and written around the fifth century B.C.E., during and after the Babylonian captivity of the Jewish people. Around 587 B.C.E. the Babylonians conquered Israel, leveled the Jewish temple in Jerusalem, and deported a large segment of the population to Babylon. In 539 B.C.E. King Cyrus the Great of Persia conquered the Babylonians and repatriated the Jewish people back to Jerusalem.

During their 50 years of captivity, the Israelites were introduced to many of the grand myths of the Babylonians. The Jewish alphabet changed, as did their calendar, and their rituals also underwent transformation. No longer could they worship a god who was close by in the temple; the temple was gone. Where was God now? They decided God was wherever the Jewish people were.

The emancipating Persians were a different lot altogether from the Babylonians they had deposed and the Jews whom they freed. They had a very different mythology. It was during the century after the Persians repatriated the Jews back to Israel that the stories of Zoroaster, the great Persian prophet, began to influence biblical thinking—but we are getting ahead of ourselves.

In the Genesis chapter 1 creation story, the breath or spirit of God moved upon the waters. To Carl Jung, the presence of water in a dream or in a myth can be symbolic of the original and undifferentiated psyche before consciousness awakens. Indeed, there is darkness on the deep waters: Something is needed to bring forth the light of consciousness, some energy must stir the water, and that energy is often a breath. Breath is life. Breathing brings to life that which was inanimate and dormant. In many ancient cultures, the word for breath and for life was the same. In Latin, *spiritus* means "our spirit" and it also means "breath." In India, in Sanskrit, the word *prana* similarly means "breath" and "life force." In Hebrew and in the Bible, the word used is *ruach*, which can mean "wind," "spirit" or "breath."

We are dealing with deep psychic images here. It is from the deep waters of the psyche that things come into the light or into consciousness. We find this in many creation myths, but notice what is unique in the Genesis chapter 1 story: God created the universe out of nothing—*ex nihilo*—not from himself. The universe is not God's body split apart, as we found in the early Babylonian story of Tiamat. Remember, Tiamat, the great mother goddess, was torn apart, and by a god who was her descendant. Also note that the biblical God is not the original Self of the Upanishad story, who split itself apart.

Notice also that God in the biblical myth gave man dominion over the land and all animals. We were ordered to be fruitful and multiply; we were told to subdue nature and make it serve us. This command reinforces the idea that we are separate from nature: We are not part of the land; we are in charge of it. The animals are there only for our purposes and have no value in and of themselves. We are given dominion over every living thing. What an awesome responsibility this myth imposes upon us!

In many creation stories, there is a god splitting something apart in order to form the heavens and the earth, and in most of these stories, God is not an impersonal force as described in many Indian stories, such as the Buddhist *Abhidharmakośa*. Rather, God is very much a person. This is more so the case in the biblical rendition: God is a personality and He is the Creator; we are His creation, and out of His own will did everything come into being.

In Western culture, our mythos is based upon this biblical story. While man is made in His image, we are not God; we are God's creation. Nature is not divine; nature is also God's creation. There is a personality running the whole show, and we are not it. According to the moral of this myth, our job is to figure out how to come into a relationship with this great personality.

✳ ✳ ✳

If we delve a little deeper in Genesis, we will find an earlier, second creation myth, one perhaps created around 950 B.C.E. [8] It is a story that scholars define more as a theology of history rather than a philosophical treatment. Regardless, there are many mythic images to be found in this second story. It is a second story of man—how he was created, why, and how he fell from grace through a great sin.

⚛ ⚛

In the day that God made the earth and the heavens, and every plant and every herb, nothing yet grew because God had not yet invented rain and there was no man to till the ground. God caused a mist to come up from the earth, and the ground was watered. Now it was time for the gardener.

God formed man of the dust of the ground. His name was Adam, which means "earth." God breathed into his nostrils the breath of life; man became a living soul.

God planted a garden eastward in Eden. In the garden grew every tree that was pleasant and good for food. There were two very special trees, as well: the Tree of Life and the Tree of Knowledge of Good and Evil.

God put Adam in the Garden of Eden to take care of it. God commanded him, "Of every tree of the garden thou may freely eat, but not of the Tree of Knowledge of Good and Evil. If you eat its fruit, you will die."

After a while God noticed that Adam was lonely and said, "I will make a helper for him." Out of the ground God formed every beast of the field, and every fowl of the air and brought them unto Adam to see what he would call them. Whatever Adam called each living creature, that was its name. Adam gave names to all cattle, and to the fowl of the air, and to every beast of the field, but for Adam himself, there was no helper.

God decided to fix this and put Adam to sleep. As Adam slept, God split Adam apart and from his side at the level of the heart, God created a woman. When Adam awoke, God presented the woman and Adam said, "This is bone of my bones, and flesh of my flesh: She shall be called

Woman, because she was taken out of Man." Now we understand why a man will leave his father and mother and will cling to his wife, so they can become joined again as one flesh. Adam and his wife were both naked, but they didn't care.

Now the serpent was the most subtle of any creature. It said to the woman, "Did God really say that you couldn't eat of every tree of the garden?"

The woman told the serpent, "We can eat of any tree, except of the Tree of Knowledge because if we do, we will die."

The serpent said, "You won't die! God knows that if you eat of the Tree of Knowledge, you will be like gods! You will know good from evil."

This got the woman to thinking: The tree did look pretty good, and what is the matter with being wise? She plucked the fruit, ate a bit, and gave the rest to Adam, who also took a bite. As if for the first time, their eyes were opened, and the first thing they realized was that they were stark naked. To cover themselves they sewed little aprons out of fig leaves.

Before long, God came looking for them, but they were afraid and hid. God called to Adam and Adam revealed himself. He admitted that he was hiding because he didn't want God to see him naked.

"Who told you that you were naked?" asked God. "Did you eat that fruit that I told you not to eat?"

Passing the buck quickly, Adam said, "That woman you gave me, she gave me the fruit."

God turned to her. "Woman, what did you do?"

Passing the buck still further, the woman replied, "It was the serpent! It talked me into it."

God first addressed the serpent. "Because you did this, you will be cursed above all creatures. You will go upon your belly and eat dust your whole life. I will make sure all women hate you."

Next He turned to the woman. "From now on your life will be hard and you will suffer in childbirth. You will want only your husband and he shall rule you."

To Adam: "Because you listened to your wife instead of me, I curse the ground you came from, because it did not speak out to stop you from committing this sin; in sorrow will you eat whatever it yields. You will live by the sweat of your brow until you return to the earth, for from dust you were made and to dust will you return."

Now God was worried. He said to Himself, "They have become like us—they know good and evil. What if they eat of the other tree, the Tree of Immortal Life, and live forever? They can't stay in the garden."

God created clothes of animal skins for the man and woman and sent them out of the garden. In case they tried to return, He placed guardians at the east gate of Eden: Cherubims with a flaming sword kept the way to the Tree of Life.

Adam decided to name his wife Eve, which means "life," because she was to become the mother of all humanity.[9]

৺ ৶

Remember the Self from our first story from India? In that myth we are all part of that original Self who split itself in twain to create us. In the Babylonian story, Marduk was the great god who split apart the Mother Goddess to form the universe, and he was the one who made man out of little piles of dust, just as God did in Genesis chapter 2. However, unlike God, Marduk brought man to life by taking a life, by sacrificing Kingu. In Genesis chapter 2, God *breathed* life into man, and along with the breath came Adam's soul. (It is interesting to notice the timing here: We do not get our souls until we take our first breath!)

We will return to the symbology inherent in this story as it applies to women when we visit the psychological functions of myths, but it should be noted here just how poorly women are depicted in this story, especially the very first woman, Eve. It is easy to see that this god intends women to be second to man in many ways. Eve came second. She came from Adam's heart, not his head; she is not his intellectual equal.

This last statement raises a very important point: When we listen to ancient stories with modern ears, we can read into them meanings that were not there originally. When we read that Eve was taken from Adam's side and not his head, it is easy to think this means she is not intellectually equal to Adam, that women are more emotional and less logical than men. We reach this conclusion because in our day, we know that the brain is the seat of thought and rationality. This was not always the map: To the ancient Greeks, for example, thinking was known to occur in the torso, not the brain. They were not sure what the function of the brain was. They knew it was important—an injury to the head could kill a man or incapacitate him—but what did the brain do? They weren't sure. One theory was that the brain was a radiator that cooled the blood. Another theory, held in both India and Greece and of great interest to yoga teachers today, was that the brain was the source of semen! Semen was produced in the brain, flowed down a central, holy channel of the spine, was stored in the testes, and flowed out from there when the need arose (which may explain why many women feel that men's brains seem to be located in their pants).[10]

If you knew that thoughts were embodied in the torso, that you made decisions based on what your heart and guts told you, then saying that woman came from man's side would not imply any intellectual superiority of man over woman. In fact, looking at the meaning of this story in Genesis chapter 2 in another light, since the soul was believed to be seated in the heart, God split Adam's soul in half and gave one part to Eve. Eve literally became Adam's soul mate. This implies that we all have a soul mate somewhere that God has created for us and out of us.

Our ability to interpret a myth in a variety of ways does not invalidate the myth, it adds to it. Claude Lévi-Strauss (1908-2009) theorized that a myth must include all the variations of the story, in the same way Freud's thoughts about Oedipus are now a part of the Oedipus myth.[11] The way a myth originally affected the people of that time and culture is not necessarily the way it talks to us now. Remember, the point of a story is not to be true for all time and in all situations, but to be useful.

Let's return to the mythic Eve: She was meant to be a helper to man, but she was the one who caused all the trouble for which man was cursed forever. Never mind that Adam willingly ate the fruit, too; he only did it to stop Eve from nagging him. (There is a story in Jewish lore that Eve had to beg and plead for hours before Adam would agree to taste the fruit.[12]) For her part in the fall in the garden, Eve was more severely cursed than Adam. Imagine having to hate snakes all the time! In their positive aspect, snakes are symbols of the continuity of life. In most of the high, ancient cultures, the goddess is often depicted with snakes. Snakes shed their skins and are reborn again and again. They are the earthly symbol of the moon, which also dies and is reborn. The goddess is the originator of life. "Eve" means "life". It is only in our Western mythology that we find snakes cursed, and women along with them.

This will not be the last time we hear about snakes, but for now just think what this myth means for women. If this story is the story that determines how you are to relate to women, how will you treat them? Even if you are a woman, notice what this story is telling you about yourself. The power of this story works at a very deep psychic level. Even if you tell yourself, "Well, I don't really believe women are that bad," if this is your guiding myth, you will act *as if* you do believe they are that bad. It is obvious that men have subjugated women throughout history, but it is equally true that women themselves have believed they were some man's property and not worthy of much.

In this myth the earth is cursed; man is forced to fight the earth in order to bring forth his daily bread. We find God against man, and man disobeying God; God against nature and nature against God; man against nature and nature against man; and woman is cursed along with nature. Quite a story!

* * *

THE SYMPOSIUM OF PLATO

In the oral traditions of Judaism, there are more to their stories than is found in the Christian Bible. From around 400 C.E. onward, a literature of commentary and expansion of the ideas and stories of the Torah (the first five books of the Jewish Bible) were developed. They are known as the Midrash. In one expansion of the Genesis tale, we learn that before God split him apart, Adam was both male and female.[13] These are echoes of the Indian idea of the original Self splitting in two— male and female—but this idea is also presented in more grandeur in this story told by Plato around the year 380 B.C.E.:

Plato called for a party, a symposium, and during the party he asked each person present to sing a song of praise to love. Due to a bout of hiccups, Aristophanes begged to be passed over the first time it fell to him to talk, but when it was his turn again he explained the power of love through a grand story.

Originally humanity had three sexes. In the sun there lived men who were the size of two men joined together. These men-men had four legs, four arms, two faces on one head looking in different directions, and they were very powerful. Similarly on the earth there lived women who were the size of two women. These women-women also had four arms and legs and two faces. On the moon, which is made of both sun and earth, there were people formed of both a man and a woman, which we called androgynous, although that word has fallen out of favor in recent times.

So powerful was the race of humans with their three sexes that the gods were worried. On one occasion the humans tried to scale the heights to the heavens so they could attack the gods. The gods debated what to do about these humans. Should they destroy them for this sin, as they did the giants of old? But if they did that, who would offer the sacrifices that the gods require?

Finally Zeus came up with a plan. He split each person apart, and Apollo stitched up the new individuals so they would be complete and healthy, although diminished. Apollo took the extra skin created by the splitting and pulled it tight to the front of the body, where he fastened it with a knot, which today we call the belly button. Zeus also moved the genital organs forward to allow the sexes to procreate and beget new humans to serve the gods.

As soon as each person was split in two, each clung to their split-apart, so great is the power of love. They would rather die than be separated from their other half. For the men from the sun, their desired half was another man and they cared not for women, while the men from the moon desired only women. For the women from the earth, their desired half was another woman and they cared not for men, while the women from the moon desired only men.

With the humans clinging tightly to their other halves, nothing was getting done. The gods realized the power of love was too strong: No one was being born, and no one was performing the sacrifices. So the gods reduced the power of love greatly and then separated the two halves far apart. Thus, to this day, men and women search for their soul mate—the one who will complete them.

⁙ ⁙

Quite the story! First, notice that man's divinity is not addressed—we don't know how man originally came into being—but man is almost as powerful as the gods themselves, certainly enough to get the gods worried. Aristotle and many other Greek philosophers were uncomfortable with telling tales about the original creation of the universe. Such stories always sounded like a stroke of divine intervention. They preferred to just assume the universe and man had always existed. What we might call God, Aristotle called the Prime Mover, a force beyond the realm of the gods and humans, or even the material universe itself, and one never involved in any of it. As a purely spiritual being, the Prime Mover could not be involved in material affairs, such as a person's day-to-day life. Even Aristophanes at Plato's party does not tell us where the first joined-together humans came from. He tells only that the sin, committed by man when he so audaciously tried to scale heaven and become like a god, had earned us the punishment of being split into two. And, if we were to try anything like that again, Zeus promised to split us in half once more!

Women in Aristophanes' story are not beneath men: they are not secondary to men. Woman did not come out of man, as is told in the Genesis chapter 2 myth; women are equal to men, and some women don't even want a man. If someone had this map as a basic template in the deep psyche, how do you think his or her life would unfold? Unfortunately, this myth of equality between all sexual orientations is not one that is well known or accepted today.

✳ ✳ ✳

A PERSIAN STORY OF CREATION

Unique to the West is this idea of sin: a fall from grace. In the East, we are part of nature and part of God. Everything comes from the same singular source, and life unfolds in an impersonal manner. Nothing is inherently good or bad, and God is not ordering anyone about. The only "sin" is to resist this inevitable unfolding. For the Greeks, the great sin of mankind is hubris, the idea that man can be as great as the gods. In the Bible, the sin is disobeying God. We are God's servants, and through our failure to obey, the earth is cursed, woman is cursed, and life is forever hard—at least, in the Christian mythologies, until someone comes along and sets things right again. The fall illustrated in Genesis chapter 2 is unusual because it is man's fault that things are screwed up. In Persian mythology there was also a fall, there is darkness in the world, and although man was not the one responsible, man can help fix things:

୭ ୫

Two great forces exist in the universe: the forces of light created by the god of light and wisdom, Ahura Mazda, and the forces of darkness created by Ahura Mazda's evil twin, the destructive mind, Angra Mainyu. Ahura Mazda is the stronger of the two; he is all-knowing but not all-powerful. He knows that Angra Mainyu can cause problems, so he bides his time, and while he waits, he creates all the things that are good.

One day, before there were any days because the sun had not yet been invented, Angra Mainyu goes out for a little walk. Cresting a hill he sees a light, a disgustingly beautiful light that annoys him greatly. In his anger Angra Mainyu attacks the wondrous light, but Ahura Mazda beats him back, and Angra Mainyu retreats to his dark abyss.

Between the two brothers is the great void. Ahura Mazda invites Angra Mainyu to a peace talk. He offers his evil brother a deal: to serve the creatures of light and in exchange live forever in peace. Angra Mainyu angrily rejects the overture and vows to turn all of Ahura Mazda's creatures against the cursed light. He retreats to his abyss, where for three thousand years he conjures evil spirits.

Ahura Mazda knows that the span of the universe, the limit of time itself, will last only twelve thousand years in total. He sees what will happen. If he tries to attack his evil brother, Angra Mainyu just might win. So Ahura Mazda bides his time and creates some more good stuff. For the first 3,000 years, both brothers create creatures of spirit only.

Ahura Mazda consulted with the spirit of humanity. Before incarnating him materially on earth, he offers man a choice: Would man prefer that Ahura Mazda protect him from evil, and evil never ends; or would man rather that Ahura Mazda let evil tempt him and challenge him, hurt him and kill him, knowing that, in the end, evil will be vanquished forever and man will be restored to his young, healthy bodies and live forever in peace? The guardian spirits of man chose the latter course, and so man chose to fight on the side of the forces of light and to oppose evil.

Now is the time for things to become tangible. Ahura Mazda first creates the sky, then water, earth, plants, animals and finally man. He creates the stars and places them in the Zodiac. He creates the moon and then the sun. He sends Gayomart and his companion, the primordial ox, Gosurvan, to earth. The period of the second three thousand years is a golden age that belongs to Gayomart. All is peaceful until Angra Mainyu rises from the depths and launches his attack.

The forces of darkness infest everything that has been created. All that was good is soiled, corrupted and darkened. Gosurvan is killed. In anguish she cries to Ahura Mazda, "Why? Where is the protector you promised for all that is good?" Ahura Mazda calms the faithful ox by showing her the spirit of the great prophet to come, Zoroaster. In peace Gosurvan surrenders her body, and from it are born the 55 kinds of grain, the 12 healing plants and all species of good animals.

Angra Mainyu attacks Gayomart and sickens him. Gayomart suffers for 30 years before succumbing. From his dead body come the eight precious minerals, including silver and gold. Through gold, Gayomart's seed is purified and from it, after 40 years, a reed grows, as big as two human beings. The reed is our first two parents, still joined together. Ahura Mazda splits the pair apart and breathes their souls into them. For 50 years they enjoy life, but something is missing; they haven't invented sex yet. One day they think, "If we open these here and put this there … ummm, that feels good," and soon babies start to appear. But Angra Mainyu confuses our first parents. He makes them pronounce the first lie—they say that we were created by evil. This is the first sin of mankind.

Our first parents breed the whole human race, but the forces of darkness make life ugly and hard. Where Ahura Mazda created new lands, fertile and well organized, Angra Mainyu created winter and excessive heat in summer; plagues of snakes and locusts; ants and anthills; witchcraft, sorcery and astrology; the cooking and eating of dead bodies and the burying of the dead; barbarians and plunder; idolatry, pride and desire; tears and lamentation; menstruation and other abnormal issues in women. All these are the works of the evil Angra Mainyu.

During these three thousand years, good and evil strive equally, neither one winning a decisive battle. At the end of this period, Zoroaster comes to earth, born of a virgin and half-divine. He creates a new religion to bring good people back to the light, and as a consequence, he is constantly assailed by the darkness. Somehow, and fortunately, Zoroaster always survives.

> The final age dawns: Over the final three thousand years, the battles between good and evil grow fierce. At the time of the final battle, the great world savior, Saoshyant, conceived when his mother bathed in a lake containing the preserved seed of Zoroaster, leads the Sons of Light against the Sons of Darkness and begets the restoration. In this final End of Days, all men, the living and the dead, are restored to life and health. Those who had sided with evil spend three days in hell for their sins, but after the purgation they, too, join the light. Everyone is saved, the good and the bad, because there is no evil anymore. Time now is finished, and for eviternity, man lives in peace.

The great prophet of Persia was Zarathustra, also known to the Greeks and thus to most Europeans and Westerners as Zoroaster. His life is shrouded to us. Scholars do believe that he was a historical figure but aren't sure when he lived. It may have been as early as the 11th century B.C.E. or as late as the sixth century B.C.E.[14] His religion became known as Zoroastrianism and was the primary religion of the early Iranians. Its influence was felt in all the Abrahamic traditions of the Near East and lasted well into the Christian era. You probably noticed many similarities in this story to ideas found in Christian and Jewish stories: the order of creation, the coming End of Days, the Sons of Light, etc.

This myth shows us that creation is meant to be good. Originally it was good, but evil was poured into it. This arising of evil was not man's fault (notice the significant difference here with the biblical story), but man is presented with a clear choice: help fight against the evil or just sit back and be overwhelmed by the forces of darkness.

There are other themes in this story that we have seen already. Notice again how in these Western stories man needs to be split apart into male and female, and a god is the one who does the splitting. Notice the dualities also: There is the dualism between good and evil, and there is difference between man and god. Man here is not divine; he is created by a creator as in the Bible, but this creator is not all-powerful. He is all-knowing, yes, but Ahura Mazda needs man's help. Man is not the servant of God, but a necessary and willing partner in the fight against evil. Man has to choose to fight on the side of right. We are here for one shot only at the End of Days—there are no grand cycles—and we only have a few thousand years for all this to unfold. There will be a restoration, and everyone, the good people and the bad people, who will have been purged of their sins by then, will live together in peace forever.

These ideas would influence other myths and cultures down through the centuries. The Jewish idea of a world messiah can be traced to this Persian myth. Remember, it was the great Persian King Cyrus who defeated the Babylonians and restored the Jews to Israel so they could rebuild their temple. Cyrus was hailed by the author of Isaiah as like unto a messiah![15] John the Baptist and the early Christians, including Jesus and Saint Paul, and their contemporaneous Jewish counterparts, the Essenes, were influenced by the Persian story and felt that the End of Days was upon them and that the Sons of Light would conquer the Sons of Darkness, personified in those days by the Romans. They also believed that the time of the apocalypse and ensuing rapture was nigh and would happen in their generation.[16] Unfortunately, they read the myth literally instead of poetically, the Roman Sons of Darkness were not vanquished, and the only End of Days would be the end of the days for the secsond temple of Jerusalem and Israel as a geographic nation.

Chapter 2: The Magic of Myth

Are we one or are we two? Are we divine or merely divinely created? Are we simply in service to a higher power, or do we have a role to play beyond one of servitude? Is the universe screwed up or just fine, and if it is all cockeyed, were we the ones who created the problem? How are we to understand ourselves with respect to the universe itself?

The cosmological function of myths shows us how to come into accord with the universe in which we find ourselves. The symbols found in the myths lay out a map which, if we follow, will make our journey easier. Remember, these symbols are not historical facts, but they are powerful nonetheless.

As we touched on with the work of Joseph Campbell, the proper way to understand a myth is metaphorically. The stories are filled with symbols that speak to us below the conscious level. In order to decide whether the symbol is appropriate today and whether we are to understand the symbol consciously given our current life situation, we need to shine a light into this darkness. Once we understand the symbol, we may find that it still works, or we may find that we would be better off finding a new myth to guide our unconscious reactions to life.

Joseph Campbell was raised an Irish Catholic in White Plains, New York. He knew the symbols of the Catholic Church very well. Like most Catholics his early images of the Virgin Mary were based on the belief that Mary's virginity was a historical fact; he later learned this is the wrong way to approach a powerful symbol. If you read the mythic images as facts, as one might find in the daily newspapers, they lose their real power. For example, if you are told that two thousand years ago, in a small town in the Middle East, a young virgin gave birth to the Son of God, you might think it interesting, but it would not move you to awe and wonder. However, if you are told that *you* have God within you and that *you* will manifest God without any help from anyone else, then the story has a very different effect. If you read the myth as a message to and about *you*, then the imagery becomes powerful. The 17th-century German mystic Angelus Silesius [1624–1677] said, "Of what use Gabriel's 'Ave Marie,' unless he can give the same message to me?"[1]

This is the magic of the myth: It is a personal power because it touches that source of energy deep within you. There is no need to take the stories literally. If you do that, you lose their power.

✳ ✳ ✳

THE MAGIC OF SYMBOLS

The seal shown here is from the ancient city of Mohenjo-Daro, a major city of the Harappan civilization, also known as the Indus Valley civilization, located in what is now Pakistan. It shows Shiva sitting in meditation. These seals were used in business to seal cargo before it was shipped abroad. The seals display a form of writing, as shown along the top, but we have no idea what the glyphs mean. There are many symbolic aspects to this little picture, but for now, notice what this early, three-faced Shiva is wearing on his head. What is that?

Horns! Now, why wear horns on your head? The crown worn by kings and gods are symbolic of the heavens. What is there up in heaven that looks like these horns? The answer is the moon: more specifically, the horns of the moon as it initially climbs out of darkness and, again, just before plunging back into it.

The moon is the symbol of the cycles of life. The moon is born out of the sun. Over the 29.5 days of its cycle, it waxes, grows strong, and then at the middle of its life, at the peak of its brightness, darkness reappears and the moon wanes; the darkness expands until the moon dies once more, returning back into the sun. Everywhere one looks, one can find this same pattern unfolding: birth, maturation, duration, decay and death—this is one of the inexorable facts of life.

The moon can also be seen as a cup that fills with life and empties again. The light of the moon is ambrosia, the nectar of the gods of Greece. In India the liquid of immortality is called *amrta*. *Mrta* in Sanskrit means "death," and it is connected with our European word *mortal* and the Spanish *muerte*. If we put the letter *a* in front of this word, like in English, it means "not", so *a-mrta* means "no-death," thus immortality.

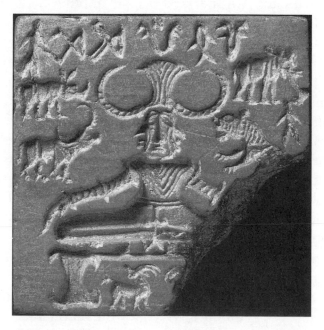

Figure 2 - Indus Seal from Mohenjo-Daro ca. ~2600 to 1900 B.C.E.

As the dark new moon emerges from the sun, it fills day by day with this amrta, the ambrosia of life. Once it is full, it starts to send the nectar down to earth as dew. In India the hot sun desiccates life; the moon at night replenishes it through the cooling dew. Thus, the moon empties so we may live.

In the practice of yoga, the symbology of the moon's liquor of immortality is mirrored physiologically within us. There is a moon center within our brains, the *chandra* center, which drips amrta. These drops of immortality fall into the stomach, the home of *surya*, the sun, where the god of fire, Agni, consumes it, just as the moon dies into the sun and is consumed each month. If we want to prolong life, we must stop the loss of amrta, so yogis turn themselves upside down. Inversions in Hatha Yoga are one means to stop this constant leaking away of life. Headstands and shoulder stands are the royal asanas, the king and queen of postures, which help the yogi live longer. This harkens back to another metaphor we have already seen: the moon's life-giving energy stored in the brain is soul food, semen. It, too, must be conserved, and in this model it is conserved through sexual abstinence, celibacy.

Do not take any of this literally, of course. The ancients didn't believe there was an actual moon in our brains dripping ambrosia that would allow us to live forever. The chandra and surya centers in our body were metaphors that worked: As long as we acted *as if* there were these centers and the nectar of immortality was being consumed inside of us; and as long as we acted *as if* turning this flow around would prolong our lives, then we could reap benefits.

Don't let the facts about the real moon cause you to lose sight of the benefits of the metaphoric moon. For example, the moon takes 29.5 days to go from full moon to the next full moon, and yet, symbolically, we say the moon takes 28 days to go through its cycle. This is not a fact: The fact is it takes

34

29.5 days, but if we act as if it is 28 days, we can come into accord with many other facets of existence. A woman's monthly cycles average to be 28 days: the word *menses*, from which we get the word *menstruation*, comes from the word *moon*. A week is seven days because there are seven wandering lights in the sky—the five planets, the sun and the moon—and each one has

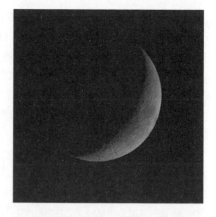

Figure 3 - The Horns of the Moon

its day. Four cycles of seven is 28, which is one cycle of the moon. The math sort of works, so don't let the facts get in the way. The sexagesimal system, with which we measure cycles of time and circles in space (from which we get 60 seconds in a minute, 60 minutes in an hour and 360 degrees in a circle), comes from the observation that a year is 360 days, more or less. Forget the fact that a year is actually 365.24 days: Just use those extra few days as holidays and don't consider them as actually part of the years, and things will be just fine.

The moon symbolizes the fact that life contains both birth and death occurring in never-ending cycles—as does the snake we saw earlier chatting up Eve in the garden. The snake throws off its skin to be reborn, just as the moon throws off its shadow to be reborn every month. The snake and the moon are equivalent images. So, too, is the bull: The inwardly curved horns of the bull are shaped like the crescent moon, one horn representing the new moon, the other representing the dying moon. It is for this reason the bull was sacred to so many ancient cultures and still is in India today: It is the metaphor of life. In point of fact, its meat and milk *were* life for many peoples. Now let's look again at that glyph from the ancient

Indus Valley civilization, which depicts a god, or perhaps it is a king or a yogi, sitting in meditation. On its head are the horns of the bull, which are symbolic of the horns of the moon. Around the seated figure are the iconic animals of ancient India: the elephant, the tiger, the water buffalo and the bull. At the bottom of the picture are deer. Each animal is symbolic and has a reason to be there.

The image has been associated with a god named the Pashupati, the lord of the beasts, and he is an early version of Shiva, although some scholars dispute this conclusion. Maybe he was just a king or a priest, but this image may be the oldest image of a god still worshipped today. He is found on many Harappan seals of this time, and he is shown in a very advanced yoga posture, *mulabandhasana*, sitting on a bench with the feet together, pointing down, which requires very open hips, lax knee ligaments and flexible ankles.

✳ ✳ ✳

SHIVA'S DANCE

Shiva has many depictions. Around the 9th ~ 10th centuries C.E., his image was condensed into dancing statues that show a skull and the crescent moon in his hair, the symbols of death and rebirth. His dance is the dance of the universe—from the smallest subatomic particles that can never be stilled to the swirling of gigantic megaclusters of galaxies in their celestial ballet, all life is but one dance. All is Shiva's *lila*, his play. It is interesting that Shiva's universe is named after a verb rather than a noun; the universe is action—forget about "stuff" and just act, move, play, and dance! Let's look at what happened when Shiva was once found dancing all alone in the forest:

ఆ ఆ

"What's this—Shiva alone? What good fortune; now is our chance! Without his armies to help him, Shiva is vulnerable. Now is the time to attack and finally kill Shiva!"

36

The priests consulted among themselves: How best can we rid the world of this arrogant god' this murderer who cut off the fifth head of Brahma, who was simply lusting after and attempting to rape his own beautiful daughter, Dawn; this philanderer who stole the virtue of our own wives while we were chasing after a beautiful courtesan that he himself sent to distract and weaken us? Pooling their black magic, the priests dug a pit from which they conjured a huge Bengal tiger, which they sent to devour the dancing fool.

Shiva did not miss a beat; his dance continued, but in the dance he slew the tiger, skinned it, and donned its skin as a skirt. Sometimes he would lay the skin on the ground to form a mat for his yoga practice. Long before rubber sheets were cut up and embossed with Lululemon logos, the skin of the tiger or perhaps a deer would form the yogi's perfect yoga mat.

Undaunted, the priests conjured again. They created a host of animals to attack the greatest god in the universe: a deer (what were they thinking!) and an elephant. But each time, Shiva easily dispatched the helpless creature. Getting desperate, the priest turned to the nagas, the serpents of the earth and the symbols of life's constant renewal, but these snakes, too, were no threat to Shiva. He turned them into ornaments and donned their coiled bodies as bracelets and bangles around his arms and ankles. The great king cobra was worn as a belt, while other cobras formed a web waving in his hair—just as the matted locks of the forest yogis fly about when they dance in imitation of Shiva.

It was time for one last, great magic. The priests drained all their hatred, all their frustrations and all their dark arts into their final creation—thedeadliest, most fearsome, ugliest, darkest, and most malevolent monster imaginable. They created … a dwarf. From their own dark hearts, they created Gimli, the son of Glóin and set him upon Shiva.[2] It was no use, however; Shiva tossed the dwarf to

37

the ground, stood upon him, and continued his dance as if nothing at all had happened. Shiva named the dwarf Avidya.

⤙ ⤚

The dancing depiction of Shiva is named Nataraja, the Lord of the Dance; the dance is called the *anandatandava*, which means the "dance (*tandava*) of bliss (*ananda*)." In this depiction he has four arms; in his top right hand, he is holding a drum called a *dumroo*, which is shaped like two intersecting cones, symbolic of the union of male and female, for Shiva is the ultimate hermaphrodite from which everything originates, just as any creator god must be. How else could generation occur if both sexes are not present? The dumroo measures the beat of the dance—the time of the universe. In Shiva's top left hand, he holds a flame, the flame that will ignite the whole universe when the time of dissolution has arrived. Shiva is both the creator of the universe, as shown by what is in his right hand, and the destroyer, as shown by what he holds in his left hand. All around the statue is a rim of fire symbolizing that final conflagration that awaits the end of the dance.

Shiva's lower right hand is raised in a universal gesture of teaching, bidding us to have no fear, for of what is there to be afraid when we are all just atoms in the dance of Shiva? The reason we do fear is that dwarf upon which Shiva dances: Avidya. *Vid* is a Sanskrit word that means "knowledge"; it is related to the Latin *video* and to the English *vision*. Remember, when we put the letter *a* in front of a word, it means "not", so *avidya* means "not knowledge" or more succinctly, "ignorance". Shiva is delivering us from the ignorance that prevents us from knowing our true nature. His lower left arm is pointing to our salvation; his arm looks like the trunk of an elephant. This gesture is called the elephant trunk gesture, because the elephant is the one who breaks new paths through the jungle, allowing others to easily go where there was no

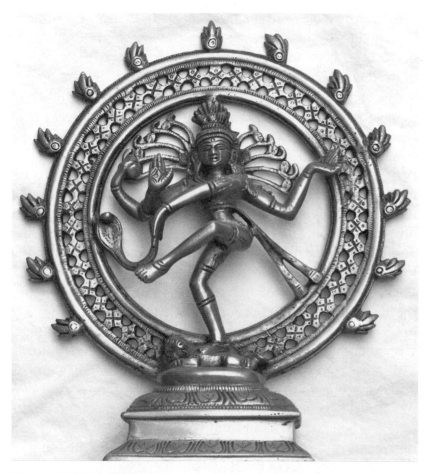

Figure 4: Shiva's Tandava

passage before. It is the teaching arm. The elephant arm is pointing to Shiva's left leg that is raised, symbolic of our deliverance from ignorance, called *moksha*.

The dance reveals the path to *satcitananada*: *sat*—"being"; *cit*—"consciousness"; *ananda*—"bliss." At the still point of the dance are Shiva's head and his serene countenance. Through mastery of the snake energy, the *kundalini* or *shakti* energy that yogis learn to control and guide through the central channel of the subtle body, Shiva has merged all opposites into simply being: male–female, birth–death, ignorance–knowledge. In this center of calm, there is the ultimate bliss of existence, ananda, and so we come to know the true meaning of the name of Shiva's dance: anandatandava.

Not shown in the statues is Shiva's ride; all the gods had their various forms of locomotion, and for ground travel, Shiva chooses to ride a great bull named Nandi. Nandi can be considered a possible precursor to Paul Bunyan's great Ox, Babe, although Babe was blue and Nandi, like Shiva, is pure white. Nandi the bull represents life and death, and he is the terrestrial equivalent to the moon. We see through many of Shiva's symbols that he is the great yogi who transcends life and death, for he is both the creator and the destroyer of the universe.

When Indians worship the bull, they are not worshipping that fact which is that particular cow, they are worshipping what the cow represents as a symbol. To say that Indians worship cows is like saying Americans pledge allegiance to a piece of cloth. The American flag is a symbol of their country, and we are to look beyond the fact that a flag is simply a piece of cloth cut into a particular shape with certain colors and geometric designs upon it. We are to see what the flag represents and put ourselves in accord with the meaning of the flag, not the fact of the flag itself.

It is easy for Western Christians to consider an Indian honoring a sacred cow as being superstitious. It's just a cow! What's the problem? Christians may laugh at the horror experienced by a Muslim when shown a cartoon depicting the prophet Mohammed. It's only a cartoon! What's the problem? But that same Christian may go apoplectic if he sees someone burn a piece of fabric that just happens to be an American flag. It's just a piece of cloth! What's the problem? It is easy to say that other people's symbols are quaint, silly or superstitious, but when our own symbols are treated as mere facts, their power erupts in strong emotions.

Our symbols have power when they represent something lying deep within our psyche. However, not all symbols have that power with all people. The cow, the moon, the snake, the word of the Prophet—these do not touch Western Christians at all, and because of this, Christians will find it difficult to understand these symbols. Carl Jung once asked, "Of what use is the image of Shiva dancing on a dwarf named Avidya to a bricklayer in Zurich?" We did not grow up with these images, so they have no meaning to us, but there are other symbols that still do powerfully speak to us.

We all have our inner maps that contain symbols. Even nonpracticing Christians in the West still have energies lurking within that certain symbols will unlock. A man doesn't have to be religious to become angered if someone criticizes his beloved Boston Bruins. A woman can be mortally wounded if her Manolo Blahnik shoes are laughed at, for she relates to and identifies with this fashion symbol. Whenever a myth is exposed as simply a fact, and often a mistaken fact at that, the power associated with the myth is released. If the myth can become consciously known, then that power may be transformed and channeled; but if it remains hidden in the deep, its eruption may cause great harm.

✳ ✳ ✳

THE SYMBOLS OF SCIENCE

Myths lose their power when they are rendered into historical facts. The metaphor must remain in order for the symbol to bridge reality and the psyche. The cosmological function of ancient myths has been challenged by the advancements of science. The early quaint and simple models of the universe we have already seen seem childish today. The notion of a three-layer universe with the heavens above, the waters below and the earth in the middle no longer moves anyone to awe and wonder. The new images of the cosmos are far grander and vaster than anything dreamed of in the past. The pictures taken by the Hubble space telescope are more entrancing than any drawings of Aristotle's view of the universe, let alone those concepts presented by biblical or Babylonian priests.

The scientific mythos of the present age tells us there is no "up there" anymore. That is not where heaven is. There is no "down there," either. That is not where the hells lie. Man himself is considered by many scientists to be a biological machine, following the programs laid down in our genes, as modified by our environment. While these theories may not move us deeply or spiritually, the modern models of the universe still play a function: They still explain our place in creation. Here is one scientific cosmological model:

⚞ ⚟

Before time was, before any place was, there is nothing we can know. Our vision fails for there is no thing to be seen. Our concepts cannot deal with things that cannot be described. Here there is a mystery from which all things come. The moment *after* becoming can be known to us, but not the moment *of* becoming itself, nor what happened before that. How can there even be a *before* when time is not yet? How can there be a *place*, when space and place do not yet exist?

Bang! And then there was something.

After this moment the history of the universe began, and it can be modeled. It is a grand model, albeit not a perfect model, for that will never be, but it is a model that works well enough to describe the last 13.8 billion years![3] In the split second after becoming, the universe was incredibly hot and dense. All the matter, all the energy that there ever will be, all that there is right now, all of space itself, was contained in an area smaller than an atom. It was too hot to stay that small—it released.

The release started time and blew space apart. After one second the universe had expanded to over thousand times the size of our solar system, and the temperature had fallen to a balmy 10 billion degrees, which is a thousand times hotter than the inside of the sun today. That was the temperature everywhere in the universe: way too hot for ordinary atoms to form. At about this time, individual protons and neutrons came into being. By about three minutes after the bang, the universe was just cool enough for the simplest nuclei to form: hydrogen and deuterium.

The universe was a soup of photons, but these particles of light were constantly being absorbed and re-emitted by the earliest atoms. By the 20th minute, matter started to dominate: Mostly ionized hydrogen, but about one atom in four was ionized helium. It would take another 400 thousand years before complete atoms could be formed. By then the universe was cool enough to allow these atoms to capture electrons.

Hundreds of millions of years after the bang, gravity drew the hydrogen and helium atoms together, and the first stars were lit. The universe was still expanding, but more slowly. These earliest stars had short dramatic lives, and from their explosive deaths, heavier elements were forged. These elements seeded the next generation of stars, like old gods giving way to the new.

After only 500 million years, galaxies were forming. There were a multitude of small galaxies, but some of them grew larger by consuming their neighbors. Giant galaxies formed—some swirling and some globular. At their hearts were monstrous black holes that consumed everything that came near. The second generation of stars grew old and died in their turn—some quietly, but many violently as super novae. From these spectacular deaths, stardust was spread across the galaxies, seeding newer stars and the planets that evolved with them.

Around 5 billion years ago, a yellow star condensed near the heart of a large spiral galaxy. It was formed of the original gas of the Big Bang and the stardust of its ancestors. Planets also formed and solidified. As this new star journeyed away from the galactic core, these early planets grew by capturing smaller rocks, boulders, asteroids and small proto-planets. One planet, the third one out from the sun, tried to capture one of these small proto-planets, but it bit off more than it could chew. The proto-planet slammed into it, fortunately at a glancing angle, and the two bodies shattered. Over a million years, the larger and smaller bodies coalesced back into spheres, and the lesser was now a captured satellite of the larger. The Earth and moon became companions that danced around the sun; they cooled. It is now 9 billion years since the bang—a home is being prepared—upon this home, life begins.

⊰ ⊱

We are stardust. That's one message we can take from this story. But we are *not* divinely created! We are just a part of the universe, a part that has evolved very recently in the grand scheme of things. Like in the Buddhist myth, there is no personality to this story; no one started the universe, and there is no grand justification for all this. It just is. The universe is unfolding according to certain laws of nature, which fortunately happen to be just right to create a universe that can contain a self-observing, conscious entity, such as us. Physicist Leonard Susskind, one of the inventors of string theory, points out that if gravity were slightly weaker or stronger, if the speed of light were different, if the force that binds protons and neutrons together were slightly off, if any of the fundamental forces or constants of the universe were just a bit different, all of this would not be, and *we* would not be.[4]

Science cannot explain *why* this has happened, only *how* it happened. There are many questions that science will never be able to answer, as we saw in the introduction. There are many wondrous thoughts about the ultimate nature of the cosmos; in an attempt to explain why gravity is so incredibly weak, at least compared to the other forces in nature, Susskind and his colleague, theoretical physicist Steven Weinberg, postulated that our particular universe is one of zillions of universes, forming a multiverse.[5] The idea of the multiverse has given weight to an idea called the anthropic principle: Our universe is the way it is because if it were any different, we wouldn't be around to bear witness to it. In this version of the anthropic principle, we just happen to be living in one universe (one of perhaps a large number of possible universes) that allows life to evolve.[6] That is an interesting thought: Our universe is not unique—it is one of many. In Hindu mythology our universe is just the dream of Vishnu as he floats on the cosmic ocean, and he is just one of countless thousands of Vishnus, each dreaming a universe into being.

Will our universe continue to expand forever, or will it collapse in a great crunch back into an incredibly tiny dot, where maybe it will re-explode and start all over again? This sounds very Buddhist in concept. Or will it die a cold death (ironically called the "heat death of the universe") as it just winds down and crawls to a stop? Maybe there are actually an infinite number of universes, with an infinite number of you's and me's. This sounds stranger than any myths we have seen so far, but it is an idea seriously considered by many scientists.[7] We don't know and maybe we can never know.

Science, remember, is not truth, but rather a process *toward* truth. The stories of science are unique compared to mythic or religious stories in one important way: A proper scientific story must be verifiable. Karl Popper [1902-1994], a philosopher of science, characterized a good scientific theory as being one that makes predictions that could be proven false. His philosophy was termed *critical rationalism*. Nothing can be proven true; no matter how many observations agree with the theory, it will only take one failure to bring the theory down. Theories are creative speculations, hypotheses that will lead to better hypotheses in time and with more observations.

A myth, on the other hand, is not supposed to be provable or disprovable; it is to be considered "as if" it were true but not actually true. An ideology that cannot be falsified is not science. This is one of the concerns over intelligent design being taught in science classes: The idea that God created the universe by causing the Big Bang cannot be proven or disproven, so it is not science. But that's OK, myths are not supposed to be science; they have a different intention altogether. Science is meant to explain us, while myths are meant to move us. Creation myths are meant to move us to awe and wonder, not to be factually true.

Myths can incorporate the science of the day to make the myth more believable and thus more powerful. A strict scientist may be jarred by the poetic sentence at the end the Big Bang story above: "A home is being prepared." That was not a scientific statement, it is anthropomorphism—it implies that someone is deliberately doing something. To prepare a home implies a preparer and intention; there is a purpose. This is not the realm of science; science does not seek meaning. It does not answer "why?" but only "how?"

There is no conflict between myth and science. There is, however, a conflict between the science that myths adopted four thousand years ago and the science of today. If the myths do not keep up with the times, they will lose their credibility and thus their power. Most people today will not believe the universe was created in literally seven 24-hour days; they do not believe the earth is a flat disk and there is a heaven up there and a hell down below. We have been up there; we have been down there. If a mythology insisted today that these things were literally true, it would lose its adherents.

While science today may not be true, it is truer than the science of ages past. We cannot know reality. As Albert Einstein once said, "Reality is merely an illusion, albeit a very persistent one." We can model it, though, and we can create maps that describe our experiences. If science can grip lightly its metaphors, how much more important is it for our mythologies to also loosen up? If we require our myths to be historical truth and factual for all people, for all cultures and for all time, it is the myth that will be lessened, not the people who chose to move with the times. But we do need our stories, and as the older stories lose their credibility, new stories are required to shape the landscape we live within.

The myths of science must keep evolving in order to be useful to us. If we try to stick to the science of a hundred years ago, we will lose all the benefits of modern thought and study. If we stick to the science of four thousand years ago, what do you think will happen? Maps are always changing, must always change, but if you don't update your map, where will you be? If you predicate all the other aspects of your mythology or religion or spiritual beliefs on the cosmological myths being "true," you are in danger! It only takes one small inconsistency to undermine the whole edifice of your belief structure.

The Cosmological Function of Mythology: Summary

The stories of the cosmos put us in accord with nature: If we act in accord with nature, all goes well; if we go against nature, we suffer. The cosmic myths answer our deep questions about how the universe came to be and why we were created, as well. These cosmological myths were the tutors of the uneducated masses, for there were no books and no access to higher learning for our ancestors. They relied upon stories told at festivals and around the campfires to explain the way things are. Today, we have science giving these lessons, with astronomers talking of the universe with the same awe and wonder the earlier stories instilled.

Knowing our place in the universe helps us to act properly toward the environment in which we find ourselves, but there are many different myths of creation. Depending upon which story you believe, your attitude toward other people, other life on this planet, the planet itself, or even your personal notion of God, may vary dramatically. There is a lesson here for the way we are affecting our planet today: global warming, removing all life from the seas, polluting the land and water. If the myths we are following are out of date, and if the way the universe works is different than what our myths are telling us, it is not the universe that needs to change—it is us. Only by becoming aware of the myths by which we are living can we hope to make the changes needed to come back into accord with nature. If the myths no longer serve us, then it is time to modernize them.

The Sociological Function

And this would be the philosophy for the planet, not for this group, that group, or the other group. When you see the earth from the moon, you don't see any divisions there of nations or states. This might be the symbol, really, for the new mythology to come. And those are the people we are one with.

—Joseph Campbell[1]

Chapter 3: Living in Accord with Our Neighbors

≈ ≈

The buffalo would not fall! The herd driven to the high cliff swerved to the left and to the right and ran down the slope of the hill and around the corral. They were escaping and the people grew anxious. The next morning the chief's daughter looked up at the buffalo milling about at the top of the cliff and cried out, "Oh—if only you would come over and feed my people, I would marry one of you!"

Imagine her surprise when, in answer to her prayer, the buffalo started to fall. Down and down they came, filling the corral with their offered bodies. From the corral the biggest bull, the chief of the buffalo, bounded over the fence and came up to the daughter: "All right my dear— off we go!"

"No wait!" she cried. "What do you mean?"

"You gave your promise!" said the bull, "and we came over for you. Now you are my wife, let's go."

The daughter realized that her sacrifice was necessary to match the sacrifice of the buffalo, so while her people were butchering the animals, she was led by the arm back up to the plain where she was to live with the herd.

After the slaughter, the chief looked for his daughter but could not find her. Reading the signs in the soil around their tent, he figured out what had happened. Alone, he went after her, climbed the cliff, and followed the footsteps of his daughter and the bull. Tired from the climb and the walk, he took rest in a small wallow.

A beautiful magpie was drinking in the wallow. Now, magpies are magical birds, so the chief asked him if he had seen his daughter. "Yes," replied the magpie, "she was being led away by the chief of the buffalo to the herd over there."

"Oh, dear magpie, would you be so kind as to fly over there and tell my daughter that her father is coming for her?"

The magpie flew to the herd and nonchalantly picked at the ground here and there, making his way slowly to the girl. Her husband was asleep; the magpie looked sideways at the chief's daughter and said, "Pssst. Your daddy is waiting for you by the wallow. He wants to come to take you home."

"Oh no!" whispered the daughter. "That is very dangerous. If my husband finds my father, he will kill him! Tell my father to wait, and I will come to him."

Presently the old bull awoke: He was thirsty. Taking off one of his horns, he commanded his wife, "Go get me some water." Obeying, she went to the wallow and greeted her father.

"Daddy, you must go back. It is very dangerous for you here."

"I am not letting you stay with these buffalo! I will take you home!"

"Not now. Wait until they are all asleep, then I will sneak back to you."

The daughter filled the horn and returned to her husband. The great bull took one sip and exclaimed, "Fee, Fie, Fan; I smell a man!"

"No, no!" cried his wife. "It is nothing!"

The chief finished his drink and bellowed loudly, stirring all the other bulls to their feet. They stampeded to the wallow and discovered the man hiding there. Feeling only rage they trampled him into the earth. So thorough was their execution, that nothing was left of the girl's father.

His wife was crying. The great bull asked, "So ... why do you cry? You mourn the death of your father? Now you know how we feel when our loved ones die for you."

"But," stammered his wife between the torrent of tears, "but he was my father!"

The bull took pity on his wife and relented. "Well, if you can bring him back to life, we will let you go and return with him."

Turning to the magpie, the girl asked, "Please see if you can find any remains of my father."

The magpie pecked and pecked and finally discovered a small piece of the chief's spine. It brought the bone to her. She covered the bone with her robe and started to chant a magic song. A form started to take shape under the robe. She checked: It was her father, all right, but he wasn't quite done yet. She sang some more, and then her father threw off the robe and stood up.

The buffalo were all amazed! The old bull said to his wife, "You may go home as I promised, but if you can do this for your own people, why don't you do this for us, too? We will teach you our dance so that when our people come to feed your people, you will dance and bring us back to life, as well."

The girl and her father returned to the tribe, where she taught the magic buffalo dance to her people. From then on, the buffalo fed the people and the people, keeping their promise, danced for the buffalo, so that they would come again next year.

ॐ ॐ

Before the dawn of history, before civilization increased the density of humanity along fertile river valleys and at strategic junctures of trade routes, survival depended upon the hunting and gathering of food. In the tropical and semitropical forests, fruits were easily plucked from trees and plants pulled up from the earth, but in the plains and boreal forests away from the tropics, it was from animals that sustenance was found. Unlike in the forest with its roots and fruits, animals do not just sit around waiting to be plucked: Animals are independent creatures with wills of their own. In order to eat animals, an accord with the animals is necessary.

The above myth of the buffalo's wife is from the Blackfoot tribe of Montana, a branch of the Algonquin nation, that migrated to the plains of America from the forests of the eastern continent around the 18th century.[2] This story clearly shows how important it is to be in harmony with one's neighbors. Joseph Campbell observed that this same accord, with different cultural inflections, was found in all primal hunting communities. It didn't matter whether the animals were buffalo or salmon, deer or ducks; the animal had to be a willing participant in the sacrifice of its own life for ours.

Life feeds on life: This is the terrible truth of life! Life in a hunting community is surrounded by death. People wore the skins of dead animals, they used their bones as tools, and they ate the meat and drank the milk of animals. They knew the animals as intimately as they knew each other. The guilt of killing an animal was as great as the guilt of killing another person. To protect the psyche from this awful realization, an accord was needed with the animals. Usually a woman brokered the accord between the totem animal and the tribe. The buffalo dance was one such ritual. Like any spiritual rite, the ritual is an invitation to participate in the original sacrifice of the god, the god here being the totem animal who willingly gives its life.

The way of life in a society must reflect the way the world is. If we are to survive, we must behave in the manner that reflects the reality of the world. But, which reality? In the time before agriculture, the reality was that some very strange neighbors surrounded us. Most were four-footed, some were very dangerous, and we were eating many of them.

Our neighbors on earth were great spirits. Usually there was an individual spirit that directed the whole species: the great bull or bear. This animal master would listen to our prayers, and if we lived properly, if we conducted the rituals correctly, it would agree to allow its brethren to feed us. There was not the great gulf between animals and humans as exists today; we were very similar spirits.

The blood of the animals had to be returned to the earth. If the blood was not returned, the spirit of the animal would not be able to come back from the earth next year. Thanks had to be given to the animal for its sacrifice, or the animal would be angry and not want to come back again.

Today, many may thank God for our daily food, but we don't think to thank the animals we consume. We are cut off from the sources of our food: We don't see the living animal with our own eyes before it gives its life to us (or more appropriately today, before we take its life); as individuals we don't slay it; we don't cut it apart; we don't tend to it before its life ends; and we don't tend to its spirit after its death.

Why should we give thanks to this anonymous slab of steak sitting on our plate? We don't even know its true name. We don't eat cows, we eat hamburgers; a pig becomes a chop or bacon; lamb becomes mutton; the deer, venison. We give thanks not to the animal itself, but to those who prepared our meal, "Our compliments to the chef!" Our stories of provenance today are quite different than when our ancestors' survival depended upon the success of the hunt.

✳ ✳ ✳

Hunting communities survived through individual achievements. In the tropics, where the forests provided food for all, anyone could pluck a banana from a tree. In the plains, not everyone could bring down a woolly mammoth. The spear points had to be shaped with skill, the stealthy approach practiced mindfully, and the quick thrusts of the spear performed with strength and timing. While there are some examples of hunting cultures that did allow women to join in the hunt, and some surprising statistics that show women were often better hunters than men,[3] it was a man's world on the plains and steppes. Women were great for dressing and cooking the meat, tending the children, and carrying the loads when the tribe followed the herd, but women were not considered essential or important, at least not by the menfolk—an attitude we will see was maintained by these cultures as they moved into more civilized zones.

The divinities in a hunting community were not the same as in the settled civilized or planting communities. For people who are on the move, no one place is sacred. Nomadic cultures had no temples where the gods could hang out while everyone came to them. But everywhere the tribe went, the sky would be there; the sky was sacred, the water was sacred, and the animals were sacred. And in the sky, sometimes the gods argued and fought, as thunder roared and lightning flashed. The great sky god, who was, of course, male everywhere save Egypt, which was a settled civilization, was asserting his dominion over everything around and below him. The great god of the nomads was this god of thunder: He was known as Zeus by the proto-Indo-Europeans who came down from the steppes north of the Black Sea and the Caspian Sea into the Aegean and Anatolia; and as Indra by those same people who went down through the Hindu Kush into the Indus Valley. For the semi-nomadic herders just north and east of Egypt, his name was Yahweh.[4]

The dates of the proto-Indo-European migrations from the north are debated. The consensus view is that these Paleolithic hunting communities of the north became Neolithic herders, and by 4000 B.C.E. they were descending southward into Asia and the Levant, westward into Europe and eventually eastward into China. There was not just one wave of migration, but perhaps four great fluxes. These northern hunters and herders were the ones who domesticated and mastered the horse. With this innovation they became formidable fighters. By 2000 B.C.E., they also invented one of the most ruthless weapons of war, the chariot, with which they conquered all the lands they invaded.[5]

These nomadic conquerers were not planters; they came out of the plains and deserts and swept everything before them. They took what was not theirs and made it theirs, as commanded by their gods. In the same way that the guilt of killing animals was assuaged by the rites and rituals of the convenant with the totem animals, as illustrated in the story of the origin of the Buffalo dance, the guilt of killing and taking that which you did not create is assuaged when you act under the commandment of God. As promised in the Bible, God will give over to you cities you did not build, wells you did not dig, grapes and olives from vines and trees you did not plant and houses filled with good things you did not produce.[6]

* * *

The end of the Paleolithic (which literally means the "old age of stone") occurred with the invention of agriculture around 10,000 B.C.E., and new forms of societies developed. No longer did survival depend upon the skills of one or two excellent hunters. Virtually anybody could be trained to plough a field, sow and reap a crop. Women and children could do much of the work just as well as a full-grown man. A new invention called *slavery* also provided unskilled labor necessary to till the land. The covenants with the animals gave way to a different sort of accord with nature.

Many myths of the early planting communities speak of a time before birth and before death, a time when sex was not yet discovered or perhaps invented. Then one day, someone is killed, sometimes by accident, sometimes deliberately, but often willingly. The sacrifice is cut up into pieces and buried, andfrom the parts grow new life: divine food. The eating of food is a partaking of divinity. It is only after this first death that sex is possible. It is only at this time that new life can occur because someone has made the ultimate sacrifice of his own life. Time for another story!

❧ ☙

It was the time when young boys seek their vision. The lad was no more than seven years old when his father put him in a hut and his seven-day fast began. He was a gentle lad, the son of a poor Ojibwa Indian who was terrible at hunting, fishing and providing for his family. They barely survived, and the sensitive boy longed to help his father.

During the first couple of days of the fast, he wandered the hills near the hut and admired and wondered at all the plants. Why do they grow so well on their own? Who plants and tends these green stalks of life? There must be, he reasoned, a Great Spirit who looks after life here. If only I could talk to this Great Spirit and ask his help for my father.

By the fourth day of his fast, the boy was too weak to go walking. As he lay in his bed, he saw a beautiful young man coming down from heaven. He was dressed in green blankets, with yellow feathers on top of his head. The stranger challenged the boy to a wrestling contest, and despite his weakened condition, the lad won. The stranger admitted that the Great Spirit, who had heard the boy's prayers, had sent him. If the boy was strong enough, a great gift would be given to his people, but he had to work to earn it.

They would wrestle three more times. Each day the boy summoned the courage and strength to defeat the green–

and-yellow stranger. After the lad won the wrestling match on the sixth day of his fast, the stranger told the boy that tomorrow, if he should win the final match, the stranger would die.

"Where I die," he said, "you must bury me. Then you must tend to the soil, keeping it clear of grass and weeds. You must water the soil, and in a few months, a great gift will be given to you." The stranger went on to explain how to cook the gift, and how to save some of the kernels for replanting.

On the last day, even though he was extremely weakened by the fast and the earlier struggles with the stranger, the boy gathered all his courage and decided that he would die before losing this final contest. He prevailed, and the stranger's life was surrendered to the earth.

The boy followed the instructions he was given and in a few months brought his father to see the place where the stranger had given up his life. Growing there were strange plants of long stalks: On top, yellow straw was growing out of green ovals. When they opened the blankets, they saw the kernels of maize. The boy realized the Great Spirit had answered his prayers and his father no longer had to rely on hunting and fishing.

⊰ ⊱

Life comes from life: This is not just the mystery of life, it is the requirement of life. Before life can be given, life must be taken. The story of a god who sacrifices his own body so that others can live is a common myth throughout the planting societies. Often the giver of that first life is a man, as in the Algonquin story above.[7] Joseph Campbell also mentions the story of a Polynesian girl who goes swimming daily, until one day a great water snake starts brushing up against her thighs suggestively. After a few days of this, the snake turns into a beautiful young man, and they make love. The snake then says that the girl must cut off his head and bury it. From this sacrifice grows the first coconut tree, whose fruit looks just like a hairy head with two brown eyes.[8]

* * *

In Egypt the story of a god who is sacrificed and buried expanded in scope to address many mythic themes. Again it is a male god who is rendered and planted, tended by his devoted wife. In Egypt, the creation roles of male and female are inverted: The sky is the great mother, Nut, and the earth is the father, Geb. Every night, Nut would descend upon Geb, bringing darkness to the land. The great sun god Ra was jealous of Nut's attention toward Geb and forbade her to conceive any children with Geb during any of the year's 360 days. Distraught, Nut turned to the moon for advice. The moon god, Thoth, created five extra days, and during these days, Nut conceived five children, the eldest and greatest being Osiris.

Osiris married his sister Isis, while the younger brother and sister, Seth and Neftis, also married. One night, Neftis, who always thought Osiris was really hot, tricked him into sleeping with her. He thought she was Isis (really?), and from such small misunderstandings generally come big problems. Sure enough, when Seth found out, he was really pissed off. He concocted a plan to get rid of Osiris and take over the great throne himself. (Coincidentally, the great throne was Isis! All future Pharaohs, who were incarnations of Osiris, would sit in Isis' lap.)

Seth had a sarcophagus built exactly to Osiris' dimensions and suggested Osiris try it out to see if it fit him. When Osiris lay down inside the box, Seth's 72 accomplices rushed over to nail the lid shut. The sarcophagus was thrown into the Nile and was swept out to sea. Isis searched high and low for the box, and finally in Syria, found it. A great fragrant tree had grown around the sarcophagus.

The tree had been chopped down to become the central pillar of the palace of the local king. Isis convinced the king to release her husband, and she brought the sarcophagus back home, pried open the lid, and lay down on her dead husband's body, conceiving a son, the great Horus, who would eventually avenge his father's death.

Seth heard about Isis' find and this time took Osiris' body and cut it up into 15 pieces, which he scattered along the Nile River. Ever since this act, Osiris' creative force causes the Nile to flood each year, bringing new life to the land. Isis was not deterred: With the help of Neftis and Neftis' son Anubis, who was conceived through her one-night stand with Osiris, they found all but one of the pieces of Osiris and put him back together again. Missing were the genitals, which had been swallowed by a great fish.

Missing his generative organ, Osiris cannot be brought back to life in this world. His son, Horus, has great power, however, and resurrected his father so that he can live in the world after this. Osiris now sits in the lands beyond and is the judge of all those who die.

❧ ❧

A god is dismembered and sown, and from the sacrifice new life grows.[9] This is an allegory, or an aetiology, if you will, of what people in the jungles and forests saw all around them, all of the time. Out of the decay and rot of old life, out of death, comes the green shoots of new life. The only way new life can be brought forth is by the sacrificial ending of what is alive right now. It was in these cultures that horrific sacrificial rituals were developed. To our modern ears, the chosen individuals must have been literally scared to death, but the scholars tell us otherwise. The ones chosen for the sacrifice went to their deaths calmly, just as Jesus went to his cross, just as the green-and-yellow stranger who surrendered his life to give maize to the Algonquin lost the last wrestling match, just as the snake gave his head for coconuts to the

Polynesians. The rituals were bloody and gruesome, but those sacrificed were rarely compelled to participate.

We find this hard to relate to, and yet we can still see this noble gesture today in the young men and women who willingly go to war at the risk of their own lives on behalf of their country and their God. Their sacrifices do not instill within our modern hearts the horror that these earlier rituals do; indeed for many, the typical reaction to the willing military sacrifice of young life is one of comingled sadness and pride, not horror or outrage.

Birth and death must come together. The rituals of death and sacrifice are chances to participate in the god's original gift to humanity. Joseph Campbell tells of a rite practiced in Papua New Guinea: When a group of boys reaches that age where they are ready for their introduction to matters of sex and generating new life, a special lean-to is constructed. A young virgin is in the shelter, and, one at a time, a boy visits her and is initiated into manhood. When the last lad is with the girl, the supports for the shelter are knocked away, and the heavy roof crashes down on the couple, killing them both. The bodies are then ritualistically butchered, cooked and eaten.[10] In the embrace of male and female, in the act of generating new life, death is present. The two young people were participating in the re-enactment of a great myth. One may well be horrified by such a ritual, but one must also admit that there is an affirmation of life in the death of the young couple. The challenge of bringing life to the greater community often trumps the lives of any one or two individuals.

✳ ✳ ✳

Problems in an agricultural community are quite different than in a hunter-gatherer tribe: Timing is key. When do we sow the seeds? When do we reap the harvest? How do we ensure the health and fertility of the animals we domesticated, especially the oh-so-useful cows, with their milk, meat and hides? The cycles of time, of the sun and seasons, are more important than the dance of the wild animals.

A calendar is needed to help regulate the life and activities of agrarian societies. The earliest cycles known to man were simple ones to follow: The rising and setting of the sun were apparent to all; the waxing and waning of the moon were obvious to every culture; as we have seen, the cycles of a woman's menses were noticed to coincide closely with that of the moon. Women and the moon became symbolically linked; they became symbols of the cycle of life and death—fertility and destruction. While the moon was symbolic of the monthly cycles, to know when the rains and the floods would come, the other lights in the sky had to be watched closely. For this, which was so critical for a civilized society, a more advanced science was needed.

The important neighbors now were not the wild animals out on the plains or lurking in the jungle; they were the stars, the planets and the two great lights in the sky. In the same way that the hunting communities sought accord with the animals to ensure their constant return, the new agricultural communities sought an accord with the heavens to assure the rains and floods that would bring new crops and maintain the new vocation of animal husbandry.

One great byproduct of agriculture is occasional surpluses; when conditions are right, it is possible for one tribe to grow more food than it needs to survive. With surpluses came wealth, power and politics. Tribes grew into extended societies. Specialization occurred. The earliest villages of hundreds of people appeared in the Middle East as far back as 5000 B.C.E along the Tigris and Euphrates rivers and along the trading routes to Turkey, where the fields of special stones provided highly desirable flint.[11] By 4000 B.C.E., cities like Ur contained tens of thousands of inhabitants.

While anyone could till a field or milk a cow, not everyone could decipher the movement of the stars. The ancient Sumerian stargazers were the first scientists, as well as the first formal priests. They assumed the role of the tribal shamans, and they took over responsibility for conducting the great rituals of the community. They created technologies that could enhance the productivity of the land: They invented writing and mathematics, calendars and horoscopes. These priests discovered that a pantomime here on earth could actually affect what happened in the heavens. Through sympathetic magic, the gods above could be coerced into doing what the priests required. All it took was a sacrifice that re-enacted some ancient event. This is no different in intent than the buffalo dance—the difference is merely in form and grandeur.

With a surplus of grain and cattle came a freedom from the farm. People who had more than they needed could trade their surplus for other goods, and they had time for other endeavors. There was time for arts and stories, for wandering and trade. A middle class arose of artisans, skilled workers and producers of goods, a group existing between those who toiled in the fields and those who ruled the society. There were always those who ruled, and the ruling chiefs of ancient tribes, the heads of families of strong, clever men, evolved into a social class unto themselves.

As communities grew from small villages 8,000 years ago along the ancient Iraqi river valleys, containing perhaps a few hundred people, into small cities of tens of thousands 6,000 years ago, power was consolidated in the hands of rulers and warriors. By 3500 B.C.E., a high, thriving and expansive civilization had appeared: the ancient Sumerian civilization.

This same evolution took place along other fertile rivers. High civilizations arose around 2500 B.C.E. along the Nile in Egypt and the Indus River in what is today Pakistan, and around 1500 B.C.E. along the Yellow and Yangtze Rivers in China. The patterns were the same everywhere; only the local inflections differed. A priestly caste of early scientists would learn the secrets of the stars and describe how life should be lived here on earth; a ruling caste of warriors would ensure these rules were followed; the middle class would manage the affairs of foods and goods; and the serving class would provide services, work the farms, and do all the manual labor required by society. One neat and tidy system based on the idea that society works best when the laws of heaven are obeyed: This was the new accord of the now civilized world.

These early scientists were not just making stuff up—they did not simply believe that the stars moved in predictable patterns—they knew the ways of the heaven because they observed them. They wrote down the facts, which anyone with some training could have noted. From these facts, these proto-scientists developed models to predict future movements. These models took the forms of stories. In the same way the earlier human communities applied personalities to the animals that were so important for human survival, these priests also assigned human traits to the powers in the sky. The stars were not just points of light high above us any more than the buffalo was just an animal on the plains. These stars were gods and angels. To Plato they were the souls of those yet to be born or reborn. The more important stars, the wandering stars described by the Greeks as "planets", were the greater gods. The moon was the goddess of birth, death and fertility. The sun was the god of life itself. The movement of the planets heralded important events such as the ending of an era, such as when Venus led the dying moon back into the heart of the sun.

This was sacred knowledge, and sacred knowledge was not for everybody. In more primitive times and cultures, the shaman or witch doctor lived apart from the tribe. He or she was not the same as everyone else. Even the chief had no command over this kind of power. It had to be kept secret; it was dangerous and potentially psychotic. The shamans' powers included the ability to talk to animals, to become an animal, to fly away, to become invisible, to know things not known to mere mortals, and to wield magic and power over man and nature. This magic was for a rare, select few. The knowledge of the stars and the revelations of the heavens were also kept to only a few. The priestly caste was always the smallest social group, the top of the social pyramid. Like all who have power, they desired to keep things the way they were. Conservatism set in. The way of society was divinely ordained and was not to be varied or questioned. The nascent scientific spirit became stifled by this conservatism; there was no quest to understand more about the ways of the universe. This knowledge, given by the first generation of priests and handed down through all succeeding generations, was sufficient.

In India this ancient priestly knowledge was sung in hymns collectively known as the *Vedas*. The word itself means "knowledge" (remember, *vid* is the root of *video* and *vision*). The language of the songs was a holy language, Sanskrit, and not a language spoken by commoners. Only the educated could learn the ways of this revealed, perfected form of communication. The oldest hymns of the Vedas are traced back almost 3,500 years, making them the oldest extant religious teachings taught today. They were not written down until almost 2,500 years ago. Until then they were memorized, which required a fierce discipline and practice—a yoga all its own. These were secret teachings. In the Laws of Manu, it is commanded that if a *shudra*, one of the lowest castes in India, should overhear the Vedas being recited, that unfortunate individual should be taken and have boiling lead poured in his ears: a gruesome death for such a seemingly minor transgression.[12]

Such severe injunctions are no different than the earliest biblical law: The laws of Leviticus and Numbers also seem harsh to modern ears. For example, when Moses asked God what to do about a man who was found to be picking up sticks for his fire on a Saturday, an act in violation of the law of the Sabbath, God said that man was to be stoned to death![13] Treat minor transgressions severely and you won't have to worry about great transgressions. The important thing in these societies is the society, not the individual. This is an important theme, one that we will return to when we investigate the third function of mythology, the psychological.

Chapter 4: The Great Cycles

The great, enveloping monster Vritra held back the giving waters as it circled the mountaintops like a great coiled cloud of snakes. For years and years it held fast, while all the lands below dried out. Life was leaving the universe. Finally, Indra, the king of the gods, remembered…[1]

"Hey!" said Indra to himself. "I have a thunderbolt here in my bag. Let's see what happens if I toss it at Vritra."

Indra let loose with his lightning, and the demon was shattered. The rains returned and life was restored. Greatly pleased with what he had done, Indra returned to his celestial city and surveyed the ruin and decay that had befallen it during the time of drought. "I will rebuild it better than before; it will be a great thing because I am a great thing!"

Indra summoned the builder, Vishvakarman, and explained his idea. Vishvakarman bowed to Indra and said, "I would be pleased to build a city and a palace worthy of your grand vision." He got right to work, and within a year the task was completed. Indra surveyed the glorious art of Vishvakarman and decided that it needed just a little bit more here and a touch more there. Another pagoda, a couple more terraces would be nice, a pond of lotuses perhaps, some more trees and towers. Vishvakarman returned to work, but every time Indra came to inspect the city, his vision expanded. In despair Vishvakarman thought, "My god, Indra will never be pleased, and being both immortals, my work will go on forever!" He decided to take his problem to a higher power.

Vishvakarman paid a visit to Brahma, the great creator of the whole world. He found Brahma sitting on the central lotus from where he sees everything with his opened eye. Hearing Vishvakarman's complaint, Brahma assured him, "Go home, Vishvakarman. By tomorrow your work will be ended." After Vishvakarman's departure, Brahma descended from his perch and knelt down at the shore of the cosmic ocean, whispering to the great slumbering god Vishnu, explaining how arrogance had overtaken Indra and that something needed to be done. Vishnu, in his sleep, merely nodded.

Vishnu dreams. Floating upon a great snake named Endless, Vishnu dreams the dream of the universe. Beneath Vishnu is Ananta, his great body soft enough to be the bed of a god, but his thousand cobra heads strong enough to hold the weight of the entire world. Ananta, which means "no end", is both Vishnu's bed and his umbrella, the umbrella that supports the world. From Vishnu's navel grows a lotus, the same lotus that opened to reveal a world-creating Brahma. At Vishnu's feet sits his wife, Lakshmi, who caresses one foot tenderly. Her touch is stimulating; without her attentions, there would be no dream.

The next morning, outside the gates to the palace of Indra, a beautiful Brahmin boy appeared and asked the gatekeeper to announce him to the king. Indra was advised that the boy is a good omen, and since it is always good luck to host a Brahmin, he invited the boy into the palace. The beauty of this young lad attracted the attention of all the children who followed closely; Indra, too, was entranced. After offering hospitality he asked the requisite questions: "Who are you; what is your name; where are you from; who is your family; and why have you come?"

The boy replied in a soft voice sounding like thunder rolling among distant hills. "I have heard you are planning a palace greater than *any* Indra has ever built before you. I had to see this for myself."

Indra was amused and decided to play the boy's game. "You know of Indras before me? How is this possible for a 10-year-old boy? Who are you?"

The boy explained, "I have seen your father, Prajapati Kashyapa, and your grandfather Marichi, and his father the great Brahma who created this world. I also know Vishnu, from whom Brahma comes to begin a world cycle. Every time Brahma opens his eye, a world comes into being, governed by an Indra; and when it is time, when Brahma closes his eye, the whole universe is washed away in a great flood of dissolution. After a brief rest, Brahma opens his eye again and another world begins, governed by a new Indra. And again when the great eye closes, everything is dissolved once more."

"After 28 Indras have come and gone, one Brahma day is complete. After 108 years of Brahma days, the world lotus closes and Brahma himself dissolves. The lotus returns into the belly of Vishnu, and a new lotus emerges with a new Brahma, with his eye opening and closing. Upon the cosmic waters are multitudes of Vishnus, each with a lotus and Brahmas rising and sinking. There may be accountants and scientists in your court, a mighty king, who claim to be able to count all the raindrops in the ocean and all the grains of sand on all the shores, but there are none who could count these Vishnus and Brahmas, let alone the number of Indras!"

Just as the boy finished his history lesson, an army of ants entered the palace, four yards wide, marching in perfect formation upon the marble floor and heading towardss Indra. The golden boy looked at the ants and laughed. Indra's mouth went dry, and the hair on his neck stood on end. It was not a kind laugh. "Mercy!" pleaded Indra. "Who are you? You sound like Wisdom itself. Why do you laugh at the sight of these ants?"

"Don't ask," said the boy sternly, "unless you are prepared to be troubled. The truth of these ants is not for everyone. There is higher teaching here that few ever come to know."

Indra felt fear but also wonder; he had to know. "Please dispel my darkness and teach me about these ants!"

"Former ... Indras ... all!" explained the boy. "For countless ages, each worked its way up the ladder of karma. They were born as plants, then as animals. Eventually each one found birth in a human womb and continued to live wisely. After 84 million incarnations, they reached the level of the gods and one day became an Indra. Then they killed the demon Vritra, the withholder of the rains, thought "what a great thing am I," and in arrogance built a fabulous city which started their fall all the way back down to the level of ants. It is through karma that one rises and falls, is born beautiful or monstrous. Pious and high deeds are rewarded in higher birth, while wickedness sinks one lower and lower. Knowledge of karma is the ferryboat to happiness and is only realized by the wise."

Indra was dumbfounded, reeling, and knew not what to say. At that point, an old yogi entered the palace. He was a curious sage: He wore a toga made from a black deer's skin, held a battered umbrella of banana leaves, and had a star between his eyes. On his chest was a very curious circle created by hair that had fallen out. Before Indra could recover his wits and courteously greet the sage, the golden boy asked, "Who are you? Where do you live? What is the name of your family and the meaning of your umbrella? And what's up with that funny circle on your chest?"

The yogi replied, "My name is Hara. I don't have a family; I don't have a house. Life is too short for all that. All I have is this umbrella to keep the sun and rain off my head. That's all I need. And as for this strange circle on my chest—it has been a source of great fear to many and perhaps a lesson for our king here. Every time an Indra dies, one hair falls out. They are half gone already, and pretty soon they will all be gone. You know, life is short! Why build a house or raise a family?"

With that, both the old man and the young boy disappeared, leaving Indra standing in stunned silence. The sage had been Shiva, and the boy, Vishnu. They returned to their homes to allow their teaching to soak in; and it did. Indra came to the realization that his work had been motivated by pride. He decided to dedicate himself to meditation, to follow the spiritual path. He summoned Vishvakarman and thanked him for his work, rewarding him with great gobs of gems and jewels. He then dismissed him; Vishvakarman's work had ended as Brahma promised. Indra made ready to head to the forest, leaving the court and palace to be managed by his son. His beautiful wife, the strength of the gods, Sachi Indrani, was distraught by the news but was unable to dissuade her husband from leaving everything behind. Useless was her beauty now. Indra's duties had been given over; there was nothing to hold him to the throne.

In dismay and desperation, Indrani sought the counsel of the palace priest, the great spiritual advisor, Brihaspati. Brihaspati kindly took Indrani by the hand and said, "Now don't you worry, my dear. Just come with me, and I will straighten everything out." They approached Indra, who bowed deeply before his guru. Brihaspati sat them both down and began to teach.

"You remember, Indra, a while back I wrote a book for you that taught you how to govern, the book of politics?" Indra nodded. "Well, I am going to write for you another book that describes the obligations of married life: of love, ethics and obligations. You may think that you need to go off to the forest to live a spiritual life, but I will teach you how you can live a spiritual life right here through commitment to your family and your wife."

Brihaspati's wisdom was convincing, and Indra decided to stay in the palace with his beautiful wife, where they lived happily ever after ... until Brahma closed his eye.

⊰ ⊱

Joseph Campbell explained the secret of the ants as"Former Indras all" in his popular TV documentary "The Power of Myth."[2] This story, which he calls "The Humbling of Indra," explains aetiologically the way both karma and the great cycles of existence work.[3] It comes from a *Purana*, which is a collection of stories that were not given by the gods to mankind in mystic revelation, but were gathered over the years by the common folk.[4] A wandering storyteller would have recited the Purana in much the same way that travelling bards in ancient Greece would entertain the people at festivals with the hymns of Homer. In India the great mythic storyteller, equivalent to Homer, is Vyasa. He is the one credited with creating most of the Puranas, and the formats are similar: Someone is explaining how something came to be to another. In this particular story, it is Lord Krishna who explains to his consort Radha how Indra was humbled. This is a nested tale, because someone named Narada, a wandering monk with magic powers, actually begins the story by asking Narayana, one of the many masks of Vishnu, to tell him what secrets Krishna revealed to Radha. This is a story within a story, symbolic of truths found within truths.

The story shows that the universe has a rhythm of its own that it follows endlessly: It comes and it goes. The gods are merely agents of this grand cycle;[5] they have no personal power to change it. The universe does not come into being because the gods *want* it to be so, but because it *must* be so. Brahma here is seen as the chief operating officer of the world, while Vishnu is the chief executive officer watching over what happens and getting involved when necessary, when the balance is threatened. Indra's hubris was a case where the balance was threatened and order had to be restored. It is then that the gods act.

* * *

It may be tempting to say that Vishnu, Brahma and Shiva acted to punish Indra, but that would involve a judgment. These gods are not personal gods as we imagine in the West, involved with retribution or seekers of justice; they are simply correctors of imbalances. There is no one, in this philosophy, who judges anyone, and there are no god-rendered consequences inflicted upon anyone after this life has ended. The law of karma takes care of that. When you drop a feather, it floats slowly to the ground; when you drop a rock, it drops, well, like a rock. A god did not decide the feather was nicer than the rock, thus giving it a softer ride down. Smoke rises— a god did not decide that, either. These things happen by their very nature. If you behave poorly in life, the consequences of your actions, your karma, will weigh your soul down, and you will find your next life lower on the ladder. Even the Buddha knew and taught this truth.

৵ ৬

A distraught man sought out the Buddha. His father had just passed away far too early. Finding the Buddha, the man begged him to assure his father's rebirth in heaven. The Buddha had to decline. The man cried and begged again. He explained his reasons for his request:

"My father was a cruel man. He mistreated everyone. I know that if I don't do something for him, he will surely be reborn in hell or worse. You must tell me how I can help him!"

The Buddha took the man to a pond and asked him to throw a rock into the water. The man did. "Now," said the Buddha, "raise the rock back up and ask it to float on the surface!"

"I can't!" said the man.

"OK," said the Buddha, "then throw a flower into the pond. Good. Now make it to stop floating and sink it to the bottom."

"I can't!" repeated the man.

"Just so," explained the Buddha. "Everything has its nature. If a soul is heavy with the actions of karma, it must sink. If the soul is light, it must float. There is no point in you or me asking the world to be otherwise: It is the way it is."

※ ※

There is no personal god judging us. God does not cause an apple to fall; it is the nature of gravity that objects must fall. No amount of prayer will stop the rock from sinking or the flower from floating. Nature does not respond to petition, and even the gods must obey the ultimate rules of nature. If you want to change what will happen to you in your next life, you must look to your actions in this life.

* * *

There is a multiverse of Vishnus, each with its lotuses and Brahmas coming and going, with each new world governed by an Indra. Cycles follow cycles. This is a wonderful metaphor for the skies: The planets, stars, sun and moon flow in mathematically predictable cycles. This is the way of the universe—there is no personality directing it, the wheel just turns. This way of life is called *Dharma*. In China it is called the *Dao*, which means the path or the way. In the West, it was also known by many names: In Egypt it is called *Maat*, which is the scale on which Osiris will weigh a man's soul at the end of his life. In Babylon it was known as *Me* (pronouncedE "may"), and in Greece, *Logos*. Jesus said that He was the way, but that personalized the power of the universe in a way that is unique to the biblical religions. The Eastern myths talk of an impersonal way of the world that cannot be argued with, bribed or changed in any way; it can only be accommodated.

Great eras come and go, but the unfolding of the cycle can be predicted and anticipated. The Indian stories explain that first there was the age of purity, known as the *Satya Yuga*. A yugas is an incredibly long period of time. The Satya Yuga lasts four times 432,000 years.[6] The term *year* here can be an actual year or a metaphoric year. We really don't know how long this is meant to be, so let's just say a yuga is a very long time. Satya comes from the word *sat*, which can mean "truth" or "being." In the Satya Yuga, men lived for 100,000 years; they had no need of the Vedas because everyone automatically acted virtuously. Men and women were born together; there was no need to search for your soul mate. The great Bull of Dharma, the cosmic cow that symbolizes universal order, stood upon four legs and was rock solid.

The great wheel spun and then came the *Treta Yuga*, which lasted three times 432,000 years. Men only lived 10,000 years because they started to forget things, and they were not quite as virtuous. The great Bull of Dharma now stood on only three legs, because the universal order was not being maintained.

The name of each yuga refers to the number on a four-sided dice. The Satya Yuga is sometimes called the *Krita Yuga*, from the root word *kri*, which means "perfected." The dice throw that shows four dots always wins: It is the perfect throw. The Treta Yuga is the side of the dice that has three dots, and remember, the bull has only three legs in that era.

The *Dvapara Yuga*, which lasts two times 432,000 years, is the age when men lived only a thousand years, and the bull is balancing on two legs. As you know, a cow cannot stand on just two legs, so a prop is needed to keep the bull balanced. That prop is the Vedas, the religious teachings. It was in this age that the Vedas were given to us, because we no longer acted virtuously on our own. Dharma is failing; things are not going the way they are supposed to go. It is like a disease infesting the universe, and if it keeps on, bad things are going to happen.

The current world age is the *Kali Yuga*, which lasts only 432,000 years. You can imagine how that poor old bull is doing now—this is the side of the dice that has only one dot. According to some mathematical scholars who think these stories are actual history, the Kali Yuga began on Feb 18, 3102 B.C.E.[7] Men have completely forgotten the Vedas, and society has gone to hell in a hand basket. The golden age of the Satya Yuga is just a distant memory. The end is nigh, the time when Brahma will close his eye and the great flood comes to wash it all away again, cleansing the world for the next grand cycle to unfold, just as the previous cycles did and just as future cycles will again. This present moment in time is not unique: You have read this page before (did you just get a sense of déjà vu?) and will do so again and again in the infinite cycles to come.

This great cycle from Satya Yuga to the Kali Yuga, called a *mahayuga*, is 10 times 432,000 years long. In "The Humbling of Indra", we learned that one Brahma day has 28 Indras, that is, it contains 28 mahayugas. Thus, one day of Brahma is 28 times 10 times 432,000 years. After 108 "years" of this, even this Brahma disappears. If you cared to do the math, a Brahma lives for about 4.8 trillion of our years! By comparison, our current scientific estimate of the age of the universe is 13.8 billion years. In contrast, biblical scholars figured out that, according to Genesis, the universe is only 6,000 years old.[8] Many maps, many myths.

* * *

In the West, the inevitable decay from a Golden Age to the woeful present age is also known, but with some significant differences. There is no grand repeating of the cycles of time as we find in the Hindu and Buddhist philosophies. Hesiod, the ancient Greek mythologist (~700 B.C.E.) in his *Works and Days* named the earliest age of man the Age of Gold. The men living in this time were a different race entirely. These men were created in the time before Zeus was the king of the gods. But how they came to be, Hesiod does not say. While death was known to these ancient men, curiously, old age was not; they neither aged nor fell sick. There were no cares at all. The earth presented food ready-made to eat, no one had to work, and after death, the ancients became kind spirits who are still present and helping us today.

The Silver Age followed with a new race of men created by the Olympian gods. This was a strange branch of humanity; people remained children in the care of their mothers for one hundred years, after which time they quickly matured and died, usually within a couple of years. This race of man died out because they ignored the duties of sacrifice to the gods and, instead, spent their time in violence. Zeus decided to wipe them out and start again, a theme we find in the biblical traditions. God regrets creating men, wipes them all out, and starts again.[9]

The degeneration continued into the next age, the Age of Bronze. Zeus personally created the race of men for this age. He fashioned them out of ash trees, which were also the favored source of handles for spears in ancient Greece. This symbolized the continued violent and warlike nature of the men of this age. No gods were needed to destroy this race of men; they did themselves in and were gone.

So far, we have seen three ages of man, just like in the Indian tradition, with each generation deteriorating. Hesiod now tells of an interruption in this downward descent, for next comes the Age of Heroes. The men of this age were not pure humans; they were the offspring of gods and women and, very rarely, of female gods and human men. These are the heroes of the epic poems Homer sung. They were the demigods of the *Iliad* and the *Odyssey*: Achilles and Hercules and their ilk. They too died and went to the underworld, all save Hercules who became a full-fledged god. After this brief, glorious interlude, the decay resumed. The final age, the present age, is the Age of Iron. No creator is given credit for creating us; we just are. Our time is the time of sorrow and hardship. When the time comes that our children are born with the grey hair of an elder, when youth never appears and we are born old, Zeus will send the inevitable flood waters and drown this final race of man.

Hesiod paints a rather gloomy picture of our past and future: Things get worse and worse, until finally we are wiped out. At least in the Indian stories, a new cycle gets started, but not in this particular pessimistic Greek mythology. The good old days are long gone. There are many modern pessimists who seem to live with this philosophy, as well You probably know some people just like this: people who believe that the best of times are all past. Everything today is miserable and will never get better. But there is another teller of classical mythology who begged to differ: Ovid, the Roman poet (43 B.C.E–17 C.E.) and writer of the *Metamorphoses*.

Ovid, writing 700 years after Hesiod, agreed with the Ages of Man, except he omitted the Age of Heroes, which he seemed to find superfluous. Perhaps Hesiod needed to explain how these demigods came to be and how they went away; Ovid, however, felt no such need. Ovid agreed that Zeus destroyed the men of the Iron Age, but Ovid put this event in the past, not in the future. Zeus did drown everyone, save for two people: Deucalion and Pyrrha. Fortunately, Deucalion was a man and Pyrrha was a woman, and we can imagine them becoming the new Adam and Eve. But remember, they are of the Age of Iron; their children would be just as bad as them. So they asked the Oracle at Delphi for guidance. They were advised to "throw your mother over your shoulders." This was a puzzle: Did the Oracle mean to dig up their mother's body and toss it about? That sounded a bit gross. They finally realized that, as children of iron, their mother was the earth herself. They threw rocks over their shoulders; the rocks that Deucalion threw became men, and the rocks thrown by Pyrrha became women.

According to Ovid, who writes much more optimistically than Hesiod, we are a new race entirely. Perhaps we are now in the Age of Stone, but this is not to say we are in the Stone Age. We are creatures of the earth, not created by the gods. Ovid said, "We show our origins in the fact that we are a hardy race able to endure a great deal of toil and trouble."[10] The Roman Ovid did write with more humor and a cheerier outlook than his Greek predecessors.

While there were several Greeks who believed in the cyclical nature of time, borrowing from earlier Sumerian traditions which may have informed the India philosophy as well, these ideas did not survive in the West.[11] From the time of Ovid through the entire reach of current Western mythologies (west of Iran, that is), the myths speak of only one round of existence. Remember, the Zoroastrian tradition said that this would all last only twelve thousand years. Ovid and Hesiod did not give such a timeline.

* * *

Regardless of how old the universe actually is, or how long you believe it has been around, the earlier realization was that everything moves in predictable cycles. We came to this realization because the stars and planets move in mathematically predictable cycles. Since this is a law of the universe, to be in accord with the universe, our life here on earth must also follow these cycles. Society and culture is set up to mirror the heavens.

Our week has seven days; there are seven constantly wandering objects in the sky. The sun has its day, obviously

Sunday, at the beginning of the week. It is a curiosity of history that we in the West now think of Sunday as part of the week*end*, but that is only because we moved the Jewish Sabbath, the day of rest, away from Saturday. After all, Jesus rose from the dead on the Sunday, not on the Sabbath, and thus for Christians, Sunday is the Lord's Day.[12] Saturday, by the way, is the day of the farthest and slowest-moving planet known to ancient man, Saturn. In Vedic astrology the planet Saturn is known as the grumpy old man of the zodiac. We start the week with the glory of light and end the week tired out and grumpy, needing a rest.

So much for the modern weekend: After the sun's day came the moon's day, Monday. It is the second-brightest object in the sky and faithfully follows the sun. And so it goes: The next day belongs to planet Mars; the English Tuesday is named after *Tiw*, a Norse god of war. In Roman times Mars was the god of war, so Tuesday in Latin is called *dies Martis*; in French, which derives from Latin, it is called *mardi*. Wednesday is named after Mercury, and the French name for Wednesday is *mercredi*, after its Latin root. In English we get the name of this day from the Germanic god, Odin or Wodin (thus Wodin's day becomes Wednesday); it is a stretch to equate Wodin to Mercury, but they were both psychopomps, which is to say, they were both gods that conducted souls to the nether world. Thursday, *jeudi* in French, is Jupiter's day, the king of the gods. In Northern Europe this was Thor's day, thus Thursday. Finally, Friday, or *vendredi* in French, is Venus' day, or *Frige*, as she was known to the Anglo-Saxons.

There are grander cycles than the week. In Egypt, when the brightest star in the sky, Sirius, reappeared after a time of absence just above the horizon before sunrise, the yearly flooding of the Nile was about to occur. The sun's path each year crossed the 12 signs of the zodiac. By knowing in which house the sun dwelt, the priests could pinpoint the best time to plant and harvest. And it was not only seeds that needed planting on a regular basis; kings, too, needed to follow the cycles of the stars—kings were also "planted" on a regular basis.

Venus circles the sun more quickly than the Earth because it has the inside track; Venus is much closer to the sun than our planet. Venus takes 225 days to complete one trip around the sun, compared to our 365 days. Time for a complicated math puzzle: If two runners were to race around circular tracks, with one track being 8/5 longer than the other, so that the outside runner took one year to traverse his course and the inner runner only took seven-and-a-half months, how long would it take for both runners to meet back at the starting point? The ancient astronomers knew the answer: eight years almost to the day. For eight years the Sumerian kings ruled, and then they were sacrificed and buried, along with their entire court.[13] This ritual on earth mirrored the ritual in the heavens; for the kingdom to stay strong, it needed to renew its leadership on a regular basis.

In *The Golden Bough* by Sir James Frazer (1854–1941), a very detailed book on mythology, he describes another celestial cycle of eight years and its mythic importance for the people of ancient Athens.[14] The struggle between the sun and the moon, between the sun god and the moon god, is symbolic at many levels. The sun is masculine and is associated with eternal life. The moon is feminine and is associated with birth and death, the coming into being and the going out of being, the cycles of reincarnation and returning again and again. Ancient priests and astrologers tried to reconcile two very different calendars, one which was based on the cycle of the moon, and one based on the yearly cycle of the sun. They didn't fit. The moon takes 29.5 days to return to completely full. This means there are 12.4 "moonths" in one year—this is not a nice round number. It takes eight years for a full moon that begins on the winter solstice to reoccur, give or take a day or two.

❧ ☙

King Minos, the ancient Cretan son of Zeus, was allowed to reign for eight years, but then he needed to take a sabbatical and recharge the batteries. He went home to Daddy and rested up for a bit, got some fatherly advice on how to run the country, and then, with a renewed mandate, he came back to rule for another term of eight years.

❧ ☙

It is interesting that prior to the Greek cultural conquest of Crete, it was the Cretan empire that overshadowed Greece. Crete was a matrilineal society, and great goddesses were the presiding deities. The moon is the symbol of the goddess, as is the bull, and Minos had a son, a Minotaur, that was half human and half bull. Every eight years, according to Frazer's reading of the myth of Theseus, the citizens of Athens had to send seven beautiful young men and women to Minos in tribute. They were fed to the Minotaur. The great hero of the city of Athens, Theseus, took the place of one of the youths and slew the monster, thus freeing Athens from the tyranny of Minos. Myths often are history in the garb of a story: Greece eventually did surpass the Cretan civilization, just as Theseus overcame the Minotaur.

This octennial cycle, matching the travels of the sun and the moon, was the basis of the quadrennial Olympics: Simply cut the time in half and have a grand athletic party every four years. This cycle is still found in modern politics. The American president has to face renewal every four years, and the maximum time he can rule is eight years in a row. Unlike old king Minos, the president does not seek Zeus' approval to rule, but rather, the modern equivalent of ultimate political power called "We the People."

84

✳ ✳ ✳

Jupiter, the largest planet in our solar system and the king of the Roman gods, orbits the sun at a much more leisurely pace than Earth or Venus: he takes 12 years to complete one cycle. In India Jupiter's cycle also governed sovereigns, as this story tells:

⇥ ⇤

The Indian City of Spices was famous for its cinnamon and other rare and exotic spices, like cardamom and black pepper. The name of the city, Kozhikode, is thought to have come from its fortified palace, but to the English it was known as Calicut, and its fine cotton products were called calico. The city lies on the Malabar Coast, down low in the southwest of India, in the state of Kerala. The kings were rich, powerful and thought to be greater even than the Brahmins, a blasphemy the Brahmins allowed grudgingly because the people bought into the delusion. Greater than the Brahmins, perhaps, but the king, known by the title Samorin, was not greater than the gods.

At a time when Jupiter was retrograde, moving backward among the stars, in the constellation of the Crab, an era was ending. The Samorin had to conduct his greatest sacrifice: He would give up his own life in exchange for the 12 years he had reigned. A great feast was arranged and a scaffold set up so that all could see the king fulfill his end of the bargain he made all those years ago. Some Samorin were fortunate enough to die before the 12 years had past, but the current king was very much alive.

The Samorin's pavilion was of finest silk, and music accompanied the rituals. His final bath was a ceremony in itself, for one must not face death unclean. After saluting all the honored guests, he went to bow in praise and prayer to his god. He mounted the scaffold, took his knife, and started the mutilation. He began with his nose—off off it came. He removed his ears and lips, throwing the pieces far away. He had to slice quickly: The loss of blood was making him faint. He began to hack off his fingers and toes. Just before passing out, he slit his own throat. From the onlookers present, one was chosen; a new sovereign elected to reign for the next 12 years.

By the end of the 17th century, kings began to modify the ritual. The golden rule has often been restated as "those who have the gold make the rules," but they can't completely disregard the will of greater powers. The law of the universe sill required a renewal every 12 years. Instead of the Samorin slitting his own throat, anyone was allowed to do the deed or at least to try, and the one who succeeded became the next king. The Samorin did not make it easy; he arrayed his guards around him for protection. The would-be successor had to fight his way through many swords in order to claim the ultimate prize. For 28 days the ritual continued. Tens of thousands of guards made sure no one would succeed, but dozens made the attempt. Some almost got through, but through the grace of Jupiter, the king survived to rule for another dozen years.

꿈 꿈

Frazer described the above rituals in *The Golden Bough* and also observed that in the Near East, the kings of old Sumer had gotten smarter; they appointed substitutes to rule for a short period of time just before the day of renewal. These substitute kings would have everything the king would normally have: great food, lots of wine, parties, and most tellingly, access to the harem. Within a week, however, they would be killed and buried with great pomp and splendor. While the heavens ruled, the rulers on earth played with those rules.

Chapter 5: Varna, Dharma and Karma

The laws of the universe are fierce, strict and meted out mercilessly. You do not and cannot argue with them. The same power that created everything dictates how everything is to be run. This is not a whim of some powerful personality. The great creator of the universe, at least in the East, was beyond personality. There was no point praying for the sun to rise in the West when it was the law of the universe itself that the sun rises in the East. No king could stop the tide from coming in. There was no point praying for that great impersonal power to elevate you from your place in society, either. A mouse is not a lion; a snake is not an eagle; the moon is not the sun; you are not a rich, powerful king—and that is just the way things are, as we will continue to discover.

Varna

꒰ ꒱

Purusha, the cosmic man, was first; he has 1,000 heads and 1,000 eyes, 1,000 legs and 1,000 feet. He is everything, and all proceeds from him. From his face, the center of knowledge and knowing, came the Brahmins, the greatest creatures in the universe, for they know. Even the gods are moved by the words of a Brahmin; sacrifice is the tool only a Brahmin knows how to wield, and without sacrifice the gods would wither. The very name, Brahmin, bespeaks their grandeur, for they are great.[1]

From the powerful arms of the cosmic man comes forth the Kshatriya—the warriors who are born to rule.

Kshatriya means "to protect or defend." What the wisdom of the Brahmins reveals to be the way of the universe, the Kshatriya are charged to make so. It was not always this way! There was a time when the Kshatriya believed they were mightier than the Brahmins: This was a time before the axe fell. An axe in Sanskrit is called *parashu*.

❦

Parashu Rama's father always suspected his wife of infidelity; he had no proof, but that was a trifling matter—he ordered his son to cut off the head of his unfaithful wife and bring it to him. Parashu Rama did not question his father, as fitting a real son, and cut off his own mother's head with his axe. Thus was he named Parashu Rama, "Rama with the Axe." His father confided his suspicions to his son: His wife had been consorting with a Kshatriya! Parashu Rama comforted his father as only an avatar of Vishnu could, by slewing every living warrior, save one. It became clear through these actions of Vishnu, in the guise of Parashu Rama, that the Brahmins are greater than the Kshatriya, and since the ending of the time of the Vedas, this has been the obvious truth.

❦

The cosmic man's legs are the source of the Vaisya, "the neighbors." The multitudes of Vaisyas are the middle class of herders and farmers, merchants and businessmen. The Vaisyas are the guts of society and support it through their taxes and tithes.

Finally, from the feet of the great Purusha comes the support upon which all else rests: the Shudra. These are the servants. They have their own religious practices distinct from the Vedic practices of the twice-born. The Shudras are not twice born: only the Brahmins, Kshatriyas and Vaisya are worthy to undergo a second birth. This does not refer to reincarnation; the first birth is from a womb, and the second is from dependency to adulthood, from being a child to being a student. The twice-born is one who studies under a guru and learns the religious obligations of society. The Shudra's practice and great aim in life is to do what he is told. In the afterlives to come, he will be rewarded, but not today, not yet.

Beneath the Shudra, below the feet of the Purusha, are those who belong to no caste at all. These are not noble beings and are given the most disgusting and menial of all tasks. They live in slums of their own and must not be touched. These are the outcastes.

The Brahmins teach the Vedas and conduct sacrifices; the Kshatriyas practice their warrior craft and protect the world; the Vaisyas serve all those above them, keep the cows, till the soil, grow crops and manage financial affairs; the Shudra provide service through their labor and fine arts. When challenging times arise, it is permitted for one to perform the functions of a lower caste, but only for that time. This is the way of the universe, and man did not decree any of this. Man simply follows along with the way things are.

ॐ ह्री

Castes are not unique to India or to ancient times. The division of humans into four levels (or five if you include the outcastes, who are not counted at all) occurred in many cultures. The French philologist Georges Dumézil (1898–1986) believed that the proto-Indo-European cultures divided society up into three parts: first, there were the sovereigns, which included the priests; second were the military; and third were the commoners. Outside of these three were the serfs and laborers, most likely formed by conquered peoples: These were the Shudra of India. We find these social divisions everywhere the ancient Indo-Europeans dominated, from India to Europe.

Societies are alive; they will themselves to continue. The members of a society are the agents that ensure the society's continuation. As such, societies do not need people who want to fulfill their unique personal ambitions; societies need people who are carved up to fit the niches society already has. Joseph Campbell suggested that we cannot blame society, for each society is in a unique situation of its own and is trying its best to continue. In his words, societies need "part people" not "whole people."[2] The more conservative a society is, the more it strives to keep things exactly the way it has always been.

The form of society developed by the "noble" rulers of India was very successful: it has lasted for over 3,000 years. In this case the term *noble* is not being used as meaning "just" or "fair" or "of high morals," but rather as the common translation of the word *Aryan*. The proto-Indo-Europeans who moved into India called themselves the Aryans, meaning "noble," "majestic" and "superior." These were not the blue-eyed blondes that the Nazis in Germany believed Aryans to be. Ironically for Hitler, Aryans were, in fact, darker in most respects than modern northern Europeans.[3] "Noble," in a scientific sense, means "aloof" and "nonreactive": noble gases do not interact with other elements, yielding a sense of being quite special, unique and unaffected by the rest of the universe. This is the attitude found among the nobility of all cultures.

* * *

Myths that provide a direction for society to follow are aetiological; they explain why the society is structured the way it is. These myths do not promise some future evolution toward a better society. It is tempting and common for modern listeners to hear an ancient myth and miss the original context. Many great thinkers of more modern times, such as Yogananda, wanted to see the roles defined in the ancient texts as being kind and generous. They wanted us to believe it was only because of ignorance that the people back then misunderstood the holy words.[4] In this view, the fact that the

Shudra were the feet of society was a good thing; without the support of the Shudra, society would fall. Similar gracious sentiments were read into the condition of women: women were to be honored at all times. While these noble thoughts are found occasionally in the ancient text, the reality of the society was that Shudras were ill-treated, and women were treated as property. This was not unique to India; almost all the high cultures of 3,000 years ago treated its women and slaves in a similar, harsh way. The Aryans were the conquerors of the earlier natives in India, and those natives, the Shudras, were ruthlessly excluded from the higher reaches of society and from the religious practices of the three noble classes.[5]

The story of the Purusha, whose arms became the Kshatriya and from whose head the Brahmins arose, is found in the oldest extant religious text still regularly read today: the *Rig Veda*. This Veda was created somewhere between 1500 and 1000 B.C.E. (although some religious scholars wish to put those dates back at least another thousand years). The idea presented here goes back beyond the Indian Vedas to the Sumerian concept of monism, where everything that exists is part of an original "one." It is found in Egypt in the Hymn to Amon-Re: "The gods' names are countless, but his name is hidden from everyone." In Mesopotamia, around 2000 B.C.E., a poem of Inanna describes her as wearing the heavens as her crown and the earth as sandals for her feet. In Greece, Parmenides (~550 B.C.E.), the philosopher contemporaneous with the Upanishadic sage Yajnavalkya, proposed that there was an original Being who was formless, much like the original Self of Yajnavalkya's story with which we started our journey in Chapter 1.[6] This original and universal Self is both transcendent and immanent. We shall have occasion to investigate these mysteries more fully later on.

There are texts that came after the Vedas which spelled out the rules of Indian society in great detail: The Institutes of

Vishnu and The Laws of Manu (the *manusmriti*). In these, the treatment of women and Shudras are quite detailed, clear and precise.[7]

- A Brahmin may have four wives, a Kshatriya may have three and a Vaisya, two. A Shudra may have only one wife. [24: 1 – 4]

- No spiritual good can come from marrying a Shudra woman. She should only be married for reasons of lust. [26:5]

- When a child is born, its name should reflect its caste. The name of a Brahmin child should signify auspiciousness; of a Kshatriya, power; of a Vaisya, wealth; and of a Shudra, contempt. [27:9]

- A woman is subject to her father while a youth, to her husband while married and to her son in old age. [25:13]

- A woman shall not stand near a window or the doorway of her house. [25:11]

- If a young girl is not yet betrothed before her first menstruation begins, and even though she is still living with her father, she is a degraded woman, and any man can lawfully take her, even if he receives no consent from the girl's family. [24:41]

- After the death of her husband, a woman is to ascend the funeral pyre and accompany him. [25:4]

While it can be argued that extracting a couple of laws from a large body of text leads to the statements being taken out of context, the treatment of women and servants as described throughout history shows the context quite clearly. Women were property and the Shudras were inferior beings. It is interesting to our modern sensibilities to know of one other warning found in both the Institutes of Vishnu and the Laws of Manu:

- No man should marry a woman whose hair is decidedly red. [24-15][8]

(There may be many people who think this is one ancient law that still makes sense, but they are simply cowards.)

The laws of ancient societies everywhere were harsh. Compare the rules in these old Indian texts with the edicts found in Leviticus, Numbers and Deuteronomy of the Western Bible. In Deuteronomy women are warned that if two men are fighting and one is your husband, and if you try to help him by grabbing the balls of his assailant, your hand will be cut off, and no one will pity you![9] Why the concern over a man's privates? Besides the obvious reason for compassion, earlier in Deuteronomy we were told that if a man has no "stones," (that was the word used) he could not attend church.[10] So, we can see that any woman gripping a man's stones with evil intent might render him incapable of ever worshipping God in public again. But even in the city of Athens, where we like to think the ancient Greeks were very enlightened, women were confined to their homes and treated as property; they had no rights in society. Marriage was an arrangement between a woman's father and the father of the groom. If the woman's father was kind, he might tell her ahead of time what was in store for her, but there was no obligation to do so.

✳ ✳ ✳

Varna is the word used to describe what is commonly called the "caste system" in India. Varna means "color," but not the color of the skin. While the darker the skin, the less beloved a person was, color here referred to the color of one's soul. There are six colors that can pour into a soul: black, grey, blue, red, yellow and white. Black is the least favorable color and white the most refined and desired. These colors refer to the karmic state of one's soul. (We will look at what is meant by "soul" when we look at the mystical function of myths.)

While the Brahmins were eventually ceded the top level within the caste system, the priests were not considered the heroes of the myths. The heroes were the *rishis*, the ancient seers and prototypical yogis. They are somewhat equivalent to Old Testament prophets and had much in common with earlier tribal shamans. The rishis were the ones who mediated between the gods and the human race, between the world that we ordinarily experience and that which is unseen and powerful. These early yogis, like their shaman predecessors, gained their tremendous powers and insight through their *tapas*]. Tapas is the heat or energy that develops through ascetic practices and severe austerities—basically through yoga (but not the yoga of the West today). If a yogi gained enough tapas, he could control the universe and overthrow even the great gods in heaven, including Indra, as this story tells:

ॐ ह

Vikra was a great yogi; his tapas came from holding one arm up in the air. This was not an easy practice. Many of his fellow yogis would stand in a pose known as the tree posture, simply standing on one leg, with hands in prayer at the heart center. The tree is not a particularly challenging pose, so to increase their tapas, these yogis would stand for eight hours at a time … on top of an ant hill … covered in honey … under the hot midday sun. This is how you build tapas.

Vikra's yoga was simple but effective. Keeping his arm raised over his head was hard for the first few days, but after a few weeks, the arm felt lighter. After a few years, he didn't notice his arm anymore, and he couldn't lower it again even if he wanted to, since it had become fused in that position. That was a small price to pay for the power he was accumulating. Soon he would have enough power to overthrow Indra himself, a fact that did not escape Indra's notice.

Indra went to the great god Shiva: "Something has to be done about Vikra! If we allow him to continue with his yoga, he will be too strong." Shiva agreed to pay a visit to Vikra to see what could be done. In the past, Shiva and other gods could easily dissipate a yogi's great tapas by sending a beautiful woman to distract him. Once lovemaking was complete, the yogi's powers were gone, and he would have to start all over again. Shiva knew that Vikra was not going to fall for that old trick. He would have to do the only thing that was guaranteed to disperse Vikra's tapas: He would have to grant him a wish.

"Hey, Vikra!" said Shiva as he manifested in front of the great yogi. "What's up?"

"My arm!" replied Vikra, pointing proudly to the withered limb.

"Yes, I can see that," said Shiva. "So ... tell me, what do you want?"

"I want," said Vikra excitedly, for his efforts were about to bear fruit! Finally, after years of practice, he was going to fulfill his mission in life. This was a mission many other priests and gods longed for but were unable to accomplish: Vikra wanted to kill Shiva! "I want ... the power to kill anything I touch on the head!"

"Is that all?" said Shiva. "Piece of cake."

With a snap of Shiva's fingers, there was a show of pyrotechnics worthy of the Wizard of Oz, with smoke and lights and a sound like thunder that ended with a small *poof*. Vikra felt the change; he felt the power within him and immediately lunged toward Shiva. Shiva suddenly realized he was in danger; he ducked and dodged, but Vikra kept coming. Shiva fled; Vikra followed.

In desperation Shiva ran toward Vishnu, the Preserver. Vishnu raised both hands and bade Shiva to stop running. "What's going on?" he asked. Shiva quickly filled him in, and as he finished the recap, up ran Vikra. Vishnu told Shiva, "Stand behind me."

Shiva did as told but was still not safe. Vikra tried to reach around Vishnu's great body to touch Shiva.

"Vikra, what are you doing?" inquired Vishnu.

"Well," came the reply, "I now have a great power, the power to kill anything I touch on the head, and I am going to kill Shiva!"

"Wow," said Vishnu, "that is quite a power—how did you get it?"

"From Shiva!"

"From Shiva?" asked Vishnu in surprise. "You know what a kidder Shiva is. How do you know you actually have this power—that it works? Have you tried it yet?"

"No," said Vikra, pausing to reflect.

"Well," offered Vishnu, "don't you think you should test it? Why not touch yourself on the head and see what happens!"

Vikra thought that was a good idea, so he did. He touched himself on the head … and he died. Thus did Vishnu save Shiva.

᭟ ᭠

This tale is illuminating on many levels. First, it was told by followers of Vishnu, and these Vaishnavites love to poke fun at the Shavites, the followers of Shiva. Remember, one of the functions of mythology is aetiological: It explains the way certain things are. If you believe Vishnu is greater than Shiva, this myth reinforces your belief. Second, this story illustrates the power that can be gained through yoga. Yoga builds tapas, and through this heat, magical powers can be obtained. Third, it illustrates the fact that what has been known as yoga throughout the ages cannot be bound to one form of practice or one particular kind of intention. There are many yogas with many quite different intentions. The story also points out that Shiva was not a god beloved by all, a fact that we will have occasion to return to. The final point in relating this story is to, of course, demonstrate that it is through these yogis that communion with the gods occurs.

The Brahmins, human or divine, are not heroes (there are gods who are Brahmins, too); they are the beneficiaries of the knowledge gained and passed down to them by the rishis. It was through the rishis that knowledge of the Vedas was revealed. *Shruti* means "heard" or "revealed." The Vedas were shruti; no one sat down to write them. It was in the extraordinary states of supreme concentration that the yogis heard the words of the gods, and through shruti the truths of the universe were learned. This is very similar to the way Mohammed had the word of Allah revealed to him while he prayed in his cave. Literature, on the other hand, was *smriti* or "remembered." The stories and myths of the common people were not revealed truth—only the Brahmins and certain Kshatriyas were privy to the most esoteric teaching. For the Vaisya, the commoners, there were the puranas: the myths, folk tales and epics recited by bards, not priests.

✳ ✳ ✳

Dharma

Societies are kept functioning through the power of the class systems, through varna, but in India two other tools were also required to keep everything in order: dharma and karma. Together, varna, dharma and karma kept Hindu society safe from any internal threats. While conquerors came from outside India and forced new ways onto society, there never occurred a revolution from within Indian society as happened in Europe during the Renaissance and the Age of Enlightenment. The conserving power of varna, dharma and karma was just too strong to be broken from within.[11]

Dharma, as we have seen, is the way the universe is supposed to work. In the story "The Humbling of Indra," we saw how the great cycles of time flow inexorably from one age to the next. In the beginning dharma works smoothly because people are following their own personal dharma. Your dharma, which is a microcosm of the universal dharma, is your role in society, your path and your virtue—it is what you were born to do. Dharma also means *virtue*. If you fulfill your role in life well, you are virtuous, and with such virtue comes power, as we will see in the story of Bindumati. Before we hear about her, however, we need to know a little bit about an Act of Truth.

৺ ৡ

Hanuman was caught; the soldiers of Ravana were tormenting him and attempting to set his tail on fire. Through the windows of her cell, Sita watched as her would-be rescuer was abused. She had been captured by the demon and taken away to his palace here in Sri Lanka. Her husband, Rama, was still seeking her all over India. Only the great friend and devotee to Rama, only Hanuman, had been able to find out where she had been taken.

Hanuman was the king of the monkeys—he was a super-monkey with super-monkey powers, but with one small defect: He had been cursed. Although Hanuman possessed many miraculous powers, his curse was that, unless reminded, he could never remember that he possessed these abilities. He had tracked Ravana and Sita to the tip of India in the south and was stymied by the open ocean. Ravana had taken Sita aboard his flying chariot to his palace that lay 100 miles away over open water. Hanuman had no idea how to get to Sita, until someone reminded him, "Hey, Hanuman, you can jump!" So jump he did. He found Sita but was found in return.

The soldiers set fire to Hanuman, but before the fur on his tail could burn, Sita said, "Let the fire be cool." She performed her Act of Truth. and the fire was cooled. Hanuman managed to escape back to Rama, who in due course came to rescue his wife from the ravenous demon.

ঌ ়

Rama is one of the 10 incarnations of Vishnu; he was sent to earth to rid the universe of the demon Ravana, whose name mutates into the English word "ravenous." Ravana's appetite was unquenchable. Through 10 years of tapas, cutting off his own head 10 times, he was granted a boon by Brahma. His request at first was for immortality, but this Brahma could not grant: all things end. Ravana then asked to have the power to never be killed by any god, demon or heavenly spirit. This he was given, but in his pride he never thought to ask for protection from mere mortal men. Thus it was that, in answer to Indra's prayers, Indra having been conquered and humiliated by Ravana, Vishnu incarnated as the great mortal hero, Rama.

This tale of Hanuman's tail being set alight is one of many in the epic called the *Ramayana* Such a story it is that in its full telling, it extends over seven books and consists of 24,000 verses. It is second only to the grand *Mahabhrata* in length and importance; these two works form the great epic poems of ancient India and are as important to the common people there as the *Iliad* and the *Odyssey* were to the ancient Greeks.

The Act of Truth that Sita performed allowed her to control the universe. If you have led your life in a way that exemplified dharma, if you always spoke only the truth, if you always followed your own personal duty as defined by society, then you had the power to command the universe by simply speaking your truth. With this background, we can listen to the story of another woman's Act of Truth: the story of Bindumati.[12]

⁂

King Ashoka was a great conqueror; he subdued all the lands along the Ganges River from source to sea. His wonderful palace sat in Pataliputra, a great city by the great river. Tired of war, he turned to the peaceful meditations of the Buddha and sent missionaries all over the Greek Empire to share the teachings. Life settled down for Ashoka, but there were still lessons to be learned. This particular lesson was to come from the Ganges herself.

One day the river started to rise: incredibly fast the waters grew higher, closer and closer to the banks that protected the capital city. In alarm the townsfolk watched the rising waters, and among them, standing on the banks of the river, were their king and his ministers. Ashoka knew that in a matter of hours, his city would be drowning. He looked to his ministers, sages and Brahmins and asked, "Will none of you speak a word of truth and make the waters go down?"

The counselors and priests looked at one another and simply mumbled. No one could perform the Act of Truth the king requested. But far from the king, at the edge of the crowd, was an old prostitute named Bindumati. Like everyone else, she heard that the king was asking for someone to speak a word of truth. She muttered to herself, "Well, I can speak a word of truth." Her friends could barely hear her but took heart. "What was that, Bindi?"

"I can speak a word of truth," she replied more loudly.

"You can!" squealed her friends, "Then quickly—speak your truth and let the waters recede. Save our city, Bindi!" Bindumati did as bade, and sure enough, with a roar, the waters backed up and then started to recede. The city was indeed saved.

At the center of the crowd, the king watched the river reverse. In amazement and delight he turned to his priests and ministers and asked, "Who did this? Who caused the river to return to normal?"

All the ministers asked each other, "Did you do that? I can't do that." Finally, through the crowd it filtered to the king's ea—it was Bindumati!

The king went down through the throng to address Bindumati: "Bindumati! You old whore! You, a wicked sinner, did an Act of Truth?" Like the crowd, King Ashoka was astounded that this old prostitute had saved them all.

"Yes!" replied Bindumati boldly. "I have an Act of Truth so powerful that if I wished, I could turn all the gods on their heads."

The king replied in a hushed and humbled voice, "How can it be that you could perform an Act of Truth?"

"My truth is simple," came the answer. "In the performance of my duty, I treat all men exactly the same. I curry no favor with handsome or rich men, and I do not refuse ugly or displeasing men. I treat the lowborn and the highborn equally. I hold no contempt for anyone and never fawn. I serve only the money that comes to me and do not judge the hands that give it. And it is through this truth that our city has been saved."

King Ashoka learned that day a valuable lesson: There are people whose dharma may be clean or unclean, but everyone participates in the ways of the universe. Virtue is found anywhere one performs his or her duty perfectly.

⚛ ⚛

Now, if this story were a Western fairytale, what would the king do for Bindumati? He would have rewarded her richly, or he would have taken her back to the palace and married her, like Cinderella. But Bindi is not Cindy, and not in India are such the rewards for these heroic acts. Bindumati was following her dharma. She had gained great virtue by being a perfect prostitute, a solid shudra. This virtue gave her the power to perform an Act of Truth, but her reward was not to be found in this life. Through her merit, perhaps, in her next life she would return as a queen, or, even better, as a man.

* * *

KARMA AND REINCARNATION

We have mentioned the word *karma* many times already; it was explained in "The Humbling of Indra" and used as an explanation by the Buddha for why a son cannot affect where his father's soul goes after death. One's actions in this life will dictate your place in the next, and your actions in past lives dictated your place today. Karma comes from the Sanskrit root word *kr*, which means "work," "action," or "destiny," and it is one of the most widely known Sanskrit words in the English world today. Most Westerners have heard of and understand karma. What is not widely appreciated is the way karma is linked to the idea of reincarnation. The two are inseparable, but they are not the same, and together they make up two-thirds of the "tripartite theory of reincarnation."[13] The missing third member of this theory is *moksha*: freedom, liberation or release from the rounds of incarnation. (We will defer the investigation into moksha to later chapters, along with the equally mystifying question of "what is it that gets liberated?")

In primal cultures it was believed that the soul of a person, his essence, departs upon death and takes refuge randomly in plants or animals. How does it get into the plant or animal? Dust unto dust! The body decays and becomes food from which new life emerges: We become plants; the plants become the body of the animals. This understanding makes some sort of sense, but it is completely divorced from any ethical concerns. It does not matter how you lived or died—you become plant food. Some cultures believed that a person continued on in the grandchildren: Thurston Howell III *was* Thurston Howell I back for another roll of the dice. (Woe to the man who had no children! How was he going to come back?) Again, the ethical idea of karma is missing; this presents a purely mechanistic view of reincarnation. There were also totemic views where a hierarchy of rebirths occurs through a series of animal forms, which culminates in another human birth. This is reflected in the view of the cycles of rebirth, or *metempsychosis*, as it was called in Greece, as described by Herodotus, the 5th century B.C.E. Greek historian:[14]

The Egyptians say that Demeter (the Greek version of Isis) and Dionysus (the Greek version of Osiris) are the chief powers of the underworld, and that [the Egyptians] were also the first people to put forward the doctrine of the immortality of the soul and to maintain that after death it enters another creature at the moment of that creature's birth. It then makes the round of all living things—animals, birds and fish—until it finally passes once again, at birth, into the body of a man. The whole period of transmigration occupies 3,000 years.[15]

The Greeks after Herodotus' time expanded this idea of metempsychosis and created a very similar version of the tripartite theory as found in the Indian Upanishads. It was so similar, in fact, that some scholars believe these two views had a common source. Perhaps the Greek ideas came from India, or perhaps they both evolved out of a more basic idea from the Middle East. We are not sure. In any case the tripartite theory was unique to Greece and India. The theory holds that it is not by chance or through the operation of some machinery of nature that your next birth is determined, but by your moral behavior in the prior life. In this philosophy, karma is firmly joined with reincarnation. But this still does not make up the full tripartite theory; one still needs to learn how to escape the cycles and avoid coming back over and over again to this sorrowful world filled with pain and suffering. Rebirth is to be dreaded and avoided.

To the Greeks karma was called *katharsis*, or purification. However, Plato described katharsis as reincarnation: "the character that is becoming better to a better incarnation, and that which is growing worse to a worser, each according to its due."[16] This sounds very similar to the Chandogya Upanishad's teaching: "Those whose conduct here has been good will quickly attain a good birth ... But those whose conduct here has been evil will quickly attain an evil birth."[17] With this tripartite theory firmly inculcated into the minds of the lay followers, priests were able to maintain a firm grip on society's structure. Followers shouldn't look for release or improvement of their lot in this life; they should just follow the rules, play the game, and in the next life they would reap their reward.

The story of Bindumati illustrates the three mythic concepts that kept India a very conservative society, functioning without social change for thousands of years: varna (Bindumati was a Shudra); dharma (as a Shudra her duty was to serve); and karma (through the merit gained by her fulfilling her dharma well, she will be reborn in a higher state). There is no room in this society for the Great American Dream; not everyone can grow up to be president, not in a society where varna, dharma and karma rule. Many sages, from the Buddha 2,500 years ago to Yogananda in the 20th century, tried to blunt the effect of these mythic strictures by teaching that one is not *born* a Brahmin, one *becomes* a Brahmin through one's actions.[18] However, the reality remained: Birth determines class, and culture, shaped by myths, determines how your life unfolds within society.

Chapter 6: Boundaries

The stratification of society into classes or castes happened in all the ancient high cultures and can be seen as an artifact of agriculture. Workers are needed to till the fields, middle men are needed to sell the excess food, craftsmen are needed to create the tools, and scientist-priests are needed to predict the future. And, of course, someone has to manage all of this; rulers are also needed—at least, they think they are, and their myths prove they are right. These rulers rise up through the right of might, with the strongest and the smartest eventually taking over. Often the strongest come from outside society from the invading armies of the herders, whether the proto-Indo-Europeans from the north or the Semites from the Arabian deserts. They come into the settled lands and by force of arms, take it over. The myths of the herding warrior tribes give permission for this conquest, as we have seen before: "cities that you did not build, you will inhabit..." The conquerors are a class apart; the indigenous conquered people are the lowest class. Boundaries are drawn and maintained through the stories and myths that explain the separation of the rulers from the ruled, the outsiders from the insiders, us from them.

"Us versus them" is an age-old problem. We have already seen how the laws that govern behavior inside society are quite different when we are dealing with people outside our society: The warriors of the deserts or plains descending upon a city do not treat the inhabitants the same way they treat their fellow tribesmen. Compare two very different sets of directives from the Bible. First,

- Thou shall not kill

- Thou shall not commit adultery

- Thou shall not steal

- Thou shall not desire thy neighbor's wife, nor his manservant, nor his maidservant, nor his ox, nor his ass, nor any thing that is thy neighbor's.

These may sound quite familiar to you: They are part of the Ten Commandments found in both Exodus and Deuteronomy. The first three are the ones that Jesus also reiterated, and to which he add added one of his own, "Thou shall love thy neighbor as thyself."[1]

Now compare the above to what is allowed in the following story—actually, not just allowed but directed:

⊰ ⊱

Now in those days, some men of Israel were committing whoredom with the daughters of Moab. This did not please God, who was already afflicting the Jewish people with a great plague. God told Moses, "Find the ring leaders for me and kill them." While Moses was relaying this decision to the judges, another man happened by the congregation with a Midianite girlfriend. This mixed couple offended Phinehas, the grandson of Aaron the priest, so Phinehas took a javelin and impaled them both. God was quite pleased by Phinehas' dedication and agreed to lift the plague, which by then had killed 24,000 Israelis.

God spoke to Moses and said, "OK, now go get those Midianites for me." Moses agreed that vengeance was required and sent his army against the five kings of Midian and conquered them. The army slew every man, regardless of whether he was a soldier or a civilian, and herded the women and children back to Moses.

Moses asked, "Why did you bring these people here? Kill every male child and kill every woman, except for the young virgins. Those you may keep for yourselves."

⊰ ⊱

The genocidal treatment of the Midians is described in Numbers.[2] The cause for the attack is the fact that God had observed some Israelis patronizing Moab prostitutes. Moab is not Midian, but let's not quibble with facts. And let's not worry about the fact that Moses was married to a Midianite woman. The point is, the rule against killing applies only to those who are within your social circle. Adultery is OK if it is raping a woman who is not of your tribe. Lest we get upset with Jewish people over this incident, know that this ancient story is not unique to the Bible; this kind of story can be found in all the warlike societies throughout history. Those who are not "us" are not human and do not have to be treated as humans. Unfortunately, this is not just an ancient mindset here is a quote from a former prime minister of Israel, David Ben-Gurion.[3]

"Our laws are not for them, and their god is not our god."

This view has been shared by colonizing people throughout history; the expansion of the American frontiers into Indian lands led to the same death and destruction of people who are not "us." The European colonization of cultures all over the world had the same devastating effect. The stories these conquerors told themselves justified their actions: The indigenous people were heathens, barbarians, uncultured and in need of a strong guiding hand lest their very souls be lost, assuming they had any souls to begin with (which was the subject of great debates).

Society's stories create boundaries; those that are outside the boundaries are not really human. They have no souls. They are totally "other." These myths arise despite the best intentions of the founders of the spiritual philosophies that the conquerors claim to follow. The Old Testament displays many horrific actions that today would be called crimes against humanity, but it also depicts much compassion and love for the downtrodden and helpless. Prophets like Amos and Hosea chastised the people and rulers for treating the downtrodden poorly. Isaiah pleaded:

> *Your hands are covered with blood, wash, make yourself clean. Cease to do evil. Learn to do good, search for justice, help the oppressed, be just to the orphan, plead for the widow.*[4]

While Jesus preached that we should love our enemies, his followers during the Crusades killed, raped, looted, and destroyed the cities of people who were not like them, just as the followers of Joshua had done to the Canaanites. Mohammed tried to set the boundaries of Islam very wide to avoid these problems of "us versus others." In the constitution of Medina that he brokered, he defined the *ummah* as including Jews, Christians and pagans.[5] The ummah is an Arabic word that can mean "community" as well as the entire Arab world, and everyone is part of it. This is a very broad boundary, but this teaching, like those of Jesus, Isaiah and others, was forgotten when it was convenient.

✳ ✳ ✳

THE NET OF INDRA

> *Imagine a multidimensional spider's web in the early morning, covered with dewdrops. And every dewdrop contains the reflection of all the other dewdrops. And, in each reflected dewdrop, the reflections of all the other dewdrops in that reflection. And so* ad infinitum. *That is the Buddhist conception of the universe in an image.* — Alan Watts[6]

The Net of Indra is a marvelous concept developed by Buddhists to indicate the interconnectedness of all life and all existence. When Indra created the world, he also created a web with a shining jewel—some say a pearl—at every intersection of the web. Within each pearl can be seen every other pearl. Not only do we reflect each other, we are physically tied to each other as well. This is summarized in the early Buddhist teaching as *anatta*—"no separate self." Everything exists because of something else.

Thich Nhat Hanh, a venerable Vietnamese Zen master, coined the term *interbeing*. We all "inter-are" with everyone else in this world. It is not possible to not be connected: There are no boundaries. The astronauts circling the moon looked back at their home, a blue white pearl floating in a sea of stars, and saw no boundaries. When we look at a globe or a map of the world, we see many lines—borders and boundaries depicting separation and differences. From space, there are no borders. All boundaries are inventions of the human imagination. These imaginary lines are starting to dissolve, and this dissolution has been accelerating over the last few centuries. New myths are arising to replace the old bounded views of the world.

✳ ✳ ✳

Chief Dan Seattle was mythically unique; he was the chief of the Suquamish people and other tribes that lived around the waters of the city that today bears his name. The new country of America was expanding and needed space. The United States of America asked the tribes to surrender 2 million acres of their land for one $150,000. This was Chief Seattle's reply:[7]

⮜ ⮞

How can you buy or sell the sky, the warmth of the land? The idea is strange to us. If we do not own the freshness of the air and the sparkle of the water, how can you buy them from us? Every part of this earth is sacred to my people. Every shining pine needle, every sandy shore, every mist in the dark woods, every clearing and humming insect is holy in the memory and experience of my people. The sap that courses through the trees carries the memories of the red man.

The white man's dead forget the country of their birth when they go to walk among the stars. Our dead never forget this beautiful earth, for it is the mother of the red man. We are part of the earth and it is part of us. The perfumed flowers are our sisters. The deer, the horse, the great eagle, these are our brothers. The rocky crests, the juices in the meadows, the body heat of the pony, and man, all belong to the same family. So, when the Great Chief in Washington sends word that he wishes to buy our land, he asks much of us.

This shining water that moves in the streams and rivers is not just water but the blood of our ancestors. If we sell you land, you must remember that it is sacred; you must teach your children that it is sacred and that each ghostly reflection in the clear water of the lakes tells of events and memories in the life of my people.

The water's murmur is the voice of my father's father. The rivers are our brothers: They quench our thirst. The rivers carry our canoes and feed our children. If we sell you our land, you must remember and teach your children that the rivers are our brothers and yours; and you must henceforth give rivers the kindness you would give any brother.

The red man has always retreated before the advancing white man, as the mist of the mountain runs before the morning sun. But the ashes of our fathers are sacred. Their graves are holy ground, and so these hills, these trees, this portion of the earth is consecrated to us. We know that the white man does not understand our ways. One portion of land is the same to him as the next, for he is a stranger who comes in the night and takes from the land whatever he needs. The earth is not his brother but his enemy, and when he has conquered it, he moves on. He leaves his fathers' graves behind, and he does not care. He kidnaps the earth from his children. He does not care. His fathers' graves and his children's birthright are forgotten. He treats his mother, the earth, and his brother, the sky, as things to be bought, plundered, sold like sheep or bright beads. His appetite will devour the earth and leave behind only a desert.

… If we sell our land, you must remember that the air is precious to us: The air shares its spirit with all the life it supports. The wind that gave our grandfather his first breath also receives his last sigh. And the wind must also give our children the spirit of life. And if we sell you our land, you must keep it apart and sacred, as a place where even the white man can go to taste the wind that is sweetened by the meadow's flowers. So we will consider your offer to buy our land.

If we decide to accept, I will make one condition: The white man must treat the beasts of this land as his brothers. I am a savage and I do not understand any other way. I have seen a thousand rotting buffalos on the prairie, left by the white man who shot them from a passing train. I am a savage, and I do not understand how the smoking iron horse can be more important than the buffalo that we kill only to stay alive. What is man without the beasts? If all the beasts were gone, men would die from a great loneliness of spirit. For whatever happens to the beasts soon happens to man. All things are connected.

Teach your children what we have taught our children, that the earth is our mother. Whatever befalls the earth befalls the sons of the earth. If men spit upon the ground, they spit upon themselves. This we know: The earth does not belong to man; man belongs to the earth. … All things are connected like the blood which unites one family. … Man did not weave the web of life; he is merely a strand in it. Whatever he does to the web, he does to himself.

"What is it that the white man wishes to buy?" my people ask me. The idea is strange to us. How can you buy or sell the sky, the warmth of the land? The swiftness of the antelope? How can we sell these things to you, and how can you buy them? Is the earth yours to do with as you will merely because the red man signs a piece of paper and gives it to the white man? If we do not own the freshness of the air and the sparkle of the water, how can you buy them from us? Can you buy back the buffalo, once the last one has been killed?

But we will consider your offer, for we know that if we do not sell, the white man may come with guns and take our land. But we are primitive, and in his passing moment of strength the white man thinks that he is a god who already owns the earth. How can a man own his mother?

We will consider your offer to go to the reservation you have for my people. We will live apart and in peace. It matters little where we spend the rest of our days. Our children have seen their fathers humbled in defeat. It matters little where we pass the rest of our days. They are not many. A few more hours, a few more winters, and none of the children of the great tribes that once lived on this earth or that roam now in small bands in the woods will be left to mourn the graves of a people once as powerful and hopeful as yours.

But why should I mourn the passing of my people? Tribes are made of men, nothing more. Men come and go, like the waves of the sea. Even the white man, whose God walks and talks with him as friend to friend, cannot be exempt from the common destiny. We may be brothers, after all. We shall see. One thing we know, which the white man may one day discover: Our God is the same God.

You may think now that you own Him as you wish to own our land, but you cannot. He is the God of man, and His compassion is equal for the red man and the white. This earth is precious to Him, and to harm the earth is to heap contempt on its Creator. The whites, too, shall pass; perhaps sooner than all other tribes. Continue to contaminate your bed, and you will one night suffocate in your own waste.

[Your] destiny is a mystery to us, for we do not understand when the buffalo are all slaughtered, the wild horses are tamed, the secret corners of the forest heavy with the scent of many men, and the view of the ripe hills blotted by talking wires. Where is the thicket? Gone. Where is the eagle? Gone. And what is it to say goodbye to the swift pony and the hunt? The end of living and the beginning of survival.

The white man's dreams are hidden from us. And because they are hidden, we will go our own way. For above all else, we cherish the right of each man to live as he wishes, however different from his brothers. There is little in common between us.

If we sell you our land, love it as we've loved it. Care for it as we've cared for it. Hold in your mind the memory of the land as it is when you take it. And with all your strength, with all your mind, with all your heart, preserve it for your children and love it as God loves us all.

One thing we know: Our God is the same God. This earth is precious to Him. Even the white man cannot be exempt from the common destiny. We may be brothers, after all. We shall see.

⊰ ⊱

Boundaries are expanding, and eventually they will disappear; they must disappear if the human race is to continue. But before this can happen, new stories will be needed—stories very similar to the myth of Chief Dan Seattle. We are all a part of the web of life, and what we do to one part of the web we do to ourselves. The web of life is the Net of Indra brought into modern parlance.

✳ ✳ ✳

Myths evolve. They are never static—sometimes we can see them evolving in front of our eyes. Joseph Campbell related the story of Chief Dan Seattle in his 1998 public television series "The Power of Myth", hosted by Bill Moyers, and in the book that followed. The story resonated deeply with the current environmental movement and reflected Campbell's belief that our boundaries were expanding: The difference between "us" and "others" was shrinking.

Amazingly, this story is not actually true! The words above were written for a movie and were not the words of Chief Dan Seattle.[8] Even Joseph Campbell was fooled. There are several anachronisms in the letter that could not possibly be true, such as seeing buffalo being killed by people in trains. It is highly unlikely the chief ever saw a train, let alone a buffalo. The cross-country railway did not reach Washington State until 1873, and yet Chief Seattle died in 1866. The systematic elimination of the buffalo didn't begin until 1870s. The letter also refers to antelopes and pinion trees, which, in fact, did not exist in the Pacific Northwest.

However, the incident that supposedly generated the letter was true enough—the U.S. government did want Seattle's lands. But his actual speech (it was not a letter) was a lament for his people. The old chief was quoted in a Seattle newspaper as saying, "Your god is *not* our god. Your god loves your people and hates mine. How then can we be brothers?" [Italics added.] Even this quote, credited to a homesteading physician who supposedly attended the speech and then wrote about it 35 years later, is of questionable veracity. There are scholars who believe there never was a speech, let alone a letter. They speculate that the writings that today's myth is based upon were the muse's songs in a physician's ear.[9]

As we have seen over and over, the historicity and factual veracity of a myth is irrelevant, as long as people believe in the story. The "letter" of Chief Seattle is now part of a modern myth of the oneness of all: The earth is precious and we are all its children. It does not matter that the myth is not true—it works! Reading the letter creates a strong emotion, and it makes one want to treat the earth and its children fairly. That is the affective power of a myth: it matches the psychic terrain creates a resonance. It molds attitudes and stimulates actions. This happens automatically, like a reflex. You don't have to think about whether you like or agree with the story—it just rings true to you. And when you hear a story that rings true, you share it. In the sharing, you start to shape the landscape of the minds around you, and then these minds reach out to others—the myth grows.

✳ ✳ ✳

Societies change. They wish not to, but change is the one constant in life. With the changes come new stories. The Reformation in Europe was a time of significant change, a change that was not occurring in the more conservative societies of Asia. The Reformation and its older sibling, the Renaissance, led to the Age of Enlightenment. Science and reason began to erode faith in the cosmological models of Aristotle and the Bible. When the cosmological functions of the Greek and Levantine myths failed to serve, then, too, the sociological functions also failed. No longer was God's law mandatory; human law became more important. Kings no longer governed by divine right, but by sufferance of the people. Indeed, a new god was born, the god we now call "We the People." With this new god came a new mythos: the myth of democracy and the rights of the individual.

Societies today are secular, for the most part (although there are many today trying to turn back the hands of the clock and re-invoke the religious rules of a bygone mythology). The laws we follow are not given by the creator of the universe but by men and women. However, societies still need their stories—people still need to know how to behave, how to fit in, how to treat others. It is difficult to see the myths we live by; it is much easier to see the myths other people live by as stories, and to smile when those people try to convince us that their stories are reality. Our modern myths are stories, nonetheless.

In the 1960s a new movement gained momentum, as people began to become aware of humanity's sheer weight of existence and its effect on the environment and our natural resources. Brave pioneering writers like Rachel Carson stood up against the conservative forces of society and blew apart the archaic myth that man was too puny to significantly affect God's earth. With the publication in 1962 of *Silent Spring*, Carson warned the world that we were killing our rivers, polluting the air, and rendering the land lifeless through the indiscriminate use of pesticides. She died only two years after her book was published, amid fierce condemnation by pesticide companies and all levels of government; she did not live to see the impact her writing had. A generation grew up willing to examine what was actually happening and to take action. New myths were created that resonated with the new cosmology, based on the new science of ecology. The letter of Chief Seattle is just one example of this new mythology built upon the new cosmology, the way of the universe.

There need not be a conflict between religion and science, but there certainly is a conflict between the proto-science of 2000 B.C.E. and the science of 2000 C.E. The religious myths of 4,000 years ago were based on the science of the day, and our modern spiritual stories, too, can incorporate the scientific understanding of our time. In order for a myth to be effective, it has to be based on something believable (but remember, not necessarily true!). The cosmological myths today are far vaster and grander than what is found in the Bible, and the sociological function of our modern myths must be in tune with this new cosmology. The change is happening, but it takes time to wean people off an old paradigm and for the new one to take hold. In 1988 the great humanitarian Mother Teresa said, "Why should we care about the earth when our duty is to the poor and the sick among us. God will take care of the earth."[10] This attitude comes from the old mythology, which is no longer serving mankind very well. A new myth, replacing the one found in the Bible, is the story of Gaia.

The Gaia Hypothesis views the biosphere as an active, adaptive control system able to maintain the Earth in homeostasis.[11]

This is the scientific definition of Gaia given by James Lovelock and Lynn Margulis. The mythic statement is more poetic: The earth is alive! Not only that, the earth, let's call her Gaia (which is the name of the Greek goddess of earth), wants us to be alive, too. To make life possible, she changes: If things get too hot, she takes action to cool us down by creating more cloud cover, which reflects sunlight away, thus cooling the Earth. If things get too cool, she takes action to warm us back up again by emitting more carbon dioxide into the atmosphere, creating global warming. Gaia loves stable conditions and seeks them all the time. This is all an over-simplification, and scientists like Lovelock don't actually believe the earth (Gaia) is self-aware and sentient as humans are, but in the poetry of a myth, such metaphors are allowed. Lovelock's point is that we have usurped Gaia's power and are making it impossible for her to do her thing. Mama Gaia, metaphorically, is very sick and is about to take her revenge on the human race, unless we change our ways.

This new cosmological myth is telling us what our society must start doing right away. Many people are listening; they get the myth and they are taking action. It remains to be seen if the changes will be in time.

✻ ✻ ✻

Our modern society is secular, again for the most part; no longer do the gods tell us how we should behave. Those old myths have lost their power, but we are never without our stories. We have the myth of democracy now. The boundaries that created classes and castes are dissolving. In the early part of the 20th century, the myth of women changed significantly. No longer were women mere property—the chattel of men; women obtained the right to vote. In the 1960s, the decade of a modern reformation, civil rights movements gave legal equality to all races. One can cry out that there is still so much more to do, and there is still a great deal of inequality to be found in the world. Still, we have come a long way, indeed, compared to the way societies were even a couple hundred years ago, let alone the horrors of the first societies in history.

Studies by Steven Pinker, a professor of psychology at Harvard, have shown that the tribal warfare of ancient times, such as described in the Bible, was nine times more deadly than the wars and genocides committed in the 20th century.[12] Murder rates in Europe during the Middle Ages were 30 times higher than today's rates. Consider all the practices that were commonplace throughout history, that are outlawed by society today: slavery, frivolous executions, torture, rape as a weapon of war, extreme punishment for minor transgressions. Pinker attributes these declines to the spread of government, universal education and literacy, trade expansion, and empathy with others. Boundaries are disappearing, and individuals today have rights that did not exist in the past. This brings us to the cusp of the third function of mythology: the psychological function and myths' import for the individual.

The Sociological Function of Mythology: Summary

The sociological function of myths and the cultural stories that are repeated and enjoyed work because they define the way people should behave within their society and toward those who are outside the boundary of the community. According to early myths, the rules of society are given by the very power that created the universe: either a personal god who gets involved in the unfolding of events, or an impersonal power that simply winds up the clock and lets it tick away. In either case, it is not your individual will that matters, but the will of God or of Dharma.

You don't have to wonder, Should I be like this or like that?—it has all been determined for you, and your duty is to do what has always been done. Those who resist are cast out; the consequences of breaking society's rules are harsh! Even the smallest transgression can be fatal. This is taken very seriously.

Today, societies have changed and continue to change, but like all societies, they are still very conservative. The changes will not come easily. Societies both old and modern require "part people," not "whole people." People today are still carved up to fit the roles that society requires. Unfortunately this often puts the individual at odds with the psychological function of myth, which we will investigate next.

The Psychological Function

When I was a child, I talked like a child, I understood the world like a child, I thought like a child. When I became an adult, I put the ways of childhood behind me.

— Saint Paul: 1 Corinthians 13 – 11

Chapter 7: The Arc of Aging

⊰ ⊱

They thought it would be improper, what with them being knights and all, it would be unfitting for them to enter the forest in a group. They decided to take no path, for to follow a path is to follow someone else's adventure: They would each enter the forest at a point of his own choosing.

An adventure is what King Arthur required that evening when the knights of his round table gathered for supper. "We must not eat until we have had an adventure." In response to his call, and so that the knights would not go hungry, an adventure appeared right before their eyes. In the middle of the table, floating above them, appeared a vision of the Holy Grail. It was Arthur's nephew, Sir Gawain, who proposed that they go off and find the Grail.

Parzival was the newest of the knights. He was big, strong, but unskilled and rough; he was not raised to be a knight. No, quite the opposite: His mother took him away from court, from the lifestyle that killed her husband, and vowed to herself that her son would not be like his father. Parzival grew up in isolation, unaware of his noble birth and of the ways of the knight. He wore only a ridiculous homespun tunic that his mother had made for him.

One day, while attending to his errands, Parzival spied a group of knights riding. His mother had not taught him about such men, so he thought they were angels—she had told him about angels. He bowed before them but learned that they were not from heaven; they were from the court of King Arthur. A lust was kindled within Parzival. He bade his mother goodbye, which broke her heart. She died as he left, but he did not know her fate until much later. He was following what was in his heart.

Parzival arrived at Camelot, untutored but of noble blood. A real knight, a great knight, dressed in blood red armor, had also arrived at Camelot and challenged Arthur's knights to mortal combat. The Red Knight's challenge was not met, so Parzival spoke up. Amid the laughter that greeted his response, there was some shame, as well. The brave knights cowered while this simple bumpkin took up the fight. Parzival surprised them all, not the least the Red Knight: In the battle Parzival killed the Red Knight and earned his armor and his horse.

Sheer strength does not make one a knight; Parzival was still raw and needed teaching. Gurnemanz saw potential in this young man and took him under his wing, becoming Parzival's guru and father for a time. Parzival learned the knightly arts quickly: He learned that a good knight does not ask questions but simply does what a knight is bound by honor and duty to do. He learned so well that Gurnemanz felt Parzival to be a perfect husband for his youngest daughter, but Parzival demurred—a wife must be earned, not given. He set off to win himself a wife and find his own path in the world.

In his wanderings Parzival met and bested many knights of renown, and each time he would send the conquered man to Camelot to serve Arthur. He was building quite a reputation at court. This simple bumpkin was turning out to be a major force in the world. One day Parzival let the reins of his horse fall slack and went wherever his steed took him. He came to a besieged castle, the home of an orphaned queen of his own age, the lady Condwiramurs, which in old French means the "drive of love."

Parzival was greeted warmly and hospitably. At night, when he had taken to his bed, Condwiramurs came to him, crying but dressed alluringly in a shift of white silk, prepared for battle. If he would agree not to wrestle with her, she would agree to keep his bed warm that night. He moved over a little to let her in. She explained that a powerful knight wanted to marry her and take her lands. Parzival suggested that he should kill the bad man in the morning. She said, "That would be nice."

And, so he did.

Parzival had earned a wife. When he returned to the castle, Condwiramurs had her hair up in the manner of a married woman; no priests were needed to solemnize this union—love is all you need. Parzival had become all grownup now. Now he had earned the right to be a Knight of the Round Table and participate in the quest for the Holy Grail.

⁂

The inflections of the cosmological and sociological functions of myths vary widely between cultures, but the psychological has much less variation, as we will discover. The psychological function of mythology puts us in accord with the inevitable arc of aging that we all traverse. From birth, infancy, childhood, adolescences, maturity, old age and death, we each have to come to terms with who we are, how we change with time, and how our roles in society and within our family also change. We look to the stories of our culture to give us the understanding we need to make sense of our changing roles.

We will finish the tale of Parzival and his quest for the Holy Grail later. Up to this point in the story of Parzival, Percival, Parsifal, or any of the many other renderings of his name, we saw a young man destined to be great, but one who is ignorant of his noble blood. This is a very ancient theme. From Karna in the Mahabhrata, to Sargon, king of Agade, who conquered Sumer, to Moses in Egypt—that which is noble is hidden. These are not meant to be historical truths but universal truth: There is nobility within *you*, but you are ignorant of it. It is part of your task of tasks in this life to discover and uncover your own birthright, the right to find your own path that will lead you to your own greatness.

Parzival's father was a king of Wales who went to fight in the Crusades. This has interesting symbolism of its own, for the writer of this version of Parzival and the Holy Grail was himself a knight, albeit not a rich one: Wolfram von Eschenbach (1170–1220 C.E.). He lived at a time when German royalty was being heavily pressed by the Catholic Church; politics was trumping sacred duty and honor. Von Eschenbach felt no compassion for the church's politics and saw in the East a nobler ethos. In his telling of this tale, the father of Parzival first took a pagan wife in the East and begat a son, then snuck away to Wales to father Parzival before going off to fight more wars and, eventually, meeting his death. His widow in Wales vowed to not let her son become like his father, so she moved to a farm and quietly raised Parzival alone and away from all temptations. This was a forlorn hope: Sons always leave their mothers to follow the way of their fathers—at least they do if they follow the rules of their society.

Societies require a rite of passage for young boys. In some primal societies, the rites are shockingly harsh and involve scarification and circumcision. A new member of the tribe is being shaped to fit. Joseph Campbell gave as an example the story of aboriginal men in Australia initiating the young boys into society.[1] When boys reach the age where the women find them hard to deal with, the men come in with yowls and screams, wearing masks and costumes, and take the boys away. The boys are taken to a sacred place and put behind some bushes; they are warned to stay there and not look. If a brave but disobedient youngster should look, he is punished by being eaten! Campbell points out that this is one way to handle juvenile delinquency. Then the boys are brought out onto the sacred ground, where men wearing the costumes of the totem animals—the dog and the cosmic kangaroo—attack them. They are circumcised and fed on men's blood: no more mothers' milk! The boys hear and see enacted the great myths of their culture. When all is said and done, each of the boys is led back to the village, where a young girl has been picked out for him. This girl, the daughter of the man who circumcised him, will be his wife.

In more modern traditions, a boy's passage into manhood is much less severe. The Catholic Church ritual of Confirmation, the Hindu investiture of the strings[2] and the Jewish Bar Mitzvah serve the function of a rite of initiation, although the psychological effect is not as profound as the earlier rites. Parzival knew no father; he had to find his own way into manhood. The first step was leaving his mother, but he couldn't completely leave her behind—he still wore the homespun tunic that she made for him so that he would look ridiculous. Her hope was that he would be shamed by the ridicule he would face and would give up any quest to become a knight. As long as he wore the homespun garment of his mother, Parzival would not truly be a man, but he put himself on the path. His initiation ritual was the battle with the Red Knight. No other knight could fight this fight for him; he had to accept the challenge. We see here the same motif as we found with the Ojibwa Indian boy who had to wrestle the god of corn: A struggle is always required, and a threshold must be crossed. Parzival passed his rite of initiation—he killed the Red Knight—but he still had much to learn. He needed a father, or at least a father figure, to teach him, and he was fortunate that Gurnemanz was willing to fill this role. This was the time for being a student; he was not yet ready to raise a family. Plus, he had to earn the right to marry. To Parzival, it did not seem proper to simply take any woman offered.

Parzival found his wife, not by plan and not by intent, but by trusting to his unconscious. He let go the reins to his horse and allowed himself to be carried by his animal nature to his future, to Condwiramurs. He still had to earn her, and once he did, the marriage was real. This union did not require any social sanction, it was sanctified by love. Here we see von Eschenbach's own feelings toward the Church. Before the power of the Church in Europe became pervasive, marriage between ordinary people was conducted without clergy; there was simply an affirmation between two people, an "I marry you." The average age of such unions was in the late teens for women and 20s for men. If any ceremony was conducted, it was a simple one done at home or in front of a church door. However, marriage for love was not the way in the high Middle Ages of Europe, at least not for those of noble birth. Marriages between the highborn members of society were arranged by families and sanctioned by society or there was no marriage, only adultery. These marriages, like the arranged marriages in India, were often brokered when the participants were very young and still only children. Von Eschenbach was not alone in feeling that society needed to resist this change and the encroachment of the Church, and we will come back to this theme when we talk about the myths of love.

Parzival is now a married man, ready to find his deeper purpose in life.

✳ ✳ ✳

THE ASHRAMA

Human beings are very unusual animals. We have the longest period of infancy and dependency of any animal, and we don't reach our physical maturity until our early 20s. We are also very unusual in having an extended middle age; we can be healthy and active for many decades after losing the ability or desire to beget children. This is true for all of humanity all over the world; there is no cultural dependency to the arc of aging that we all follow, but there is variety in the mythic representations of these stages. Different cultures offer different maps and models to help us deal with the transitions that come with growing older. These are all part of the psychological function of mythology.

In India there are four main stages of life that men follow, known as the *ashrama*:

1. *Brahmacarin* or "the student": this is the time to learn;

2. *Grihastha* or "householder": this is the time to raise a family;

3. *Vanaprastha* or "departure to the forest": this is the time for yoga;

4. *Sannyasin* or "the renunciate": this is a time of returning to teach others.

It should be pointed out right at the start that these are the idealized life stages, and not everyone needs to follow them. It is OK for someone to stay in stage 2 for their whole life, in fact it was suggested that most people should stay there: Imagine the chaos if everyone left their homes and headed to the forest. And guess who prefers that we stay in the household mode? The priests and the conservative agents of society! If everyone pursued a path of leaving the household life for spiritual freedom, it would not be good for society. This is one of the important lessons we learned in the "Humbling of Indra" myth. Remember, it was the palace priest, Brihaspati, who convinced Indra that he did have to go to the forest.

The first stage of life (brahmacarin) is characterized by obedience: The child must learn to obey his elders, especially his guru. The student is an empty vessel into which is poured the teachings of his master. Absolute faith, *shraddha*, is required. There is no room for interpretation or questioning: What you are told is truth, and you do not argue with it. Strict celibacy is also very important. To have sexual relations with someone would break the intimate relationship with the teacher, and a harsh punishment would befall the student. It is during this period that the child learns the vocation he will practice for the rest of his life. With the investiture of the sacred thread, the student is given a new umbilical cord, tying him not to physical life, but to the spiritual life as demonstrated by his teacher.

The true guru, according to the Kula-Arnava-Tantra, is the one who reveals the Self.[3] According to the Indian saint of the 18th century Sri Ramakrishna (1836-1886), the guru is like a tiger:[4]

☙ ❧

Once upon a time, there was a tigress, heavy with pregnancy and very hungry. She came upon a little herd of goats and sprang upon them. In her exertions, she caused the birth of her little cub, but unfortunately she died in her labor. The goats, being kind and nourishing creatures, raised the little tiger as one of their own. He grew up learning the way of goats. He learned to eat grass and bleat like a goat.

One day a big male tiger came upon the little flock and also pounced. The goats scattered, as did the now-almost-grown little tiger. The big male tiger noticed the young tiger running away and so chased after him. When he caught the youngster, he asked him, "What in the world were you doing with those goats? Surely you weren't living with them!" The youngster said in reply, "Baahhhh."

The big tiger was horrified. He thought, "I have to fix this!" He picked up the smaller tiger and took him to a pond. In the still waters he forced the youngster to look at their reflections. Towering over junior the old fellow said, "Look! Look at your face. You look just like me. You are no goat; you are a tiger. You have to learn to be a tiger."

Next the teacher took his ward to his cave, where there was a leftover leg of a gazelle. He threw some meat to the youngster and said, "This is proper tiger food. Meat! Not grass. Eat!"

The youngster demurred; he had been a vegetarian up until now. But following the command of his new teacher, he finally took a taste of the meat and discovered he liked it. He could feel energy and life flowing through his veins.

"Finally," said the teacher, "you are like me! Come, let's go into the forest and live like true tigers."

❊ ❊

The guru is the archetype the student emulates. Through his submission to the guru, the student identifies with the teacher, becomes exactly like the teacher, and thus passes on the traditions that created the previous generation of gurus.

All societies mold their young into proper members of that society. Recall Joseph Campbell's observation that societies need part people, not whole people. India was no different in this regard; however, in the modern Western societies, children are more likely to be allowed, or required, to choose their own vocations. "What do you want to be when you grow up?" Vocation aside, how you are to act within society, even in the West, is still quite prescribed: You are to be a good citizen and consumer, you should not make waves, and you are to perpetuate society's culture when it is your turn to raise a family. As we will see, this is exactly what our current myths are still trying to teach us.

* * *

Back in India, after being a student comes the stage of being married—grihastha. This can happen quite suddenly when an arrangement is made between the two families. The bride and the groom most likely have never met. With a bang (and Indian weddings have wonderful fireworks with many loud bangs) you are hurled into the second stage of life. It is time to leave the stage of dependency and enter one of responsibility. You are now expected to earn a living, raise a family, bring forth sons, and take care of your parents. Not only do you have to earn enough to continue the standards of living your father provided, you must also continue to support the priests and pay for their rather expensive sacrifices. The Brahmins continue to be your spiritual guides, doctors, counselors, wizards and lawyers.

Now comes that very interesting transition that not everyone longs for—vanaprastha. It is time to drop the masks that society asked you to wear and head to the forest. In ancient Greece actors held masks in front of their faces to depict the role they were playing. In Latin these roles, these masks, were called *personae*. You are not your mask; you are not your persona; you are just acting. Time to take off your mask. When your son is old enough to take on the responsibility of leading the family, your work in the world has ended. Now you head to the forest to work on your own development. This is the time to do yoga. This is not the Hatha yoga popular in the West today; this is a fierce practice of dropping the world entirely. This is the stage that is beyond the joys and obligations of living in the world, beyond pleasure, (*kama*), and achievement, (*artha*). This is even beyond dharma, the obligations of caste and culture. This is the time of moksha, release from the bondage of the world, when you drop your persona or ego completely and find your Self.

Sannyasin, the final stage, is one of returning to the world, but what returns is not the person who departed earlier. The one coming back is empty of everything; there is nobody there. The renunciate has dropped all desires, all fears. This person is the wandering beggar or mendicant, the *bhikshu*. He is no longer bound by any cares of the world; he may be naked (clothing depicts one's caste, but he has now gone beyond any caste) or clothed in simple cloth, often the color of a burial shroud—yellow or dark orange, signifying that his former life is dead. Perhaps he is just wearing the bark of a tree. He has no residence or favorite place. He is totally free now, although this freedom does not mean that he is free to do whatever he wants; rather, it is freedom *from* wants. A better translation of the word *moksha* is "liberation": liberation is freedom *from* something, in this case freedom from aspirations or fears. This is the final stage of life. Thus prepared, death holds no terror, for there is no one who dies.

Joseph Campbell discovered in a trip to India that while women can go to the forest and men should go to the forest, few actually do. Again, this is a suggested path. Joseph asked several Indian women why they didn't go to the forest, since they were allowed to follow their husbands there. The answer was quite interesting: Girls grow up having to answer to their fathers. When they are married, they have to answer to their husbands. When the husbands go to the forest, they answer to their sons. For their whole lives, women are told what to do. Finally, when their sons take over the husbands' role as head of the family, there comes into the family a wonderful creature known as a daughter-in-law. At last there is someone whom the mother can boss around. Most women are waiting for the day they become the mother-in-law, and they are not going to miss this by going to the forest.[5] Carl Jung thought the reason women don't go to the forest is simply because they are too full of life! In the forest life is desiccated and drops away. Women, from whom life springs, are not fit to go to the forest and to waste away. Leave that to the dried-up old men.

✳ ✳ ✳

The Indian mythology relating to the arc of aging is not quite the model we follow in the West. Consider the phases of life as it unfolds for us living in the West today: We can break these down into at least six distinct ages:

132

1. Infancy: a time of total dependency on our parents;

2. The early student years: from about age six to 12;

3. The late student years: inhabited by creatures known as teenagers;

4. The work and family years: the time of reproducing and rearing young;

5. Middle age: the time of being a grandparent and wise elder;

6. Retirement and departure: the time to leave it all behind.[6]

We are born completely helpless: We cannot feed ourselves, we cannot walk or dress ourselves, and we even lack control over our bowels and bladders. For the first six years of life, we are totally dependent on our parents. This is a time when we learn how to be fully functional animals—to run, jump, speak, and talk. We are downloading massive amounts of information about our families and the rules of relating to others. As the Jesuit Ignatius of Loyola (1491-1556) once observed, "Give me the boy, and I will give you the man." It is in these first few years that a person's basic mythos is laid down: This is the base map that he or she will follow throughout life.

In the first six years of life, our mind is in a hypnotic state; there are no alpha waves created in the brain until around the seventh year. Alpha waves are found in states of calm consciousness.

We have learned through electroencephalogram studies that children only experience delta and theta waves; these are dreamlike states where the imagination of the mind and the reality of the real world are mixed together, undifferentiated.[7] Delta and theta waves indicate that the brain is acting below normal adult consciousness, the state of hypnosis when one is super-suggestible. Directives and statements can be downloaded directly into the unconscious mind without any conscious pre-evaluation.

When a child is young, before his brain begins to produce the higher frequency waves of alpha and beta waves, he is open to the story unfolding around him. He is in the midst of a living myth, and the people around him become symbols and inflections of archetypes; the morality of his society is displayed and absorbed. He is swimming in mythic waters from the very first. He has left the waters of his mother's physical body and now swims in the waters of the mother culture. These stories shape his mind until he is ready to layer on top of this landscape another level of mind, of awareness, which we call the conscious mind.

From six years of age onward, we are able to generate alpha waves in the brain: We become self-conscious. The earlier landscape is submerged beneath the mind's new awareness, but the earliest layer is still there, formed purely of stories that were absorbed in the first years of life. An unconscious database was built that governs our basal reactions to life, and now, on top of that, we can start to discern for ourselves what is real and what is imaginary. Now we are able to develop critical thinking skills, but this comes too late to influence the maps we have already had implanted in our minds. The early myths, or imprints, or belief structures, if you prefer, are there to stay unless something very significant occurs that allows us, or helps us, to change them. We begin with stories, we grow up with stories, and when we are older and recognize that some of the stories don't work anymore, we need to replace them with new stories that do work. But these stories need to talk to our hidden mind, we need to dive into the deep and rearrange, renovate, and transform what is down there.

Around the age of six is the time a big change occurs—the biggest moment in our young lives so far: We experience our first day of school. Our teachers are no longer just our parents and family, we are given over to the gurus of the school system. It is not just one person we must trust and respect; each year we are given a new teacher and soon multiple teachers within each school year, as specialization occurs. We are not given individual instruction, we are part of a group—a class that learns together. We are being developed and broadened, molded into members of society that society, through its formalized school system, has decided fits best. By about our 12th year, our brains start to produce beta waves.[8] Beta waves occur when we concentrate, when we are active or busy or feel anxious. It is time for another transition: Another rite of passage is upon us.

In primal societies, as we have seen, the rites of passage from childhood dependency to adult responsibility are quite profound, dramatic and life altering. In the West, the rituals are tame by comparison. The student is still in school when the transition is occurring. The transition is demanded by biology, although in the West we wait for chronology to decide when we should undergo the ritual. The body is changing: around the 12th year puberty happens. The child is growing into a person capable of reproducing. For girls this change happens distinctly and suddenly; for boys it is a long, drawn out affair. It is for this reason that boys need a ritual more than girls do. In the West, there are very few rituals or myths remaining to help demarcate this transition from boy to man. This period is marked for most boys solely by the change in the school system: The ritual is simply the graduation from elementary school to junior high. The second stage of learning is upon us, and we enter a very different environment than the childlike security of elementary school. High school can be a frightening and sublime place. Without a good map to follow, we become confused.

In past eras, the puberty rituals occurred at an age that is too young for modern society: More ripening is needed today. In earlier centuries and in very different cultures, a girl of 13 would be old enough to marry; her first period would be enough proof that she had become a woman. Today a lad or lass of 13 is hardly ready for such responsibilities.

While in the West students have the freedom to choose the field of study they can pursue, there is no choice that study they must. Everyone must stay in school; dropouts have a grave disadvantage in society. In the middle of the student years, we leave childhood behind and enter a distinct time of life called the teenage years. This is a stage is unique to the West. In older cultures we went straight from the child-student to the adult-householder. In the West the teen years have great mythic importance. It is during this stage of life that the opposite sex becomes noticed and objectified. There is that mysterious other person you feel so strongly attracted to. Courting rituals have to be worked out. Your family may have an opinion about whom you should be attracted to, but they are not going to find your spouse for you. What map are you going to follow now? Probably one described in stories told among your friends and in magazines, books and movies—peer pressure is heavy. Unfortunately, the myths available to teenagers today are not very deep or skillful, because they tend to objectify the sexual aspect of relationship at the expense of deepening understanding of the nature of relationship. The myths are shallow and focus on eros or kama: pleasure.

Finally, graduation! The child is grown and ready to take on the full responsibilities of an adult—to get a job. There are a few modern rites of passage here, but they are mostly passive. The high school graduation ceremony, obtaining a driver's license and the right to vote and drink are the modern hallmarks that one is now an adult. But, get a job? Not so fast!

In the 1930s and earlier, few would finish high school; it was more important to learn a trade, because that is what guaranteed you a job. By the 1950s a high school diploma was necessary to get a good job. By the 1990s a high school diploma was no longer a guarantee of anything better than a MacJob: working in the service industry for minimum wage. University education was now required to earn a decent living. This gradual inflation of time spent being educated delayed the final assumption of adult responsibility. The time of youth was being extended, and this is mirrored in the myths of society.

Youth is king and must be served; the mythos of the baby boomer generation included the belief that the best time of life is found in youth. To have a young, strong, healthy body that was free from disease and was beautiful and attractive and desired are the aims of life. In 1965, the rock band The Who had a hit song called "My Generation" in which they sang, "I hope I die before I get old." This was the decade of the generation gap and the adage "Don't trust anyone over 30." To be old, weak and wrinkled is not only uncool, it is a tragedy to be avoided or masked at all costs. We need not look far to find these myths on full display: music videos, movies, airbrushed models in magazines, the latest hi-tech gadget—all these are aimed at the young and are designed to get those who used to be young to act young again.

Over that last few decades, the average age to graduate from the school system has gone up, as has the average age to marry and to have children.[9] We long to be teenagers forever. Joseph Campbell paraphrased a teaching of Freud when he said that a neurosis is simply having feelings of dependency when one ought to be having feelings of responsibility. So the neurotic person goes to the therapist, who basically tells him to grow up! That is all that is needed.[10] But in the modern West, this growing up takes longer and longer. Some drag it out forever; they wish to forgo all the other stages of life. This is a forlorn hope presented by unskillful myths. You can choose not to participate in the stages of life, but time and biology will force them upon you. If you are not ready for them, or if the map you have chosen to follow does not show you the way, you will be lost, confused and suffer psychic harm. You could crack-up or have a breakdown. You may decide not to grow up, but you cannot decide to not grow older.

After the student stage has been left behind, the next stage is the working world/householder stage: marriage and family, mortgages and career. This is a long stage. Because children do not reach the age of responsibility now until their late teens or even late 20s, the stage of being a parent has expanded into the 50s and 60s, a time when traditionally one became doting grandparents.

✲ ✲ ✲

Middle Age and the Wise Elder

Thank god for grandparents! A study of South American hunter-gathers showed that in primal societies, it takes more than two parents to raise children.[11] A child consumes calories provided by the parents without contributing many calories in return. It takes an additional 1.3 adults to look after children beyond what the parents can provide: enter the grandparents. Middle-aged adults provide an important repository of knowledge, skills, experience, and labor that are required by society. The fact that humans have an extended period of life beyond the time we are able to reproduce new humans is not an accident or a fortunate mistake; natural selection has chosen us *because* we have an extended middle age.

It may seem strange to think of it this way, but menopause is a good thing for women and society. When people can no longer reproduce children of their own, their time is freed up to help others with rearing young. There are few animals like us in this respect, but Orcas also experience menopause, and their life cycle is very similar to ours.[12] The success of our species owes a lot to the reality of grandparents and extended middle age. The sudden ending of our fertility may be shocking, and our current myths do not prepare us well for this, but it is liberation. In the words of David Bainbridge at the University of Cambridge, "[menopause] liberates women and their partners from the unremitting demands of producing children and gives them time to do what middle-aged people do best—live long and pamper."[13]

What do the current Western myths say about aging? It is not cool. Fight it. Rage against the wrinkles you see in the mirror, tuck this and nip that. You are getting older—what a catastrophe! Botox! These prescriptions, proffered by advertisers hawking beauty products, simply mask the reality of a body that is growing older. There are other myths to follow: There are myths and stories about people who are gracefully old, about wise elders.

In our tradition, the elders were honored because they were the ones who had the knowledge. Long ago there was no written knowledge. We passed on our laws and our knowledge through the oral tradition. And the old people were the keepers of this. They were the ones who had lived longer and experienced more things. They knew what to do if a big storm came or something like that. They were the ones who had the answers. See, it might have been a hundred years since such a big storm or drought had come. And these were the people who had the knowledge in that area. No one else had it. You couldn't just get the information out of a book; you had to get it from one of the old ones. So that's where the respect came in.

— Nundjan Djiridjakin, senior male clan leader of the Australian Bibulmun Aboriginal tribe[14]

We have all experienced the benefits that wise elders provide. When you were young, surely there was a Mrs.

Macintyre in grade 3, or a Mr. Gregory in high school, or a Brother Guy who helped you through a troubling period, who gave you a steer in the right direction or gave you some self-esteem when the rest of the world was kicking you in the teeth. The classic hero myths that Joseph Campbell cited in his book *The Hero With a Thousand Faces* often include an elder who helped the hero in his quest. These are the fairy godmothers, gentle kings or powerful wizards who look out for us. We also find them in the modern hero movies such as *Star Wars*, in which wise elders Obi-Wan Kenobi and Yoda guide young Luke Skywalker. Likewise, Harry Potter's Professor Dumbledore and Sirius Black are two wise elders who guide the main character in his quest and growth.

These myths of the wise elder point in two directions: When we are young we *tune in* to the wise elder, but when we are older we *turn into]* the wise elder. There is a time to be a Luke Skywalker or Princess Leia, Harry Potter or Hermione Granger, to be Frodo leaving the Shire to do great deeds, but there is also a time to be Galadriel or Elrond. We can look at these stories as glorifying the bravery of youth and the need to do great deeds, but these stories also tell us how to be old, wise and useful.

There was good reason the founding fathers of the United States of America in 1789 assembled a second chamber of government called the Senate. This was the place where wise elders could assist and, if necessary, restrain the "fury of democracy," fury being a trait of youth.[15] James Madison (1751-1836), the fourth president, commented, "The use of the Senate is to consist in proceeding with more coolness, with more system, and with more wisdom, than the popular branch." That is a function of age. Aaron Burr (1756–1836), America's third vice president, said of the Senate, "This House is a sanctuary; a citadel of law, of order, and of liberty; and it is here–in this exalted refuge; here if anywhere, will resistance be made to the storms of political frenzy and the silent arts of corruption."

The U.S. Senate was inspired by the British House of Lords and the ancient Roman Senate, but there was another influence at work, as well: the Iroquois Confederacy. Historians are divided as to how much the Iroquois government was in the minds of the founding fathers when they drew up their own designs, but Benjamin Franklin did write, "It would be a very strange thing, if six Nations of ignorant savages should be capable of forming a Scheme for such a Union ... and yet that a like union should be impracticable for ten or a Dozen English Colonies."[16] The government of the Iroquois nations had an established senate as well, formed entirely of women! No Iroquois treaty was binding unless 75% of the men and 75% of the women elders ratified it. A chief could be demoted, even impeached, if the mothers of the tribe so decided; it was a process known as the "knocking off the horns." A chief's insignia of power was the antlers of a deer, and without these horns, he became just a private person again.[17] What is notable is not whether the Founding Fathers did or did not borrow from the Iroquois ideas about governance, the role of women in government, and the need for a sober second body of elders—what is interesting is the fact that they could have!

The point is that youth is not the only valuable or desirable time of life! We can drop the current myths that idolize youth and return to the myths of the wise elders. Getting older is neither a problem to be solved nor a mistake. It is a required part of life; our species survived because people lived into middle age. To quote David Bainbridge again, "Middle-aged people tend to be better at developing long-term plans, selecting relevant material from a mass of information, planning their time and coordinating the efforts of others—a constellation of skills that we might call wisdom."[18] Middle-aged elders may have slower cognitive abilities, but what is most useful at this stage in life is the ability to think differently, not quickly.

* * *

The infant becomes a student, the student an adult, the adult a parent, the parent a grandparent, and then follows a period of decay. The last stages of life await us: retirement and departure. Powers are lost; what was easy is no longer possible. We fumble. It is time to get out of the way. In the West, we do not choose to go to the forest as is suggested in India, but often a choice is made for us—we are sent to the "home," where we can spend our last few days with others like us. It is a lucky Westerner who dies in his own bed; for our last few days we are sent to a hospital to battle against the inevitable. If we are fortunate, we may be sent to a palliative care ward. We end as we began, unable to feed or dress ourselves, with no control over our bladders or bowels. We slip out. The slipping away is supposed to be helped by our myths, which for some no longer work, but for many still provide great solace and comfort. It is at this time that many come back to the myths they rejected in earlier life, the stories that were implanted in those earliest years of hypnotic suggestibility.

Immigrant families living in the West may have four generations living under one big roof, which seems very odd to Westerners, although very natural for Easterners. Easterners don't send the grandparents away; in the West we hire people to look after our parents when they get too old and become a burden to us. Or, if we can't afford to hire someone, we suck it up and do our best. All our friends commiserate with us and tell us how great we are to look after our own parents, as if it was something unique and unusual. Our current Western myths state quite clearly that individuals should fend for themselves as best they can and be independent right up to your last breath. What a tragedy it is to have to rely upon others when you are old and infirm.

There was an advertising campaign in Canada called Freedom 55 that offered investors an early chance to retire. The myth showed people, quite young and lively looking, enjoying the good life: travelling to exotic locales, golfing, dining and dancing. Life looked great, and the people weren't a burden to their children. That is the myth of freedom in the West: Freedom means you are able to do whatever you want. However, this is not the vision of freedom *from* wanting that is promoted in the myths of the East. Of course the reality for most who do retire is quite different, and it becomes evident that these current Western myths do not serve us well. They are illusions claiming that this is what life *should* be like, but is not. These myths serve only to alienate those who find that their golden years are not so golden, with the trips to doctors and hospitals, the fear of retirement pensions ending before they do, the feeling of burdening their now elderly children. These feelings belie the myths, and the result is a sense of failure. Our myths are no longer helping us transition through this last, great psychological stage.

Joseph Campbell recalled a time when the Barnum & Bailey Circus had a problem: Their feature attraction, the tent of freaks and human oddities, was too popular. People were coming into the tent but not leaving. Circus coordinators needed a way to get people out nicely, so no one was offended. They came up with the idea of posting an elaborate sign that read, "This Way to the Grand Egress." People were curious and wanted to see the Grand Egress, but before they knew it, they were outside the tent and couldn't get back in. [19]

This, according to Campbell, is the function of the myths of the last stage of life. We create a story about a happy hunting ground, or a loving sky-guy up there above the clouds, or some other pleasant metaphor of the land beyond this life.

Curious and relieved that there is some place to go to next, we leave this tent and we are out. For some, these old myths still work—and if yours work for you, then feel free to keep using them. For many, the old maps don't ring true and fail to show the way. The new cosmology denies the possibility of a heavenly abode "up there." A better story is required.

꿍 꿍

This was the night that Siddhartha Gautama was destined to go backward and become the Buddha. Remember that original Self of our first creation myth back in the first chapter? The one who first thought "I" and became afraid? The one who thought "I" and became lonely and wished for an other? The one who then, out of fear and desire, became many and lost awareness of itself in confusion? On this night Siddhartha Gautama would reverse those steps and make his way back to the state of oneness; he would go past confusion, desire, aversion, and past even ego, the false sense of "I."

He decided to sit beneath a grand tree—not just any tree, but the tree that seemed to him to be perfect for his meditation. Siddhartha chose the immovable spot upon which all the Buddhas before him had sat. The tree was the axis of the world, and everything revolved now around the Buddha-to-be. Only the tree and he were still, while the rest of the universe remained in motion.

A young girl approached Siddhartha. Long ago she received a prophecy that one day a great sage would come and sit beneath this tree. She had been preparing for this moment. Her father was a rich king with many cows. Every day the girl and her maids took the milk of a thousand cows and fed it to a hundred cows. From the hundred cows she took milk and fed it to just ten cows. From these ten cows she took the milk and fed it to one chosen cow. Now from this one cow she took milk in a golden bowl and brought it to the Buddha-to-be.

Siddhartha smiled and accepted the gift; he drank the milk and returned the bowl to the princess.

"Oh no," said the princess, "I cannot take back what I have given. The bowl is yours."

Siddhartha replied, "I have no need of a golden bowl. Tell you what: Let's toss the bowl into the stream beside us and see what happens. If the bowl floats, it will be a sign that upon this night, I will become enlightened."

Siddhartha tossed the heavy bowl into the water, and to the girl's amazement, it did not sink! Not only that, as it floated, it went backward against the stream and toward the source. Counterintuitive and surprising was the action of the bowl, just as counterintuitive and surprising would be the revelations of the Buddha. He would often say that his teachings go against the stream, and the way to understanding is to enter the stream itself. The bowl was going backward, just as Siddhartha Gautama himself would go backward that night. This process became known as *pratiprasava*—an involution back toward the source.

Night was falling, so Siddhartha settled into his favorite posture. With legs crossed and spine straight, with head and chest erect, hands folded in his lap, he became perfectly still. He vowed that on this night he would either achieve awakening or die: It was all or nothing. He began by watching his breath, allowing it to simply come and go, until there was no breath, no breather, no watcher and nothing to watch. Subject and objects dissolved. What was left was neither nor both.

Watching from the heavens, the gods gathered. Like all living things, they were not enlightened; they were merely gods, and with growing excitement they waited for the sage to awaken. But not everyone wanted this. There was one who constantly moved against the world—the trickster, the adversary. The Hebrews call the one who opposes, Satan; the Greeks call the one who obstructs the path, Diablos; to the Buddhists the enemy of freedom is known as Mara, the killer. Mara was not going to stand by and let the world savior easily realize his true nature.

Mara turned into Kama, the god of pleasure, and sent his three lovely daughters against Siddhartha: Desire, Fulfillment and Regret. They were sensuous, beautiful women, who danced and teased Siddhartha, offering much if he would only stand up and come with them. But there was no one there; the Buddha-to-be paid them not the slightest notice, for he had gone beyond desire and longing. He had gone backward passed the point where the original Self had felt yearning for another. In shame the daughters of Mara retreated.

Mara turned himself into Yama, the lord of death. With his huge army of ogres and demons, he approached the silent sage. "You! You are sitting in my spot. Leave now or I shall destroy you."

But there was no one there: Siddhartha felt no fear because there was no subject to be afraid. He had gone further backward past the point where the original Self thought "I" and felt fear. Yama launched his army, and their weapons flew toward the Still One, but as they came closer, the arrows and knives turned into flowers that fell softly at Siddhartha's feet. Yama's great elephant bowed down to the Buddha-to-be, and the army retreated.

Mara finally played his last card: he became Dharma, the god of duty and virtue. Approaching Siddhartha he admonished him, "Why are you sitting here neglecting your family? Don't you know that your father the king needs you? You are born a prince, a Kshatriya—born to rule! Why do you ignore your responsibilities? Your young son is seven years old—where is his father? Son and mother are both cruelly abandoned: How can you sit here? Go back to your home and do what you were born to do!"

In reply the Buddha-to-be simply touched the earth with his right hand, and in his defense the Earth herself spoke. "Leave him alone! Through countless lifetimes, he has given of himself to the world, and now at last, the Buddha is about to awaken, to help all beings everywhere have the chance to be free."

Mara withdrew, but this was not the last time he would come to test and tempt the Enlightened One; do not think that enlightenment is the end of struggle. Mara's poisons of greed, hatred and confusion are subtle, and he will use them again and again, as long as life remains.

֍ ֍

Notice how in this story, the earth is far from cursed as we saw in the biblical creation myth; she is an important partner in the Buddha's enlightenment. She defends the Buddha from the curses of the dark side of life. Metaphorically, our own original, basic nature can rise and help us deal with our shadows when they threaten to knock us off life's path. All it took for the Buddha to call upon her was a simple, humble gesture: touching the earth. This was not an exalted expression of power or grandeur (those are manifestations of the ego, of the dark side within) –he reached down, not up. There is the key lesson for us: When assailed by doubts and temptations that would move us off the path we know we must follow, bow low and touch the earth.

Chapter 8: The Goals of Life

The Brihadaranyaka Upanishad, in which the story of creation by the original Self is found (given at the beginning of Chapter 1), was written probably around 800 B.C.E. The Buddha lived around 500 B.C.E., and his teachings took the philosophy of the early Upanishads further. In the myth about the night of enlightenment, we saw how the Buddha went against the stream of the Upanishadic teachings to the place where there was no one to be affected by the poisons of life. The myth also beautifully illustrates what became known in India as the purusharthas: the four aims of life. Ramakrishna often called these the four fruits:[1]

1. Dharma: the virtue of fulfilling your duty and obligations in life

2. Kama: desire, the seeking of pleasure and the avoidance of pain

3. Artha: competitiveness, the struggle for achievement

4. Moksha: liberation from all the above.

On the night of his illumination, the Buddha dropped the first three goals, resisted their temptations, and arrived at the fourth goal, moksha. The first goal, dharma, was his last temptation. We know all about dharma—we have seen how even Indra must follow his dharma and rule the universe. We have seen how a lowly prostitute must follow her dharma and serve the money that comes to her. Dharma is the way of the universe, and by following one's own dharma, virtue is gained. At least that is the view in orthodox Hinduism; the Buddha disagreed, as do all who leave the world to seek freedom. But just running away from home and responsibilities is not enough. There are other aims of life that must be transcended, as well.

KAMA

Kama means pleasure and love. The goal of kama is the obtaining of physical desires: the promise of the god Kama's three lustful daughters, who tempted the Buddha on the night of his enlightenment. One of the most well-known, perhaps infamous, texts of India is the *Kamasutra*, the book of sexual pleasure. It is easy to think of the *Kamasutra* as simply an early version of the *Joy of Sex*, but it is more, offering a complete description of how to live with your spouse graciously. Recall that it was Indra's Brahmin guru, Brihaspati, who promised to write this text, which allowed Indra to follow a virtuous path while staying with his wife, Indrani.

Love and sex are so easily confused and misunderstood. In the West two myths of Eros have come down to us from ancient Greece. In the first, Eros is one of the original powers of the universe. Hesiod in his *Theogony* described how out of the void of Chaos came Gaia (Mother Earth), Tartarus (the space under the Earth, which becomes the underworld in due course) and Eros (sexual desire). Hesiod places sex here among the first gods of the universe, because without the desire to procreate, how can anything be created? It was in later myths that Eros was demoted to be the son of Aphrodite, herself the goddess of sensuality and desire. Aphrodite is the female embodiment of kama; so powerful is she that all the other gods are subject to her games, even Zeus.[2] Her son in the Roman versions of these myths becomes the god of love, Cupid, who in modern times is simply a cartoonish figure with his little bow and arrows. His power, however, is real and needs respecting. Even the original Self of our opening story felt this urge to merge, and from this union came everything. Like the Greek gods, the Indian gods are also not immune to the power of lust, as we will see in this story:

❧ ❧

Parvati could not get Shiva to pay even the slightest attention to her. He was in one of his moods again. Long ago, in another lifetime, Parvati had been married to Shiva, but in despair caused by her father's disrespectful behavior toward her great husband, she cast herself into the sacrificial fire, hoping to be reborn of proper parents. She chose her new parents well: Her new father was Himavat, the great mountain range. But now that she was back, Shiva was locked into a deep meditation, oblivious to the world.

Indra also wanted Shiva to stir, because a demon named Taraka was making life rather difficult. Brahma had made one of his rash promises; he granted Taraka immortality in reward for his yoga practice. Taraka used his invulnerability to conquer and wrest tribute from the gods. Ah, but Brahma tricked him: There was one who could kill Taraka—a son of Shiva. The problem was, Shiva had lost his wife and was completely celibate and removed from the world. Indra thought that Parvati was the answer.

To assist Parvati, Indra asked Kama to go with her to the cave where Shiva meditated. Kama, the god of desire, lust and love, and the wish fulfillment that was carnal gratification, brought his bow and quiver of five arrows. Kama was also called Puspabana because his arrows were flowers. He bore a noose to snare and bind his victims and a hook to drag them closer. Not easily do people submit to the power of love.

There was no other choice: Parvati had tried the ascetic lifestyle that Shiva perfected, but her yoga did not stir him. Kama fitted one of his arrows to his bow and shot Shiva in the heart. This, Shiva did not appreciate; he opened his third eye, and a brilliant flash of light consumed Kama. The world had lost lust and love—but Shiva's next vision was of Parvati. Kama's arrow worked its magic and Shiva fell.

Parvati cried in anguish when she saw Kama destroyed. The other gods watching were also shocked. How could life continue if there was no power to love in the world? Men would no longer embrace women, and there would be no sons to carry on the traditions of sacrifice. The only good news was that Shiva was awake and in love. Parvati beseeched her lover to bring Kama back. Shiva, happy to see his beloved again, agreed, but it was not possible to bring back Kama's physical form. From then on, only the spirit of Kama has existed. His presence can be felt but not seen, which makes his power even more surprising when it manifests.

⅋ ⅋

The *Kamasutra* was not created out of hedonism. Life was highly proscribed in the conservative society of India. A wife was given, not chosen. The heart was not involved. The arts of lovemaking, of enjoying married life, of relating to a wife or to a husband did not come naturally in such a restrained culture. Instruction was needed. Kama was an aim of life, a goal to work toward, and if done well, it was quite pleasurable.

The Eastern idea of kama deserves some consideration, as it contrasts to the way pleasure is dealt with in the West. The sages of India knew that life was hard, the requirements of society very strict, and without some good times, there would be no reason to live. Pleasure in the West can conflict us: On the one hand, it feels nice to make love, to have a beer on a hot day, to enjoy the pleasures that life has to offer; but on the other hand, pleasure is seen as sinful and undeserved. Eve ate the apple, enjoyed it, shared it, and suffered because of it. Pleasure should be deferred to the life hereafter: "Seek your reward in heaven not on earth." Pleasure is either too much, hedonistic and an escape from life, or it is sinful and a path blazed to hell. The Indian view is much more balanced. Pleasure is rightfully an aim of life. Lust is to be avoided, but pleasure is not; lust is the attachment to pleasure, so drop the attachment, but keep the pleasure. Enjoy life: The gods know it is hard enough; you don't need to make it worse by denying what few pleasures there are.

This is an interesting point to consider: The question is, which map do you follow in your life? Is pleasure a guilt-ridden sin or a source of comfort? How do you feel right after you do something pleasurable? Were you "cheating" or did you "deserve it?" Or was it just nice and nothing more or less than that?

✳ ✳ ✳

ARTHA

Artha means "thing or object": stuff to be acquired in order to live well. This spans a range of material goods that can be possessed, enjoyed, won or lost. Things are needed in order to raise a family and meet the responsibilities of being a husband and father, the head of a family, and the supporter of the priests. The goals of artha are the achievement of riches and worldly possessions, of profit and career, of climbing the ladder and keeping up with the Joneses.

Kama and artha are animal instincts that appear early in human life. Kama is simply the desire for things we like and the aversion toward things we don't like. Artha is the competitive urge: what others have, we want. Little Johnny is playing happily in his preschool class until he sees Julian picking up a toy truck. Johnny immediately wants that toy and takes it away from Julian, pushing him down in the struggle. Watch crows fighting over a scrap of bread and you will see artha. This is described as *matsya-nyaya*, the Law of the Jungle, or more literally, the Law of the Fishes: big fish eat little fish. That's life! (And if you are a little fish, you better be a fast little fish!)

Given that that is the way life is, what are you going to do about it? You are going to go out and try to eat as many little fish as you can. *Artha* has informed the politics of India since the earliest days. Do you remember in the story of "The Humbling of India," when Brihaspati reminded Indra of an earlier book he had written for Indra? Artha was the topic. The *Brihaspati Sutra*[3] was the artha equivalent of the *Kamasutra*. The closest Western book on the philosophy of power might be Machiavelli's *The Prince* published in 1532.

Jesus once observed that it is harder for a rich man to enter heaven than for a camel to pass through the eye of a needle.[4] Not very encouraging! In the East, however, artha is a fundamental part of life: we need to achieve to thrive; so how do we square Jesus' warning with the struggle to survive? There are two legendary rich men who may provide us with maps to having both riches and peace. The first of these is Joseph of Arimathea:

⊰ ⊱

Joseph of Arimathea was a wealthy man and an important man. He was a member of the Sanhedrin, a powerful Jewish council to whom questions of law that could not be decided by lower courts were put. While the devout Joseph waited for the coming of the kingdom of heaven, he came across Jesus of Nazareth and found it no longer necessary to wait. He became a secret disciple.

When Jesus died upon the cross, Joseph took a great risk: He approached Pontius Pilate, the Roman governor of Judea, and begged him to release Jesus' body. Pilate, upon being assured by his guards that Jesus was indeed dead (one guard punctured Jesus' side with a sword to check whether Jesus was still alive or not), agreed that Joseph could have Jesus' body to properly bury him. This was the custom: Any family member could take the body of an executed man and offer it a proper burial; Joseph, however, was not a relative of Jesus, so he took a big chance in asking for the body.

Joseph, as a rich man does, had built a beautiful tomb for the day of his own inevitable demise; this tomb he gave to Jesus. He anointed Jesus and clothed him in fine linen. He entombed the body of Christ and had a boulder rolled across the opening of the tomb, sealing it in. He had given his place to Jesus and was accosted by the high priests for this act. They imprisoned Joseph, but in the morning when the priests went to question him, they found the prison cell empty, the locks still in place. Joseph later explained that Jesus had come and taken him safely home, and he had slept that night in his own bed.

Joseph of Arimathea was no longer welcomed by his peers, so he left Jerusalem and Judea; he left behind his wealth and went to the West. He went as far to the West as he could: He settled in Briton. Hundreds of years before Rome became a Christian empire, Joseph taught the teaching of Jesus to the Britons. He brought one other important item to the British Isles: a wooden cup—the Holy Grail that Joseph had used to catch the blood of Jesus after He had been stabbed in the side by the soldier's spear.

ॐ ॐ

There are many versions of the myth of the Grail. In some stories Jesus gave the cup to Joseph when Jesus rescued him from the prison cell of the high priests. In other stories the Grail was the cup that held the wine Jesus drank on the night of his last supper. By the 12th and 13th centuries, with the Cistercian monks' retelling of the myth, the Grail had become a chalice of life similar to a cauldron found in early Celtic tales that was endowed with great powers. Again the Grail is calling to us, and again we must defer this particular adventure for a little while.

The story of Arimathea is a legend, which is a different kind of story—not quite a myth, but still able to move us. A myth classically deals with gods and demi-gods, and Joseph was a real man (at least according to the Bible). Legends deal with flesh-and-blood men and women. While mythologists may argue over the differences between myths and legends, for our purposes we do not need to put such a fine point on it: They are all stories. The thing with legends is that they grow over the years. Did Joseph really come to Britain? Did he really bring the cup of Christ with him? We will never know the historicity of these tales, but again the power of the tale is not in its truth, but in its effect on people. The legend of Joseph of Arimathea shows that a rich, powerful man can do good in the world and can gain the love of God.

There is an Eastern counterpart to Joseph of Arimathea, one who predates him by over 400 years: Anathapindika.

꒔ ꒦

"Thus have I heard: One time the Blessed One was staying at Savatthi in the Jeta Grove, in Anathapindika's Monastery..." So start many of the stories about the Buddha. Anathapindika's real name was Sudatta, but he gained his nickname because of his generosity. *Pinda* are alms, and *anatha* referred to the unprotected—thus Sudatta was called the great benefactor, Anathapindika.

Anathapindika was a banker. Banking was not considered the most honorable of professions even 2,500 years ago, but Anathapindika knew the proper use of money. He constantly helped the downtrodden and poor; one needed only to ask for assistance and it was provided.

One day while visiting his sister, who was married to another rich banker, he found his brother-in-law busy preparing a great feast. Anathapindika asked, "Who is getting married?"

"No one," came the reply.

"Well then, is the king coming to dinner?"

"No."

"So for whom is this great feast being prepared?"

"The Enlightened One!" was the unexpected reply.

A real, live Buddha was living nearby, and Anathapindika didn't even know it. He grew tremendously excited and drew all the information about this Buddha out of his brother-in-law. Anathapindika was so excited that he couldn't sleep, so well before the sun rose, he was out of bed and walking toward where the Buddha was staying. He didn't know the way, but a kindly spirit guided him right to the Holy One. The Buddha had begun his mission of teaching just one year earlier, so it is understandable that Anathapindika had not yet heard of him. He made up for lost time: He listened intently to the discourses the Buddha offered on the nature of life and the causes of suffering.

With great humility Anathapindika approached the Buddha and asked if he could prepare a place near his own home in Savatthi where the Buddha and his monks could spend the rainy season. The Buddha agreed but cautioned, "Enlightened ones do love their solitude." Anathapindika understood the Buddha's words and agreed to find the perfect site for the retreat; in fact, he already knew the perfect place.

There was one small problem, however. The perfect park was owned by Prince Jeta, the son of King Pasenadi. Anathapindika approached the prince, but he was unwilling to sell the forest. Anathapindika persisted, and with each new approach, he increased the offer till finally, in jest, Prince Jeta said, "If you were to cover the whole forest floor with gold, then perhaps I would sell it to you."

Anathapindika quickly said, "Agreed!"

He went to the park with wheelbarrows full of gold foil and started to cover the ground. It took 18 million pieces of gold to cover the floor of the forest, but even then there was one small plot still bare. Prince Jeta said, "That's enough. Let me gift this area to the Buddha myself, and I will erect a wonderful gate here to protect the monastery and keep it quiet."

On top of these 18 million gold pieces, Anathapindika spent another 18 million pieces building huts and furnishings. He spent a further third fortune funding the upkeep of the monastery. Jeta Grove became the favorite retreat of the Buddha and his *sangha*; he spent many rainy seasons in seclusion within this marvelous park.

Anathapindika was aptly named—he could refuse no one, but such largess has a cost. He suffered severe financial losses when he loaned a fortune to investors who never repaid him; he lost another fortune in a ruinous flood; he had already invested three fortunes buying, building, and supporting the hundreds of monks who lived in the Jeta Grove monastery. Anathapindika was broke, but still he continued to give what little he had: He shared his morning gruel with whoever asked for it.

A house spirit grew upset with Anathapindika and his inability to say "no." The spirit complained to Anathapindika, but the banker would have none of it, and he banished the spirit from the home. The spirit wandered around the city; finding no new home, he eventually appealed to the king of spirits for help. All he got was advice: "Go get the debtors to repay Anathapindika, and go find the treasure that was washed away by the flood, and you will be forgiven." The spirit did all he was directed to do and restored Anathapindika's wealth.

One day the Buddha was visiting a village in which lived a miserable old miser. The people of the village approached the Buddha, asking what they could do about this very rich man who helped no one. The Buddha did not reply but went to visit the miser, and he asked the scrooge,

"What would you call a man whose hands were always clenched into a tight fist, never able to open?"

"A cripple," replied the miser.

"And what would you call a man whose hand was always open, never able to hold on to anything?"

"Deformed" was the reply.

"Just so," continued the Buddha, "and one who knows this knows how to live life properly, neither giving too much nor clinging too tightly to what they have."

The man was old, but he was smart enough to understand the Buddha's teaching; he became a model citizen and much beloved by the villages for his kind support of the poor. The Buddha later told Anathapindika, "There are few rich men who know how to balance the pleasures of life profitably and responsibly."

While Anathapindika lay dying at the end of his long life, he asked for Sariputta to visit him. Anathapindika was too humble to ask for the Buddha, but Sariputta was the most venerable monk, second only to the Buddha in understanding and clarity. He counseled Anathapindika through his final hours of life. As death approached, Anathapindika dropped all his attachments; like a monk, he no longer cared about profession or possessions. He was leaving it all behind. In this state of complete openness, he understood the teachings that Sariputta offered, and with his final breaths, Anathapindika entered the stream. This was the same stream the Buddha travelled backward along on that night beneath the tree of illumination. Anathapindika became an arhant, a worthy one who defeated the foes of greed, hatred and confusion and was reborn in Tushita heaven, the abode of the bodhisattvas.

৯ ৶

MOKSHA

Moksha is explained by Georg Feuerstein as liberation, not from a place, but within the mind, or rather *from* the mind: "Liberation is said to be the dissolution of the mind upon the obliteration of all aspirations."[5] Heinrich Zimmer offers a more extensive definition that captures moksha's vagueness: "... from the root *muc*, 'to loose, set free, let go, release, liberate, deliver; to leave, abandon, quit,' (all of which) means 'liberation, escape, freedom, release; rescue, deliverance; final emancipation of the soul.'"[6]

While Joseph Campbell travelled through India in 1954, he asked a question that puzzled him. What is moksha? Is it release from ignorance or release from the world? If it is release from ignorance, then release from the world may be misguided and unnecessary. He had the chance to ask Ananda Mayi, a great Indian saint. Her reply was that when one was enlightened, the question no longer mattered. Campbell could only bow to her in response.[7] Despite the saintly answer, his question is still a good one: "Should I stay or should I go? Sure, after I achieve moksha the answer is obvious, but before then ...?"

We find a mystery surrounding this fourth aim of life. The first three aims are evident and found in everyday activities—the attempt to fulfill desires, avoid pain, achieve goals while still trying to fit within the social rules. But few are those who go to the forest. If the myths tell us what to do, why is it that so few do go to the forest? Is it misguided to go there, as Joseph Campbell wondered? And of those who do go, Ramakrishna warns, many just fake it. There are three kinds of renunciation, according to Ramakrishna: feeble, intense and "monkey renunciation." Feeble is slow—this is not the real way to be free; intense is like a sharp razor, and one quickly cuts through all delusion. This is the way Ramakrishna recommended. But there is another quality of renunciation, he warns, called "monkey renunciation," which is just a temporary fleeing of troubles in life, and then a return when you feel better.[8] That is not real liberation; that is just taking a vacation.

Renunciation, Ramakrishna advises, is giving up of gold and women, which is to say, going beyond artha and kama. But, as with Indra, it is not for everyone. For those followers who just can't bring themselves to leave the world, Ramakrishna offered this parable.[9]

ॐ ঃ

A disciple was wondering whether the world was real or not, and if not, what happens to all of us who are living in this world. The master, reading the disciple's state of mind, answered:

"Suppose there was an office clerk merrily going about his daily life who was suddenly arrested. He is thrown in jail. While in jail he lives the life of a prisoner but when released from jail, what does he do? He goes back to his life as a clerk and does what he always did. The knowledge of freedom he now has does not change his actions in this world. He simply lives in this world as a free man."

ॐ ঃ

Recall that it was Freud who remarked, "Myths are public dreams, and dreams are private myths." Carl Jung learned that we can look at a dream in two ways: We can ask *why* we had this particular dream, the cause; or we can ask *what is the purpose* of the dream, the reason.[10] The question of why is aetiological: Dreams have a cause, and what is that cause? Myths, too, are aetiological; they can be seen to explain why certain things are the way they are in society or in life. The purpose of a dream or a myth is a deeper, more mysterious question. What is the reason this dream has surfaced? What is it trying to correct, balance, direct or make happen? Myths can also have a similar purpose. While everyone may be aware that they *should* go to the forest to free themselves from the first three aims of life, the urge to retreat to the forest is coming from the deep psyche and is its attempt to establish balance.

Jung explains that dreams do not tell us what we are doing is right. This is an important point—our conscious mind always assumes it is making good, rational, right choices. The dream arises from the hidden landscape, and, if life is unbalanced, the purpose of dream is to bring balance to the conscious view of life.[11] A dream may be arising to help us achieve wholeness, to change the way we are living. The imbalance of seeking the first three aims of life is offset by the fourth. The number four represents wholeness—the four corners of the world encompass the whole world.

Jung fabulously said, "To round itself out, life calls not for perfection but for completeness."[12] Think of what this means for you: You are not here to be perfect; you are here to be whole! What a liberating realization.

✳ ✳ ✳

ॐ ॐ

The Buddha walked mindfully around the beautiful park. His morning alms had been eaten, his bowl washed, and he was free to just soak in the beauty of this moment. Part of this beauty appeared before him in the form of a very agitated man, who in anger began to verbally attack the Buddha.

The incensed man was a farmer. It was the time of the harvest, but his son had just run away. Where did the young man go? To the Buddha! He had heard the Buddha give a talk, and as a result, he up and quit the world; he joined the sangha, shaved his head, donned a worn-out old robe, and left his family in the lurch. How could the Buddha allow sons to leave their fathers? How could he encourage them to shirk their duties? Without his son, the father and the rest of the family were suffering greatly. The Buddha should be ashamed for what he was doing:

corrupting the youth and changing the way society had always been.

The Buddha stood calmly still and listened deeply to every word the farmer threw at him. After many minutes of abuse, when the farmer finally ran out of steam, the Buddha asked, "May I speak?"

"Of course," replied the farmer, "I would love to hear what you have to say for yourself!"

The Buddha began with a riddle. "Imagine a man gave a gift to a friend, but the friend did not accept it. To whom does the gift now belong?"

The farmer answered quickly, "The gift remains with the giver."

"Just so," said the Buddha, "and this gift of anger that you have brought me, I am sorry, I cannot accept it. It remains yours."

ॐ ᳍

Society would not function properly if everyone shook off the dust of the household and sought the open road as the Buddha (and Jack Kerouac) suggested. This renouncing of the world can only work for society if it occurs at a time when the man was no longer contributing much or at least had found a replacement who would continue the work in his stead. Hindu society allowed for renunciation at the appropriate time of life, but the Buddhists and many other yogis were leaving too soon. This could not be tolerated. This was a conflict that persisted for many centuries: When was the right time to leave the world? The answer depended upon the philosophy, the map that one followed. The sage Shankara said that a Brahmin is very lucky, for only a Brahmin male can achieve moksha.[13] By this, Shankara allows only Brahmins to go to the forest; everyone else stays in the world. Their chance will come in some other lifetime.

Chapter 9: The Soul Question

Moksha means "liberation." There is a question that begs to be asked about enlightened, liberated or awakened masters: What is it they are enlightened *about*, liberated *from* or awake *to*? And while we ponder that mystery, just *who* is it that wakes up, is enlightened, or is liberated? Maybe it is more appropriate to ask *what* is liberated, awakened or enlightened. What is this thing that I call "I"? Not surprisingly, there are many answers to the question "who am I?" and many maps. This is the great soul question.

* * *

In the early 1300s, Dante Alighieri (1265-1321) wrote a comedy; that is to say, he wrote an uncommon story in the common Italian language, a story with a happy ending. This was in contrast to a tragedy: Tragedies were written in Latin and were high stories with a tragic ending. Dante called his epic poem simply the *Comedy*, to which later readers appended the adjective "divine." Thus we have today Dante's *Divine Comedy*, an allegory and a presentation of several myths of his time.

An allegory is a story where words are used but other meanings are intended. Myths can be seen as allegories, but there is much scholarly debate over the exact nature of allegories.[1] Since we are speaking of Dante's allegories, let's allow him to define the term for us, which he does in an earlier work, the *Convivio*.

The first [sense of a story] is called the literal, and this is the sense that does not go beyond the surface of the letter, as in the fables of the poets. The next is called the allegorical, and this is the one that is hidden beneath the cloak of these fables, and it is

a truth hidden beneath a beautiful [lie] ... Indeed the theologians
take this sense otherwise than do the poets; but since it is my
intention here to follow the method of the poets, I shall take the
allegorical sense according to the usage of the poets."[2]

Works of literature are stories, and, while mythologists
may caution against reading literature as myth, the stories
still work on us. Stories that attract us resonate with the
symbols of our deep unconscious landscape. We enjoy them
for the same reasons that myths speak to us: They reflect
ourselves back to ourselves. Or as B. P. Reardon observed,
"Stories can seep through the cracks in our consciousness."[3]
So, in other words, Dante's poem, or any allegorical work, is
not literally true. But that is exactly our whole point about
myths – they are not true, but they work and have deep value.
Dante advises us to read his story "as if" it were true and let
the other meanings soak in.

There is a point to be made from the *Divine Comedy* about
the way Westerners look at the "self" (as opposed to and
distinct from the "Self"). To see this point, we will indulge
ourselves in a small sampling of the first portion of Dante's
journey, with a brief summary of his trip to hell and beyond,
which begins on the evening of Good Friday:

ৰ্ঙ ৡ

The woods were dark and the way hidden. Dante tried
to climb up toward a mountain to see better the direction
he should follow. Three times he tried to ascend, but three
times he was blocked by the wildness of animals. A leopard
first scared him off the path, then a fearsome lion; then a
skin-and-bones hungry she-wolf denied him passage. This
was not his way. Filled with sleepiness Dante backed off,
disconsolate. As he descended deeper into darkness, a
shade appeared before him and asked, "Why are you
coming this way? There is nothing but misery below."

Dante explained that his way was blocked, though he
would like nothing more than to mount the heights and

see the light. The shade understood and offered the only wisdom available: "If you can't go up, then you must go down—down, through and then out. I shall guide you."

Dante appreciated the gesture but wanted to know who his benefactor might be. He was told, "I was a poet of old and sang songs of Troy and the founding of Rome before the Emperor whose seat is on high was made known to me."

Dante recognized the soul of his favorite poet, Virgil, who lived just before the coming of the Son of God. Dante was happy to throw himself on Virgil's mercy. "Tell me, please—how did it come to pass that you are here just in time to help me find my way again?"

Virgil explained, "Three ladies, most blessed, are concerned about you. It was through the grace of the Holy Mother, who saw your plight and dispatched Saint Lucy. Lucy ran to another, whom you knew in life and who is greatly esteemed in the highest reaches. Out of compassion for you did fair Beatrice come down and implore me to find you and help you in your waywardness. Though I felt unworthy to be in her presence, I hastened to do her bidding."

Beatrice! Dante had first fallen in love with her when he was but a boy and she a girl one year younger. His heart had burned for her glance and smile; her occasional rebuke was the greatest pain. She married another, but that was no matter; his love was not carnal. When she died, still so young, a huge hole in Dante's heart was ripped open—a hole so big, not all his poetry could fill it, and neither could marriage and subsequent children. Beatrice was looking out for him from on high, but to find her again, he must descend lower.

Virgil led Dante to hell, and through hell to the mountain of Purgatory, which is found on the opposite side of the world from Jerusalem, at the very tip of the Antipodes. It was after passing through hell and Purgation that Virgil would have to give way to Beatrice, for Virgil was not blessed: He had lived in a time that knew not the truth, and clung to lies and false gods, though through no fault of his own. Like many whom Dante would soon see in the first circle of hell, which was the circle of Limbo, Virgil was a good soul and suffered only from the lack of the Beatific Vision. He did not know God and had never in his life heard of Jesus. Still, he saw briefly in Beatrice, just as Dante had, what the Blessed One was like, and that was enough to move him.

To Limbo, then! Across the dark waters of the river Acheron, Virgil guided Dante to the place of good men and good women, whose only lack was being born too soon or born too far away to have heard the gospels. In this first of nine great circles of hell, they suffered no ills beyond a great longing to see the face of Glory. Dante was surprised to recognize so many famous and wonderful people: There he saw Homer, the greatest poet before Virgil; he saw Horace, Ovid and Lucian—great writers and poets. He saw Electra, who gave birth to the race of Romans, and Hector and Aeneas and other great heroes of antiquity who helped create the city that would become the seat for God's representative on earth—Rome. Dante saw Plato, Socrates, Diogenes and the great Aristotle—the philosophers of the Classical Era; he saw much and many, too much for this short tale to recount.

Dante followed his psychopomp through the rings of hell and past realms where punishment was exquisitely crafted to fit the personalities of the damned. There was a circle for the lustful, the illicit lovers whose sins were of the body not of the heart. There were hells for the gluttons, the hoarders, spendthrifts and all those who were anally retentive in life. For those who could not control their temper, the wrathful hell circle was far worse, and yet there was still worse deeper in. Frauds, panderers, blasphemers and their ilk found punishment suited to their crimes. Fire burned the feet of those who sold holy sacraments, positions in the church, and dispensations; fortune tellers and sorcerers had their heads twisted halfway around so that they had to walk backward to see where they were going; corrupt politicians and power brokers were being boiled in pitch.

Throughout his journey, Dante kept meeting people he knew in life: Friends, teachers and so many enemies—he could name them all to Virgil—all ended up here where their actions brought them. While Dante could not bring himself to console them, out of compassion he chatted to them about what had been happening back home. He realized that it was by choice and not chance that everyone ends up in exactly the place they deserve; it is hardly a judgment—we all sink or float to exactly the place where our soul finds its buoyancy.

Past the titanic giants who fought against Zeus, half buried and bound by iron and by their pride, past a lake of ice that contained the souls of traitors, to the very center of the earth, they stole past Satan himself who, despite having three faces, did not notice the two poets. Completely passive was Satan, locked as he was in the lake of ice, save for the tears he cried and his mindless chewing on the bodies of three sinners: the greatest of all the traitors, Judas of Iscariot; and Brutus and Cassias, the murderers of Julius Caesar. The two poets clambered down Satan's body and passed through the center of earth.

Now at last Dante could start his ascent; he had reached and passed through the icy core of the world and up was the only direction left. Virgil guided Dante until the vault of heaven opened above and strange, new stars could be seen. He stood now upon the opposite side of the earth itself, and before him was the great island mountain of Purgatory from which four great rivers flow, forming the oceans of the world.

❦

There are many symbols we could analyze and many maps we could draw from the travels of Dante in his fantastic voyage. Taking a Jungian perspective, we can look at the frequent use of the number three: the three wild animals that initially block Dante's ascent to God; the three women who send Virgil to rescue him; the three faces of Satan and the three traitors who exist at the core of being; and of course the most famous trio of all, the Holy Trinity of God the Father, the Son and the Holy Spirit. Threesomes are not complete, they are not whole—a fourth is required. There are not three corners of the world; there are four. The cross of Christ has four arms, not three. Even the Holy Trinity of the Catholic Church has been deemed incomplete by some thinkers, being composed only of three male images. The trinity lacks the feminine, which is why eventually the Church deigned to allow worship of Mary, the Holy Mother.[4] Dante's search for redemption is a search for his missing wholeness.

All the symbols are representation of Dante's own psyche: his own wildness within symbolized by the wild animals; the love and compassion within represented by his anima figures of Beatrice, Lucy and the Virgin Mother; the three aspects of Satan and the three aspect of God. These are all part of Dante, and these parts struggle together within. It is by following his wise elder, his *senex*, as Jung would term the old poet Virgil, that Dante is led through his inner darkness and back to the surface. But it is Beatrice, his beloved anima figure, who will escort him higher to the bliss of the divine. However, in the last of the three segments of the *Divine Comedy*, the vision of paradise, which we have not related here, Beatrice gives way to a man, the mystic Saint Bernard, who brings Dante to the final vision of the three circles of light, which is God the Father, the Son and the Holy Spirit, all inter-reflecting. Dante ended his story with this vision of the Three.

Symbolically the dark woods Dante is initially lost within is the deep, hidden psyche. The animals are the dark terrors that prevent ego from taking the easy way out; he has to go through this experience. Virgil was a historical person, taking on the godlike role of the psychopomp, a Hermes or Thoth, who guides the souls in the afterlife. Dante was a devout Roman Catholic, who couldn't have a god serve him (there is only one God!), so his guide is a man, albeit a man of power: a Roman, notice, not a Greek.

It would be very interesting to continue to pour over this map in greater detail, but this is not why we viewed Dante's poem. We could examine the chaste love he felt for Beatrice, but that will wait for our exploration of the myths of love. The main point for us of this story is the fact that Dante *recognized* many of the people he saw in hell. Dante recognized people in Purgatory and in Heaven, too. Dante borrowed deliberately from ancient Greek myths, and there we find that the heroes who visited Tartaros, the underworld realm ruled by Hades, recognized the shades found there. Hercules, as just one example, went to hell to bring back the hellhound Cerberus; it was the last of his 12 heroic labors. While there, he chatted with old friends and freed one of them. This idea of recognizing people in the underworld goes back even further than the Greek myths. About 1,000 years earlier, a Sumerian myth tells how the hero Gilgamesh summoned from hell his best friend Enkidu. Enkidu described the condition of those in the netherworld, including the plight of Gilgamesh's parents, who were condemned to drink muddy water.

In our Western philosophy, the view is that each of us has a unique psyche. Remember that *psyche* is the Greek word for "soul". The common view in the West is that we are bodies that have souls, and when we leave the body behind, the soul remains. The soul retains the ability to reason and remember.

Our personality remains intact: We know who we are, who we were, and others can also recognize us. While we are born blank and equal, we die unique and individual. This is not the view in the East! What is meant by "soul" is very different there. They have different ways to answer the fundamental question of "Who am I?" as we shall see in this little vignette.

⊰ ⊱

You are walking down the street. What a glorious day! Wouldn't it be nice to take a ride along the ocean and up into the mountains? If only you had a car. You've been meaning to buy a car. Looking at the cars driving by stokes your desire to acquire a set of wheels. Ah, but look! A "For Sale" sign in the window of a parked car!

You approach the car. It looks nice: great color, newer model, good lines. Peering in the window, you see the bucket seats you always wanted, and you also see that the keys have been left in the ignition. Perhaps a little test drive is being offered? The door is unlocked, and you get in.

The smell is wonderful: rich Corinthian leather. The dashboard is space-aged modern and even has wireless for your cell phone. You connect your phone and turn on the car. Now things start to happen: The sound of music surrounds you. The engine purrs. You put the car in gear and start to drive.

It doesn't take long before you can feel the car on the road. You know exactly where the tires are; you can parallel park without using the Braille method. Your senses have expanded, and you feel everything the car feels … you have become the car.

At a stoplight, you look out the window and see some teens on skateboards practicing moves. One of them loses control of her board, and it flies toward the car. It hits the front fender, creating a big scratch! You roll down the window and scream at the girl. Frightened, she picks up her board and runs away. Fuming with anger at being hit and scratched, you drive away muttering curses.

In a little while, you have calmed down. You are on the sea-to-sky highway and enjoy the view of the ocean to your left and the sight of towering snow-capped mountains to your right. Life is good again. You keep driving.

⊰ ⊱

This little vignette[5] symbolizes an ancient Indian view of our true nature, a view perhaps originally espoused in the Samkhya and Jain traditions. Hundreds of years before the Buddha, Indian philosophers began rejecting the traditional Vedic view of religion. In the new philosophy, what mattered most was not the powers that were "out there" all around us, personified as gods, but what was here inside of us. The revolutionary Upanishads were exploring the idea that it was the spark within each of us that mattered. Many scholars call this spark the *reincarnating monad*.

Heinrich Zimmer explains, "... in our Occidental concept of the 'soul' we have mixed up, on the one hand, elements that belong to the mutable sphere of the psyche (thoughts, emotions and similar elements of ego-consciousness), and on the other hand, what is beyond, behind or above all these: the indestructible ground of our existence, which is the anonymous Self ... far aloof from the trials and history of the personality."[6]

While one branch of reasoning leads to the idea that our monads are all part of the original universal divinity, there are other views that what is within is unique and separate from everything else in the cosmos. To use our modern metaphor, we are the *drivers* of the physical vehicles, we are not the vehicles, and we are separate and unique from all the other drivers on the road and their cars.

Our original Indian creation myth that explained how we are all part of the original divine Self is a nondualistic myth. Eastern philosophies love this idea that we are all one; however, there are competing, *dualistic* views that show we are not all one ,we are not part of nature, and each of us are single beings of pure consciousness, called *purushas*. This was the philosophy underpinning Samkhya and Jainism, and we will examine these two views in detail, right after reviewing what is meant by *purusha*.

Remember the cosmic purusha, the original man we have seen before? He is the original Self from which we all came: From his head came the Brahmins, from his arms the kings and warriors, from his legs the middle class and from his feet the servants. The term *purusha* literally means "male", referring to a man, and it is used in a variety of contexts, which leads to some confusion. In some schools there is only one cosmic purusha; he is also known as Brahman, or Ishvara, or paramatman, or the Prajapati, or by many other names. Distinct from this nondualistic philosophy, in Jainism and in Samkhya it is taught that there exist an infinite number of individual purushas, each omniscient, eternal and totally unique.[7]

※ ※ ※

SAMKHYA

Samkhya means "to count," or "to enumerate": it can also mean "discrimination." This word was applied to a philosophy that arose around or before the time of the Buddha—it is impossible to precisely date when it began. It is considered to be the oldest of the six *darshanas* or systems of Indian philosophies. The definitive texts describing Samkhya weren't written down until hundreds of years later, but their antecedents clearly existed by 500 B.C.E.[8] In this viewpoint our individual monads are simply and exclusively pure consciousness. You may have gotten some sense of this at one time or another in your life when you gazed at your hand or your body and just observed it; you may have felt that you were not your body, you were the thing that was watching your body. You got a taste of simply being consciousness.

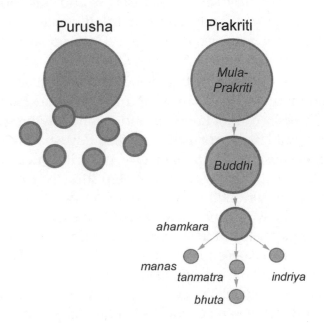

Figure 5. The Ontology of Samkhya

The Samkhya philosophy begins with looking at the two great divides upon which the model is founded: *purusha* (the reincarnating monad) and *prakriti* (nature) as shown in this graphic. Keep this little diagram in mind as we describe the differences between these two categories.

There are countless individual purushas, each one infinite, eternal, omniscient, unchanging and unchangeable. There is no single purusha that sits hierarchically above any others (we will explain that one big bubble later). There is no creator god or puppet master pulling any strings; there are gods, but the gods are just purushas as well, trapped in their Lamborghinis while the rest of us drive our Ford pickups. Purusha is pure consciousness, so it follows that prakriti is unconscious. Prakriti is everything that is changing. Prakriti is not just the physical aspects of the universe that we can sense; it is our very senses themselves and our thoughts, memories, desires, and even our intelligence. Prakriti is everything that is that isn't conscious. Consciousness resides only in purusha, or more properly, as purusha.

Purusha, pure and distant, is beyond subject and object. One cannot understand purusha, for that would make it an object. Purusha cannot know or understand anything either, for that would make purusha a subject. Purusha simply just is. But, because of the presence of prakriti, purusha gets attracted to nature in the way you were attracted to the car in our earlier story. In another, older analogy, purusha is attracted to prakriti the way a man is attracted to a beautiful dancing girl: he cannot help but try to get closer. And then the disaster occurs—purusha becomes trapped inside prakriti. This is the key moment and the key mistake of our lives, and it happens over and over again. We see the car and we climb inside. Like Brer Rabbit when he touches the Tar Baby, purusha gets more and more entangled in prakriti. Soon the purusha forgets that it was ever separate and ceases to struggle to regain its freedom.

Prakriti is completely inert, like a flower closed up upon itself at night: but once the sun rises, things start to happen. An evolution occurs within the prakriti: this is depicted in the graphic above. The first thing to appear out of the natural foundation of *mula-prakriti*, which simply means the root prakriti before purusha comes near, the flower before the sun touches it, is *buddhi* or our awakened intelligence. Buddhi is intuition, or cognition, but it is not consciousness. Because of its great intelligence and luminosity, it is often mistaken for consciousness, just as our car can sometimes seem to have a mind of its own: buddhi can seem to be conscious, but it is an illusion. Only purusha is conscious.

From buddhi evolves *ahamkara*, the "I-maker." Ahamkara creates the sense of self (with a small *s*), and here Westerners often make the mistake of calling this *ego*. But as we will see, this is not what is meant by ego as it is defined in Western psychology; ahamkara is the sense that I am my car. In this respect, ahamkara pretends to be purusha (which is a Self with a big *S*). So now your car starts to act as if it's the boss. Perhaps here our analogy begins to break down, but you probably know some people who seem to be owned by their cars or other belongings. A small scratch on the fender can send them into great angst and frenzy. It is at the level of ahamkara that subjects and objects arise. "I" becomes the subject, and the rest of the world provides the objects. At this level individualism arises, because inherent in the subject/object duality there is separation.

From ahamkara evolves *manas*, the mind, and the 10 senses (the *indriyas*). Manas here is the lower mind. It is often described as the 11th sense. Of the 10 senses listed, five we are very familiar with. These are called the cognitive senses: listening, feeling, seeing, tasting and smelling. The remaining five are the conative senses, the senses of action: speaking, grasping, moving, excreting and reproducing. Also out of ahamkara arise the five elements (*bhuta*) and the five energy potentials (*tanmatra*). The elements are space, air, fire, water and earth. The five energy potentials, more subtle than the elements, are the energies through which the senses function: They are the energy potentials that give rise to sounds, feelings, sights, tastes and smells.

Samkhya provides an ontology, a cosmological map of being. With the 24 principles of prakriti, Samkhya provides a map of the inner and outer universe. This is a map blazed by those who have gone before us—the pioneers we call psychonauts. But this raises one more question: How do we follow this map? What is the practice of Samkhya Yoga?

The union of purusha and prakriti was a horrible mistake; this unfortunate marriage should never have happened. The only remedy is a fast and thorough divorce! Like Brer Rabbit, the only way to be freed from the Tar Baby is to be thrown into the briar patch where we can scrape off prakriti and finally free ourselves. The briar patch is the practice of yoga, and there are many forms of yoga to choose from.

Samkhya Yoga and its close cousin Classical Yoga are *not* about union. The Classical Yoga of Patanjali's Yoga Sutra, compiled around 200 C.E., is about getting a divorce as quickly as possible. If you don't do it now, you will have to come back again and again, suffering countless new lives, until you finally get that divorce and are free at last.

Liberation is freedom. Remember, when we hear the word *liberation*, we should enquire, "Liberated from what?" In this case we are seeking liberation from prakriti. This state of freedom is called *kaivalya,* which means "aloofness, aloneness, or isolation." To obtain this form of moksha, one must separate from the body because, despite all its wonderful qualities, the body is made from prakriti. Separation is needed from the mind as well. In some philosophical departures from this earliest Samkhya teaching, kaivalya was seen to be, not the state of separation of purusha from prakriti, but rather non-identification of purusha as prakriti. The renowned Yin Yoga teacher, Paul Grilley, explains, "Kaivalya is not isolation from prakriti; kaivalya is realizing the Self is not dependent on any aspect of changeable prakriti for its existence."[9]

However, in the earliest Samkhya traditions, true liberation cannot be obtained while embodied. Remember, prakriti is not just the physical manifestations we see in life; memories, thoughts, emotions and even intelligence are all prakriti and need to be left behind. Only after leaving the body-mind in all its facets can one be truly and finally liberated. This is known as *videha mukti,* which is disembodied liberation. But, if the purusha is not cleansed of all its attractions to prakriti, then death is just the beginning of a new cycle, and the purusha once again becomes joined to prakriti.

To achieve lasting, eternal liberation, the Samkhya yogis employ discrimination and renunciation. Discrimination (known as *viveka*) is a knowing that is gained partly through reasoning. Renunciation is a moving away from everything that binds us to this life. Viveka, which can also mean "discernment or separating out," is knowing the way of the universe, not just intellectually, because the intellect is still prakriti, but at a deeper level. Viveka develops an inner knowledge that discerns the ephemeral from the actual, separating the apparent nature of the world from its underlying reality. While it is gained through reasoning, viveka also develops the will to renounce all that is unreal. While similar to Classical Yoga, Samkhya practice does not use as the main tool for liberation *samadhi,* which is a deep ecstatic absorption of the mind into itself.

Samkhya was a masterpiece of modeling the ways of the universe. The adoption of its cosmological structure by the Classical Yogis and Buddhists testifies to its power. However, the practice of Samkhya and its underlying dualistic philosophy were the basis for its eventual demise. Classical Yoga moved away from Samkhya and replaced the emphasis on viveka with the practice of samadhi. Later yoga schools, starting with Tantra, followed the Buddha's path of renouncing the fierce renunciation practices of the Jains, Samkhya and Classical Yoga paths. Eventually all that was left of Samkhya was the cosmology.

There were several logical problems with the original Samkhya philosophy. For example, how can there be countless individual purushas, each one all-powerful and eternal, without each purusha running afoul of all the other purushas? Samkhya's strict adherence to its pluralistic purusha was one of its major downfalls. Later generations of philosophers and yogis tried valiantly to fix Samkhya by extending it so that it wasn't dualistic, and they would try to claim that the original writings were misquotes of the founders of the philosophy. Historians begged to differ. Other philosophies simply copied the ontological theory proposed by Samkhya and dropped the distasteful duality; they liked the way prakriti was described, but they hated the idea that we each had our own unique and separate purushas. Another problem was Samkhya's atheistic nature—there is no creator god in this cosmology. Every purusha is equal and equivalent to every other purusha. The final problem with Samkhya was its strict dualism. If purusha is distinct from prakriti, how can it ever become entangled in the first place?

In the fertile period, around 500-600 B.C.E., ideas were being developed and exchanged between many fields of inquiry. Samkhya philosophy informed pre-classical yoga, which borrowed from Jainism, which also influenced both Samkhya and Buddhism. Each philosophy borrowed, tested, adopted, and discarded ideas and practices from each other. We will never know which philosophy originated which concepts, but one religion embraced the dualistic nature of reality firmly: Jainism.

* * *

JAINISM

Vardhamana, of the clan Jnata, was born at a very early age in the northeast of India, a region now called Bihar, and at a very interesting time. It was late in the sixth century B.C.E., a time when society had grown rich enough to allow many young men to leave their homes and wander the countryside, living only off the alms that they could beg from those who chose to stay in the world. Vardhamana's father was a prosperous Kshatriya, devout and pious, a worshipper of Lord Parsva, the 23rd in a long line of Jinas, the Jain heroes. Like his father, Vardhamana honored Parsva.

⛧ ⛧

Parsva had through countless lifetimes progressed upward, being born an elephant, a man, a king, a god, an Indra—the greatest of the gods—and finally a world savior. In his last incarnation, Parsva achieved perfect isolation and freedom, and upon his death his *jiva*, which we in the West might inaccurately call his soul, floated upward beyond the realms of men and gods, above even the highest heaven, to the place known as *isat-pragbhara*: "slightly tilted." There he abides in perfect isolation and introverted-awareness.

⛧ ⛧

Vardhamana was the second son: in his 30th year his parents passed on. Thinking this was a good time, he begged permission from his elder brother and left the world: He left behind riches, a wife and a young daughter. He had always been pious and studious, a devotee of Parsva, but now he got to live the life he was born to live. He became a Jain monk. For 12 long and hard years he perfected his practice of tapas, of strict ascetic practices. He discarded his clothes and went naked in all seasons and in all weather. You see, clothes come from living beings; he could not wear the fibers of plants any more than he could wear the skins of animals. Finally, Vardhamana achieved *kevala*, total isolation from without and integration from within. He was freed from earthly bondage and would be reborn no more. From this point on, he was like a spinning top without any new karma to extend the time of his spinning. Momentum alone kept him in this world for another 30 years. He became known as Mahavira, which is to say, the great hero, the 24th and final Jina of this present age.

As the latest and last great world saint, Mahavira began to teach. Walking everywhere, he spread the knowledge of the ancient Jinas, but he adapted for the times in which he now lived. His followers numbered in the tens of thousands; men and women of all castes were drawn to him, and he made no distinctions. To the earlier four precepts of ethical behavior fit for Jains he added a fifth. The vows were now:

1. *Ahimsa*: Cause no harm.

2. *Satya*: Speak the truth.

3. *Asteya*: Do not take that which is not yours.

4. *Aprigraha*: Detach yourself from things, places and people.

5. *Brahmacarya*: Practice celibacy.

In later centuries these five precepts would be repeated in the Classical Yoga schools as the *yamas*, or restraints for living among others. Mahavira also added three spiritual objectives that his followers must cultivate, and that would also be adopted by the Buddha:

i. Right View

ii. Right Knowledge

iii. Right Conduct

Mahavira's followers cleansed the stains on their jivas through the fierce adoption of these practices: They plucked no living thing and would only eat fruit that had fallen from the vines; if they fell in water, they rolled onto their backs and floated to shore, never moving so as not to hurt the molecules of the water; if wet, they would not wipe off the moisture, as that, too, could hurt the atoms of water; they swept the ground where they walked and limited the number of steps they took each day to avoid harming any insects; and they never drank at night in case a small bug had fallen into their cup. Intention was irrelevant; even if one intended no harm but accidentally sat on an ant or breathed in a mosquito, the jiva (the reincarnating monad) was stained.

When this life was ended, the jiva rose of its own accord to a higher incarnation. Even the gods die and have to be reborn. Life is just a play, and each player dons a mask for the performance. After all the possible roles have been acted out over and over again, why act anymore? You are not the mask! You are the actor, not the role, so give it up. Pleasure is always fleeting, even the divine pleasures of the gods. Cleanse the jiva through pure living and leave this material world behind. Follow the way of the Jinas, those victors who have won freedom.

Mahavira obtained his final release in his 72nd year; like Parsva and the others before him, his jiva had become completely transparent, identical to theirs. The huge statues carved in his honor look exactly like the statues carved in honor of the other Jinas: naked, aloof and indifferent. Mahavira's jiva floated up to the roof of the universe that, like a great umbrella, overlies all the worlds. There he experiences no feelings, no thoughts; in his tremendous isolation, he is completely indifferent to the world, untouched by prayers or acts of worship. He will never more be involved. Gods may be petitioned to intervene, show favor to one or strike down and curse another; they are far from free from the world. The great Jain saints are forever beyond all of that.

It is likely that Jainism has its antecedents far back into the pre-Vedic Dravidian culture. It clearly pre-dates Samkhya and Buddhist philosophies, although it did evolve, as all philosophies do, and it was not the only ancient school in India.[10] In Jainism we find a dualism that would be adopted into the Samkhya philosophy; the reincarnating monad known as the jiva became purusha, and everything else, called ajiva in Jainism, became Samkhya's prakriti. Everyone has his or her jiva, unique and separate from all other jivas. Your jiva has always existed, will always exist, was uncreated by anyone or anything. Unfortunately, it is stained or colored by its association with the world of nature. The Jains believed that the only way to clean the tarnish from the jiva is through fiercely adopting ahimsa: non-harming. Even breathing harms the molecules of the air; therefore, masks are worn to protect the air, to avoid inadvertently swallowing an insect, and to protect the soft tissues at the back of your throat. The most extreme Jain saints would cease walking, because every step harms some microscopic creature and crushes the atoms of the earth. Eventually the saints would just sit at the side of the road and wait for death to take them. This is a complete renunciation of the world and all its attachments. It is a pessimistic retreat from the world. It is hard to relate to, but perhaps an analogy will help us understand the concepts of jiva and karma:

ॐ ह्

Think of your favorite coffee cup. If you are an avid addict of coffee, chances are there is a very noticeable stain in your cup. You may have friends who have the exact same cup, and they, too, will have their stains. The stain is your karma; your mug is your jiva. The coffee mug itself is pure and unaffected by the stains, but the stains prevent the mug from being returned to the store where you bought it. To return the mug, you must first remove the stains. To purify the cup, you must first stop staining it any further: You must give up your attachment to and love of coffee! Not easy. Then you must start to wear away the stains through compassionate cleaning of the cup, by drinking only pure water. It will take some time, maybe many lifetimes, but eventually your cup will be like new, and it can then be returned to whence it originally came.

ॐ ह्

How different this view is from our Western view of our soul. Dante, Hercules, Gilgamesh and many others who visited hell recognized people there. This is not possible in Eastern hells; the purusha, or jiva, or atman as it is sometimes called—the the reincarnating monad—is simply a perfect coffee cup, unfortunately stained by the actions we have performed while we play our role on the stage of the world. In the West we believe our soul is immortal and will never die, although, strangely, we also believe it had a beginning. Our souls are created brand new when we are born; the Eastern purusha has always been and will always be. For us in the West, we are unique and new: We have never been here before, we have never faced this situation in our life before, we are tested, and our souls are affected and changed by what we do in this life. In the East, we have been here many times, and we will be here again many more times. If we want to get off the merry-go-around called *samsara*, the ever-spinning wheel of birth and death, we need to clean up our act; in fact, in the Jain view, we need to stop acting entirely.[11]

Jainism is *transtheistic*, a term coined by Heinrich Zimmer that means it goes beyond the gods.[12] Sure, there are plenty of gods around. The unorthodox beliefs in India such as Samkhya, Jainism and Buddhism did not deny the existence of the gods; they simply posited that the gods are as confused and trapped as we are. There is a place we can go to that lies beyond the ken of the gods. The ones who have gone beyond are known as *Tirthankaras*, which means the "makers of the river crossing."[13] Beyond the gods are these special "souls," also known as the *jinas*, or victors: the guys (and they were all men) who have obtained release (moksha) and who have succeeded in achieving total isolation from the material world.

If you look at the Samkhya diagram we saw earlier, you will see there are many purushas, but one in particular was drawn bigger than the others. This represents those

Tirthankaras who are no longer attracted to prakriti, or ajiva as it is called in the Jain philosophy. In the Classical Yoga as described by the sage Patanjali, there is only one purusha that is untainted by prakriti, and his name is Ishvara. The word *ishvara* means "lord or foremost ruler."[14] In the Yoga Sutra, Patanjali defined this term: *purusavisesa isvarah*—Ishvara is a special purusha that was "at no time embroiled in the play of nature."[15] Confusingly, Patanjali also says that Ishvara was the first teacher. But how can purusha be completely separated from prakriti and yet still affect others who are bound by prakriti? This same dilemma arose in Jainism, too: Why pray to the Tirthankaras if they are forever beyond caring about us? If these special jivas or purushas are beyond this world, if they are beyond being able to interact with us, why even think about them? How can they possibly help us?

꩜ ꩜

Lord Parsva was confused. In this, his next-to-last incarnation, he was a great and powerful king. His first minister suggested that a religious celebration was in order to mark the occasion of his great victory over the surrounding nations. When Parsva began to pray to the statues in the temple, this doubt arose within him: "Why pray to an image? These statues are not conscious. How could praying to images do any good?"

The wise saint Vipulamati was in the temple at the same time as the king and read his thoughts. The sage enlightened the king: "Images affect the mind even if they are not conscious themselves. Place a red flower in a pure glass vase, and the glass will become red. Place a yellow flower in the glass, and the glass becomes yellow. Your mind, dear king, is like the glass. Be careful of what you place in it."

Vipulamati offered a parable: "There was once a beautiful courtesan who died in the prime of her youth. When her body was laid upon the pyre, a horny man gazed upon

184

the body and yearned for it. He thought to himself, 'If only I could, once in my life, lay with such a beautiful woman!' A dog was also looking at the corpse thinking, 'What a waste of good meat. They are just going to burn the body.' A yogi also watched the cremation and thought, 'It is so sad that she wasted her life in the pursuit of pleasure instead of seeking true knowledge and liberation.' There was but one body, but in three minds there were three feelings. Any image can affect the mind, and the effect will be in accordance with the nature of that mind."

"By contemplating the pure ones that have gone before us, our minds are purified. Images of the Tirthankaras can prepare the mind for nirvana and lead us to eternal freedom."[16]

᠄ ᠃

The Tirthankaras and Ishvara are role models we can look up to and model ourselves after. Do not expect them to become personally involved in your life, though. They are not like Jesus; these are not personal gods, and they can't get involved. Getting involved would recontaminate them. They are special, aloof and untouchable, but they are also great examples of how you could live your life.

* * *

Around 2000 B.C.E. the great Harappan civilization, strung along the banks of the Indus River, collapsed. Climate change led to drought, and perhaps overgrazing and soil depletions also caused the crops to fail and famine to arise. The people of that great civilization had to move or die, and so move they did. To the West there were the remnants of the Akkadian empire struggling to survive between the two great rivers of the Tigris and Euphrates. The climate there was no better, and drought was a curse upon their land; a massive migration westward over highlands and desert was not a viable option. Fortunately there was another great fertile river valley to the east, the Gangetic Plains. An Asian fertile crescent existed, linking in a grand arc the lands of the Indus, the Punjab and the Ganges River. This arc was an easier path to follow than the road westward.

Indologists like Heinrich Zimmer think that the Indo-Europeans that lived along the Indus River migrated eastward, overrunning the indigenous tribes settled along the Ganges banks. The indigenous people were the Dravidians, and their culture was as ancient as the invaders, most likely far older. The warrior people came in their chariots, with their Brahmin priests and thunder-hurling god and won the battles, which is exactly the same story told of Semite invaders from the Arabian Peninsula, led by their priests and their god of lightning, defeating the indigenous people of Canaan. The Dravidians were conquered, subjugated and debased. Usually, conquerors absorb the conquered into their own culture, but in the north of India, a reverse assimilation occurred, slowly and over centuries. Not all the Dravidian tribes were conquered, and not everywhere were the Indo-European mythologies adopted. A fusion developed.

We saw earlier in the myth of Parashu Rama that the Brahmins, through the will of Vishnu, conquered the Kshatriya warrior kings, proving that AryanBbrahmins were the greatest caste of all. This myth may be based on an early struggle between the priests and the warriors, or it may reflect the time of the Indo-Europeans coming into the Ganges region. As noted, not all the native tribes were vanquished. It is interesting to note that the proto-Indo-Europeans of the Near East and Europe—the the Persians, ancient Greeks, Celts and Germans—never developed yoga. The retreat to the forest, the deep introspection and getting out of life, was unknown in the earliest westerly cultures. Indologists believe the Indian branch of Indo-Europeans absorbed these practices from the earlier Dravidian culture. No Indo-European worshipped the goddess, as was done in India before the Indo-Europeans arrived. In the early Vedas, Vishnu and the earliest forms of Shiva did not have the full breadth that they would acquire after the Indo-Europeans moved eastward. Two pantheons came into collision, but the newer gods did not displace nor replace the older ones, as happened everywhere else. Instead, a curious comingling occurred.

The people of the Vedas assimilated many of the teachings and philosophies of the indigenous people whom they conquered. Mircea Eliade lists several of the mystical themes and rituals that came into Hinduism from the earlier, pre-Vedic cultures: the devotional cults, puja and bhakti; the elevation of the goddess to near-equal standing to the gods (Kali and Shiva became equals); fertility cults and worship of the lingam; shamanic techniques that became part of yoga practices.[17] Zimmer states, "... Jainism retains the Dravidian structure more purely than the other major Indian traditions—and is consequently a relatively simple, unsophisticated, clean-cut, and direct manifestation of the pessimistic dualism that underlies not only Samkhya, Yoga and early Buddhistic thought, but also much of the reasoning of the Upanishads, and even the so-called "nondualism" of the Vedanta."[18]

It is interesting that in the Greek mythologies, the newer generations of gods defeated and replaced the older. Chronos fought and defeated his father, Ouranos, replacing him. Zeus defeated Chronos, and, when the reign of the Olympian gods usurped the earlier Titans, no one bothered worshipping the Titans anymore. This is the way it normally goes: The new gods defeat the older gods, symbolic of an assimilation of the old into the new. This is the Western view of progress! Individual assertion does make a difference: Zeus defeats his father. Each generation learns from the past and improves upon it. Ouranos, for example, tried to prevent his sons from coming out of their mother's body; Chronos discovered that didn't work, so he swallowed his kids as soon as they came out of their mother's body; and Zeus discovered that didn't work, so he swallowed the mother before the next generation could be born.[19] Each generation learns from the prior and adapts.

Not so in India. Indra, the counterpart of patriarchal Zeus, became subservient to Vishnu, who was an inflation of an earlier Dravidian deity, the sky god Vin.[20] In the East, the Indo-European gods were not the next generation replacing the older gods; these Vedic gods were assimilated into the older existing culture of the Dravidians, and the Dravidian gods eventually prevailed as the greater gods. Vishnu and Shiva have no counterpart in Greece. There is no progress of positive evolution in the East, just a downward spiral, as the yugas unwind.

In our story of Mahavira, the last Tirthankara of the Jains, we saw that Vardhamana did not create a new world religion. He was a reformer of what was already extant: the Jainism of the Dravidians. What Mahavira taught was not rooted in the Vedas. By contrast, the Buddha did create a new religion. Like Vardhamana he was not a Brahmin; they were both Kshatriyas. The Buddha also broke away from the Vedic beliefsby negating the need for priests, sacrifice and caste, but what he developed was absorbed eventually into Hinduism.

The point to realize in this brief history is that the idea of a pure, undifferentiable but unique, reincarnating monad is today uniquely Asian. There was a time in ancient Greece when philosophers developed, or perhaps acquired from India, a similar understanding of the reincarnating monad, but this map did not stick in the West. Our Western concept of soul developed much more along Zoroastrian and Biblical lines: the soul with personality. We can see this difference starkly displayed today in the two very different ways people react to the concept of reincarnation.

In the Eastern philosophies, reincarnation is something to be avoided at all costs. To live again and again in this sorrowful world is unbearable. True joy, bliss, ananda is obtained only when we are free from the cycles of rebirth. In the West, however, among those who believe in reincarnation, such as the followers of Orphism and Pythagoras in ancient Greece to New Age believers, the reaction to the idea of reincarnation is Great! Wow! I get to return and do this all over again; no need to fear the great terminator, for I'll be back! We are comforted with the thought that we won't really die when this body fails us.

The difference in these two attitudes toward reincarnation is the emphasis on *what* it is that is reincarnated. In the West we dearly hope it is our *personality*, our ego, which survives to the next life (or the afterlife for those who don't believe in reincarnation). We are drawn to stories of how someone can remember her past life, hoping this means that something of the person we are now will still be around in some future incarnation. In the Eastern view, nothing natural survives from one life to the next. By "natural" we mean nothing of nature, of prakriti, and this includes our memories and personalities. What returns is the reincarnating monad, stained by the karma of our prior lives.

Chapter 10: Matter Versus Spirit

What is mind?

No matter.

What is matter?

Never mind.

— Bertrand Russell's Grandmother

Samkhya created a philosophical problem when it insisted that purusha is pure consciousness and everything else is prakriti. If purusha cannot actually be affected by prakriti, how can it become trapped by it? How can it even sense or be conscious of anything at all? To sense something you must somehow come into contact with it via some sort of sense organ. For example, our eyes sense light because light affects the photoreceptors in our eyes, the rods and cones, which in turn send a signal to the brain, and only then do we become conscious of what we see. If purusha is pure consciousness and is thus unaffected by the material world, how can it be conscious of anything at all? This dilemma exists in every philosophy that postulates spirit and matter are completely separate qualities: How can spirit ever exist within matter, if it is so pure as to be not contaminated by matter?[1] Some sort of bridge is needed to connect the two realms. In some models of Tantra, these bridges are the chakras, but we are getting ahead of ourselves. We will come to Tantra when we look at the mystical function of myths.

The ontological model that Samkhya postulated explaining the nature of prakriti was attractive to many other schools of philosophy. These schools adopted the cosmology of prakriti but rejected the unsupportable and unpalatable doctrine of the duality between purusha and prakriti. In the later Vedantic philosophy, the split between purusha and prakriti was healed by bringing them together in the body of Brahman: the original Self that split apart into both spirit and matter. As we will see, Tantra Yoga also merged purusha and prakriti into the ultimate Shiva, which is actually Shiva/Shakti, two sides of one coin. There is no duality; we are all part of Shiva and his consort, Shakti. Shakti is the objective side of reality, the stuff that we sense, and Shiva is the subjective side, the stuff that senses. They seem two, but they are really one.

According to Vedanta we are all part of the *universal atman*, called the *paramatman*, and so is everything we see. Everything is divine. With these newer philosophies, there was no problem for our reincarnating monad to interact with the material world, because everything has some degree of consciousness. Even a dead brick will make a noise if struck by a hammer. There is a primitive form of consciousness, present even in inanimate objects, that will react to events.

Despite the claim that duality is an illusion, it is a very persistent illusion. Vedanta and Tantra and many other schools tried to do away with duality, saying we are all part of the one, and it is only our ignorance that prevents us from seeing this truth. However, the fact remains that my particular particle of conscious awareness does seem to me to be awfully separate from that grand vision of oneness. If we are all one, and if the practice of yoga or other spiritual methods can liberate my monad from this dualistic delusion, why is it that all monads are not simultaneously liberated when just one monad succeeds? If we are all one, if one is free, why aren't all free? Remember the quote cited a moment ago by Zimmer: "so-called 'nondualism' of Vedanta"? He put *nondualism* in quotes to show that, despite the claims that we are all one with the greater existence of everything, it is not always expressed that way. We have our atman (small self), but Brahman is supreme (the great Self).

Vedanta literally means "the end of the Vedas." It is the completion of the earlier religious thought in an analogous way that Christians believe the New Testament to be a completion of what got started in the Old Testament. The books of Vedanta are the Upanishads, which includes one real gem, the Bhagavad Gita. In this philosophy we are taught that each of us has a soul (for lack of a better English word) called the *atman*. Unfortunately, this atman is hard to see, for it is hidden; thus the first part of the spiritual practice is to uncover who we are at our very core. The atman is what is immanent within us. In the other direction, we discover that our atman is actually part of a larger being called Brahman, which, for lack of a better word, might be called God or the transcendent. Brahman is everything; it is that original Self that we were introduced to in the first chapter. The problem is, we don't realize we are Brahman, so we have two challenges spiritually: to recognize our inner nature, which is atman, and to realize that our inner nature is identical to the divinity of the whole universe. The practices of purification, rituals, chanting, fasting, meditation, devotion to the gods, all of which have their counterparts in various forms of yoga (bhakti yoga, jnana yoga, hatha yoga, mantra yoga, raja yoga, etc.), help us to dispel the illusions that prevent us from realizing our true nature. Once we have seen through these veils of Maya, the illusions she casts over us, then we are liberated. What we are liberated from are the cycles of death and rebirth.

On the surface Vedanta is a nondualistic philosophy because atman is brahma and all is one, but it is hard to avoid slipping back into a dualistic philosophy, even if we would like not to. We are told that we are all part of Brahman, but we suffer because we don't know we are part of Brahman. We seem to be dual: we have a body and a soul (or atman or monad or whatever you want to call it), but we don't really. Because of this ignorance, we will keep on being reborn and re-dying. But whose is this "me" that is born, and what dies? I get reborn out of my ignorance of my true nature, which is Brahman, but Brahman suffers no such ignorance, so if he is me, and I am he, how can I be ignorant while he isn't? Why am I reborn when he knows me, who is he? Confused? You are not alone. We are entering realms where logic does not apply and here words cannot go.

My atman puts on bodies and takes them off again, lifetime after lifetime, like an actor playing first this role and then that role. This implies a duality between our body and our atman. But, if our atman and our bodies are identically part of Brahman, how can it be said that one is taking on the other, when it is all just one? The feeling that we are minds that have a body, or we are atmans that have a mind and a body, is overwhelming and dualistic. We find this stated in the West all the time; our primary belief is that we are spirits that have a body, or perhaps bodies that have a spirit. In the West, we are used to this dualism because it is in our heritage, but dualism does keep coming up in the East, too.

The points raised above are not new; scholars and theologians have encountered them and countered them, generating counter-counter responses, and the whole debate has cycled on for centuries. If you wish to dive into the waters of duality versus nonduality, be prepared for a whirlpool that will suck you in deeply. When faced with head-spinning conundrums, the best recourse is to listen to a story. Here is a favorite of Joseph Campbell that may help.

༄ ༅

Laghu was lost in thought: Guruji had been explaining to him the truth of truths—that he, Laghu, was God! The illustrative saying from the Chandogya Upanishad was repeating itself over and over in his head: *Tat tvam asi!* That are thou! You are it!

Guruji had recited a story from the Chandogya Upanishad in which a father was teaching his son. It was a story about the most secret knowledge—that we are divine. The son, Svetaketu, did not understand, so the father, Uddalaka, one of the greatest ancient Indian philosophers, told him to fetch a fruit. Svetaketu went and got an orange and presented it to his father.

Uddalaka said, "Peel the orange."

Svetaketu peeled the orange.

"Now break the orange into pieces."

Done.

"Now break open a section and take out the seed."

This Svetaketu did.

"Now, cut the seed in half and tell me what you see."

Svetaketu gazed at the center of the opened seed in silence: He didn't see anything. He shrugged his shoulders and said, "What? I don't see anything!"

"Exactly!" trumped his father, "and that are thou! You are that nothingness. Just as a huge orange tree can grow from the nothingness you are looking at, comes all things. You are it!"

This is the key mystery of the Upanishads. You are it! All the gods, all the heavens, all the demons and all the hells are *within* you; they *are* you! Your job is to follow their footsteps, like a herder following the footsteps of a lost cow, until you come to this realization.

Laghu kept saying to himself, "*I* am God. I am *God*]! I *am* God." He wandered aimlessly down roads and onto a narrow jungle path, lost in "tat tvam asi." Coming the other way along the path was an elephant. The path was narrow and the rider of the elephant cried out to Laghu, "Get out of the way!"

"Get out of the way?" thought Laghu. "But I am God! Why should God get out of the way of a mere elephant?"

He kept walking and the mahout kept shouting, louder and louder. Finally at the critical moment, with its great trunk the elephant lifted Laghu and roughly deposited him in the bushes. The mahout and elephant continued on their journey, unperturbed by the whole incident, but Laghu was dismayed and distraught. He brushed himself off and, ignoring his injuries, hurried back to Guruji.

"Guruji!" cried Laghu as he bowed before his teacher, "please explain to me how this could be."

"What?" replied Guruji.

Laghu related his story and explained his logic. "You told me that all things are divine, that I am divine, too, and that I am God. How could it be that God was thrown to the ground like that?"

Guruji shook his head, laughed, and asked Laghu, "It is true that you are God, but why didn't you also listen to the voice of God telling you to get out of the way?"

≈ ≋

The Buddha knew all about the philosophies of duality and nondualism and the various explanations about our true nature. These ideas were all around him and quite current in his time. It is natural that his disciples would ask his opinion. Remember his response? "Don't think about it!" It does you no good to waste your time to puzzle out whether we have a monad that survives our death and is separate from our body, or whether it dies when the body dies. Knowing whether existence is inherently dual or nondual will not help you become a better monk, nor will it lead to ultimate freedom. They are both concepts, not truth.

Now wait a minute—not truth? Reality surely must be one or the other. Either reality is all one, and our spirit and bodies are joined together in some ultimate ocean of being, like so many raindrops and snowflakes melting into the sea, or our ultimate nature is consciousness and not matter, because matter is forever distinct from spirit. We can't have it both ways or neither way. This is funny, because that was exactly the puzzle facing scientists in the 19th and 20th centuries when they tried to discern the true nature of light:

⁓ ⁓

Sir Isaac Newton (1642–1727) theorized that light was corpuscular—it was made up of numerous tiny, individual particles. This was a pretty good theory, and it held up for over a hundred years, until a physicist named Thomas Young (1773-829) proved that light actually behaved like waves. If we were to direct a beam of light through a tiny hole and toward a screen, the light would be spread out on the screen in a diffraction pattern, the same way waves are diffracted around objects in water. The wave nature of light was also demonstrated in a famous double-slit experiment, where the light rays travelling through one slit interfered with light coming through another slit. There is no way particles could create the alternating bands of light and darkness that arise in the interference pattern. The fact that light can be polarized also proves that it is not made up of particles, so it was obvious that light was actually a wave.

Ah, but not so fast. In the late 19th century, Heinrich Hertz (1857-1894) discovered something known as the photoelectric effect. Hertz showed that light could eject an electron from the surface of an object. This could possibly happen if light was a wave, but the amount of the light (the quantity or brightness) required to free the electron was shown not to be important: the frequency (the energy or color) of the light was. By using higher frequencies of light, more electrons were emitted regardless of how much light was striking the surface, implying that light was actually a particle, an individual particle carrying with it an individual packet of energy, which is proportional to its frequency. In the early 20th century, Albert Einstein (1879-1955) explained the photoelectric effect by theorizing that these particles of light, called photons, came in discreet bundles of energy, called quanta; electrons only react to photons that have the right quanta of energy to excite them. (It was this piece of work, not his theory of relativity, that earned Einstein his Nobel Prize!) Now it became obvious that light is quantized and particular.

But, this is a puzzle. How can light be spread out and at the same time be concentrated in one place? Can light be a duality of wave *and* particle? Or is it nondual and only one *or* the other? It turns out the answer is … yes. If you choose to measure light as a particle, you will discover that it is a particle. If you choose to measure light as a wave, it will act as a wave. It is almost as if light knows what you are trying to do. If that is the case, how about we try to trick it and measure both qualities at the same time? It turns out, we can't. There is no way to experimentally measure both the wave nature of light and its particle nature at the same time. This has become a central concept in quantum mechanics and is its most mysterious aspect: Light is both a wave *and* a particle (it is dualistic) until you measure it, in which case it is only a wave *or* a particle (it is nondualistic.)

੩ ੬

The universe, it seems, doesn't care if we can't wrap our minds around its mysteries. Given that it is a fact of the universe that things can be both A and not-A at the same time (in defiance of the ancient Greek principles of the Laws of

Thought where things must be either A or not-A), what can we say about the whole debate about duality versus nonduality? And within the nonduality camp, what can we say about our spirit being personalized or depersonalized? One of the major premises of this book is that none of these models are truth! The scientific model that says light is a particle is not true, and neither is the model that says light is a wave. Myths, maps and models are never truth, but they can prove useful.

The advocates of Vedanta and our nondual nature have presented us with a model of the universe that is not true, but it is useful in many situations to act "as if" it were true. The Samkhya and Classical Yoga advocates who believe our individual monads are completely distinct and unique and unaffected by the material world are also not telling us the truth. But their maps, too, are useful in some cases. If we can see all these stories and viewpoints as *representations* of the way Reality is (whatever Reality is) and not Reality itself, then we can consciously choose whether to employ that model or not. If it works for you, use it. When it doesn't work, find another story that does. There is no need to argue that one map is right and thus the other must obviously be wrong. Of course, there is value in debating the internal consistencies of the various philosophies. It is through the rigors of debate and cross-examinations that models become stronger, more robust and thus more useful. This is a strength of science— the continuous re-examination of its theories. But don't lose sight of the fact that these are all just models in the end.

* * *

The mystery of consciousness has not escaped the attention of science; many great minds have tried to puzzle out what the mind is. Since the time of Newton, scientists viewed the universe as a huge machine that was hugely complex, to be sure, but a machine nonetheless. This view also prevails in neurobiology: The mind, or consciousness, is simply an emergent property of the complexity of the brain. Just because we haven't figured it all out quite yet does not mean there is a separate mind beyond the brain. Without the brain, according to this model, there is no mind.

This viewpoint contrasts distinctly with the old idea of a spiritual homunculus, a little man sitting in the brain (or the heart) pulling all the strings. According to the Upanishads, this little guy is about the size of your thumb and is subtle.[2] He is not physical, which is why you can't find him in an autopsy. Scientists shiver when they hear this, because how are we supposed to find and study something that doesn't physically exist? And if it doesn't physically exist, how in the world can it affect the brain and cause anything to happen? Here we have that old chestnut again: If spirit is truly distinct from matter, how can it affect matter? Note that we are not talking about spirit as energy; we know how energy affects matter and vice versa, and we also know that matter *is* energy, thanks to Einstein's little equation. What is meant by spirit is not energy. If it was, we could measure it, and we would have detected it by now.

There is a great debate raging between the materialists and the spiritualists even in modern neurobiology. The materialists insist that the sense that we have a mind is just an affectation of biology; the spiritualists believe that there does indeed exist something outside the brain that influences our actions. It is not our intention here to resolve this debate or even contribute anything new to the discussion; rather, let's just look at the two points of view, remembering that neither model implies truth! Which view you find useful may depend upon your intentions.

My fundamental premise about the brain is that its workings—what we sometimes call "mind"—are a consequence of its anatomy and physiology and nothing more. — Carl Sagan[3]

The Astonishing Hypothesis is that "You," your joys and your sorrows, your memories and your ambitions, your sense of personal identity and free will, are in fact no more than the behavior of a vast assembly of nerve cells and their associated molecules. As Lewis Carroll's Alice might have phrased it: "You're nothing but a pack of neurons." — Francis Crick[4]

Man no longer has need for the "Spirit"; it is enough for him to be Neuronal Man. — Jean-Pierre Changeux[5]

Despite our every instinct to the contrary, there is one thing that consciousness is not: some entity deep inside the brain that corresponds to the "self," some kernel of awareness that runs the show, as the "man behind the curtain" manipulated the illusion of a powerful magician in The Wizard of Oz. After more than a century of looking for it, brain researchers have long since concluded that there is no conceivable place for such a self to be located in the physical brain, and that it simply doesn't exist. — Michael Lemonick[6]

Wham! Take that, spiritualists! It is pretty clear that matter is all that matters and never mind the mind. These quotations were compiled by the authors of *The Spiritual Brain*, Mario Beauregard and Denyse O'Leary.[7] Their view is not in agreement with these materialists' sentiments, but they presented them in their book so that they could refute them:

As soon as one begins to understand subjective and objective, mental and physical phenomena as relational instead of substantive, the causal interactions between mind and matter become no more problematic than such interaction among mental phenomena and physical phenomena ... the demand for a mechanistic explanation of causality has long been rejected in various fields of physics, including electromagnetism and quantum mechanics. — B. Alan Wallace[8]

All we know about consciousness is that it has something to do with the head, rather than the foot. — Nick Herbert[9]

Consciousness and other aspects of the mind, which can influence neural events, can occur independently of the brain, generally through aspects of quantum mechanics. This view is associated with neuroscientists John Eccles and Wilder Penfield as well as philosopher Karl Popper. — Mario Beauregard and Denyse O'Leary[10]

In this last quotation, we are told that it is to the mysterious and almost mystical agency of quantum mechanics we need turn to explain the unexpected. There are a lot of spooky things that go on in the quantum world. Action at a distance is just one, and it is the one that most spooked Einstein: Two particles can be "entangled" and separated by a vast distance. Because they are entangled, what happens when we observe one particle instantaneously affects the distant cousin-particle. Einstein showed that nothing is instantaneous in this universe, because everything is in motion relative to everything else, and this affects our frame of reference. Time is relative to the speed at which we are moving, so how can two events be instantaneous in all frames of reference? And, furthermore, he showed that no communication can exceed the speed of light, so these two distant particles cannot possibly communicate instantaneously with each other. And yet they do! Spooky.

Something is at work in the universe that our intellect cannot wrap its head around. We don't have good intuitive maps that help us navigate in the quantum world, and many spiritualists use this quantum loophole as a way out of having to prove their assertion that mind is separate from brain. But the materialists still have a valid objection. Just because they cannot prove the mind comes from the brain does not mean the mind doesn't come from the brain. Their inability to prove their position does not automatically prove the contrary position. The spiritualists still have to offer their own proof.

* * *

There are many contexts in which the debate between duality and nonduality arises. We have seen in the creation myths there are nondualistic philosophies that posit man came directly from the body (or mind) of a god and is divine, and there are dualistic philosophies that posit a god created man, and man is not divine, only divinely created. It is instructive at this point to stop and ask yourself once again, "Which map am I following?" Do you believe I/you are divine, or simply divinely created? If we believe that we are divine, and so is everyone and everything else, we may see others differently, and we may behave differently than if we see everything as a plaything created by a remote power.

That we are divine is an attractive supposition: since I am made of the same stuff as you, and since we are both divine and just different aspects of God, we should naturally treat each other with love and respect. But does it play out that way in reality? In Vedanta and Hinduism, the idea that we are all divine is widely held. The Brahmins are divine and so are the outcastes! Yet, knowing this, India is home to some of the deepest divides between rich and poor. The number of beggars in the crushing metropolises of India beggars belief. If all is divine, why do the divine wealthy members of Indian society permit the divine poorest members of their society to suffer so greatly?

Joseph Campbell commented on this during his journey to Asia in 1955. He noticed the Western Missionaries did more for the poor than did the Indian rich or middle classes.[11] The Christians' dualistic view that we are all divinely created and not divine seems more able to generate compassion for the poor than the nondualistic view that all is God. The great humanitarian organizations of the world are Western inventions: the Red Cross and Red Crescent, the YMCA, the Salvation Army, Doctors Without Borders, and so on. Why are there no Eastern organizations of similar reach? The answer may be found in the previously described view of karma: these poor unfortunate lower castes of people are poor and unfortunate *because* of actions they themselves committed in prior lives. They are reaping what they sowed, and it is only through their suffering in this life that they will be elevated in later lives. There is no point in helping them now. The map of nondualism when combined with the myths of dharma and karma turn the otherwise beautiful sentiment of "all is divine" into a repressive tool that keeps the vast majority of people under the thumb of the powerful elite. India is struggling today to change, but to effect this change and treat everyone as divine, the myth of dharma, varna and karma must be greatly modified. That map no longer serves!

To return to the topic we have been examining, mind and body, let's ask:ils our mind completely separate from our body, or is there a connection? We can also substitute the word *mind* with *spirit*, or *soul*, or *purusha*, or *reincarnating monad*, etc. Are they the same as the body or different? We have seen stories that symbolize a dualistic viewpoint and stories that are nondualistic. Samkhya, Jainism and Classical Yoga posit that mind and body are quite distinct. Western religions also posit that soul and body are distinct: These are dualistic views. The Biblical traditions believe that God puts a soul into each and every body; it is not there naturally.

Nondualist Tantra and Vedanta say, "No!" The mind and body are not different; they are found together in the original Self, called Shiva/Shakti or Brahman; we just think they are different because of ignorance caused by a deceiving goddess named Maya.[12] Many neuroscientists and philosophers of science also take the nonduality position, but spin 180 degrees away from the spiritualists. There is no difference between mind and body because mind is the illusion created by the body, more specifically by the brain. The brain's activities do the same thing as Maya, by presenting an illusion of separateness where there is none. So, there is one branch of nondualism that says the mind and body are the same because the body is a manifestation of the ultimate spirit of the universe; while another branch argues that mind and body are the same because the mind is a manifestation of the ultimate matter of the brain.

Again, our point is not to prove which model is true, because none are. We are not going to even try to qualify which map is more accurate or useful, because that depends upon your intention, on how you want to use these maps. It is useful that scientists are debating these issues; that is bound to lead to better maps in the future. It is enough for us to see if these stories can help us with our own passage through the inevitable arc of aging. Which story helps you come into accord with your own personal and inevitable journey? Let's leave the last word on this topic of the nature of mind and matter to Joseph Campbell and see which map he preferred.[13]

⋅⊰ ⊱⋅

One day Joseph Campbell was lecturing in a hall and wondered how best to explain consciousness to his students. He looked up at the ceiling for inspiration and came up with an enlightening analogy.

"Look up," he said, "at all those lights. Now, we could say we are looking at 'the lights,' or we could say we are looking at 'light.' We can notice each individual lightbulb, or we can pay attention to the totality of light in the room. Now imagine one of those bulbs burns out. Does the superintendent come in and say, 'Oh my, that was a very special bulb!' Does he take it out and put it on the fireplace mantle and build a little shrine to it? No, of course not.

What is important is not the bulb but the light that shines through the bulb."

"Now, I look down at all of you, and what do I see? Bulbs of flesh and bones called heads. The brain is the vessel of consciousness, not the source of it. Imagine a lightbulb that could repair itself; it would have to have some consciousness to know when it is not working well and then direct the repairs. This is what our bodies do, but still the lightbulb would not be the source of the light or the energy that flows through it."

"If a lightbulb burns out, does this mean the electricity is no longer there either? No, the source of energy is still there, but the vehicle is gone. The source of energy remains, just as we remain even after the body is gone. We are the source. We are the light, not the bulb."

❧ ☙

Chapter 11: The Individual in Society

Gotta Serve Somebody — Bob Dylan (1979)[1]

Serve Yourself — John Lennon (1980)[2]

Kama & Artha: I want.

Dharma: Thou Shalt.

You gotta choose!

Selfishly serving the "I want" urge is the devil's choice, according to Bob Dylan, and society in general would agree with him. Serving the Lord serves society. Recall President John F. Kennedy's exhortation: "Ask not what your country can do for you—ask what you can do for your country!" This is society claiming pre-eminence over the individual. And yet, in the American Founding Fathers' minds, there is the right for each individual to the pursuit of liberty and happiness. There is a place of conflict arising here between the psychological function and the social function of mythology. Which map is operating in your life: Bob Dylan's or John Lennon's? Or is it sometimes one and sometimes the other?

The way the individual is trained and expected to behave is vastly different between East and West. The roots of this difference go back thousands of years; however, with the movement of the Middle Eastern influences into Europe during the early Christian years, an attempt was made to synthesize these two very distinct mythos. It has not been a completely successful fusion. We can understand the Eastern view of the individual's role in life with two illustrative stories: one from India and the other from Israel. First, the story of Krishna and Arjuna from the *Bhagavad Gita: the Song of the Lord*:

THE BHAGAVAD GITA

Here on the Kurushetra and the Dharmashetra, the field of action and the field of duty, two great armies are about to meet. On one side of the field are arrayed the five sons of Pandu, the Pandavas, and their friends and allies. Opposing them are their evil cousins, the Kauravas, the hundred sons of the blind king Dhritarashtra, led by the usurper Duryodhana. This is a cruel and divisive struggle; one that pits a great family against itself. Thousands of soldiers have taken arms, with beloved uncles, friends and teachers on opposite sides and the outcome uncertain.

On the morning before the great battle begins, the most perfect warrior of the age, Arjuna, wanted to go into the middle of the field for a final look around. His good friend Krishna drove him there in their chariot. Brave men are lined up on either side of the battleground, waiting for Arjuna to unleash the carnage, but Arjuna's courage fails him. His bow drops from his hands, and he asks his friend to take him far away from this place. He cannot begin this fight: By the end of this day, many whom he loves and holds dear will be lost. He will not be the cause of their deaths.

Krishna remained steadyand upbraided Arjuna. "Where does this great cowardice come from? You are a warrior, a Kshatriya! Your purpose in life is to fight, so get in there and do your job, do your duty!"

Arjuna just can't. He has no heart or stomach for the slaughter. He would rather quit and be called a coward than kill and take innocent people's lives. Krishna saw the compassionate source of Arjuna's misgivings and began to talk some sense into him.

"You think that you will kill anyone?" said Krishna. "You are simply the vehicle through which I act. Do you blame the bow for launching the arrow? Your life is one of action: act! Do not be concerned with the outcome or the cause of your action. You do not control anything. Whether you will be successful or whether you will fail is not decided by anything you do. I and I alone determine the play of events."

For many long years, Arjuna and Krishna had been good friends, but this was the first time Krishna had ever spoken in such a voice. "Who are you, Krishna," Arjuna asked, "to claim such power? What do you mean when you say that *you* decide who will live and who will die?"

"Who dies, Arjuna? You cry over men who need no tears. The wise do not grieve for the departed, for whoever is has been before, and whoever was will be again. Never was there a time when I was not, when you were not; and never was there a time when all that you see was not. The body is put on and taken off again like a set of clothes, but the self which dons and discards the body is everlasting. Fight, mighty Arjuna! That is your duty in this world."

"The war upon us now," continued Krishna, "is a just war. This is the highest honor a warrior can obtain—to fight in a just war. If you were to shirk this duty, you would fall into grave error. You have benefited greatly from being of the noble warrior caste; now that it is time to pay the price, you cannot run away. Your only right now is to act. What you intend is what brings you credit, not the results of your action. This, dear Arjuna, is called *Yoga*—abiding steadfast in equanimity, remaining balanced and without attachment to success or failure."

"The results of all actions are given to me, Arjuna. Act without consideration for yourself. Dedicate yourself to this higher cause, and transcend your own sense of self."

"Who are you?" repeated Arjuna. "Your words cause my hair to stand on end. You sound divine and wise, and I would follow your guidance, but I remain confused. Your words are filled with wisdom, but is not wisdom superior to action? Should I not better retire and ponder what this all means rather than stay and act rashly? Please explain more clearly."

"Arjuna, I have created many paths for many people. There are those who should sit and meditate; this is the wisdom path of Jnana Yoga. There are those who should sing and dance and expand their hearts; this is the joyous path of Bhakti Yoga. There are those who should act and dedicate their actions to me; this is the path of Karma Yoga."

"Imagine the world if I, like you, refused to act! If I did nothing, all the worlds would perish, and chaos would ensue. It is only the unwise who act with attachment to their actions; those knowing my true nature act and leave to me the result. Know me, Arjuna, and be not afraid to do your duty."

"I would know you, Krishna. Please show me who you are."

With his mere mortal eyes, Arjuna could not see nor comprehend the vastness of Krishna. He was given a great gift—Krishna granted him divine sight. Now Arjuna perceived the lord of the universe in his true splendor, and it was a sublime, horrifying, awe-full sight. His whiskers stood on end, and a thrill of fright trickled down his spine. He saw a great gaping maw with armies flying toward blood-stained fangs. He saw his cousins' broken bodies crushed in the mighty jaws of death. He saw whole planets being consumed, stars being extinguished. The universe itself was being constantly devoured and then vomited forth again. The vision was too much, and with a soft cry, he asked for mercy. Krishna removed the sight and appeared before Arjuna as the average man: completely normal and unremarkable in every way, save for the fact that his skin was a lovely dark blue. Arjuna's old dear friend was back once more.

"Arjuna, I come whenever the law of universe is diminished. When dharma falters, I create myself in a bodily form. He who knows me is free to abandon his own form and, coming to me, is never reborn again. It is impossible, dear friend, to relinquish actions, for even the decision to not act is an act. It is only possible to relinquish desire. Give up any desire and attachment, and do what must be done. It is better for a man to follow his own dharma poorly than to attempt to follow another's dharma well. Arjuna, you must take up your bow and live your life as you are meant to live it."

Arjuna, the perfect warrior, finally understood. "My confusion is gone, thanks to you, Krishna. All uncertainty is banished. I am resolved once more, and I will do your bidding."

ॐ ৯

Krishna, the avatar of the great creator god Vishnu who had come to lead mankind through the chaos of the age, teaches Arjuna the law of dharma: You are born to your role in life – do that! There is no room here for "I want." Your bliss is found in surrendering your whole life to the will of God. God revealed himself to Arjuna, and Arjuna bowed under the revelation.

The Bhagavad Gita, compiled somewhere around the time of Jesus Christ, is rich in metaphors and allegories and was considered by the enlightened thinkers of the 19th century to be the most sublime text of all time. Thoreau and Emerson referred to it constantly. Mahatma Gandhi called it his mother.

Despite this high praise, the metaphor of a war, even a just war, is today a tough one to relate to. Many women find that the medium of the story, war and violence, does not sing to them, but the conflict between action and inaction, of doing what you ought to do and what you want to do, is clear. This mythic story definitively tells us to act as we must, as society commands us to, and not to worry about the consequences of our actions. As long as our motives are just, the means will justify the ends.

✳ ✳ ✳

THE STORY OF JOB

Compare the teaching of Arjuna by Krishna to the lesson God taught Job in the Old Testament.

❧ ❧

God and his boys were hanging around one day when Satan happened to stroll by. God hailed Satan: "Hey, Luci, where have you been? Haven't seen you around for a while."

Satan replied, "You know, I've been down on earth walking about, seeing the sights."

God knew all right. "Did you come across my man Job? Isn't he something? He is just perfect: He adores me and always behaves himself."

Satan smiled to himself, sensing a chance at some mischief. "Well, sure I know Job. He's the guy you gave seven sons to, a few daughters, thousands of camels, goats, cows. He is a rich man, no wonder he loves you—who wouldn't? I bet if you took away all those good things, he would end up cursing your name."

God said, "I'll take that bet! You go on down there and do your worst, but Luci … don't do anything to Job. You'll see. He'll still love me even after you're done."

Satan got to work. That night, when all the sons and daughters of Job were having dinner together at the eldest brother's home, the house was destroyed by a great wind. Everyone died. While Job was being given the terrible news, another messenger came and told him that raiders from several tribes had come and stolen all his camels, cows and goats and killed all the servants who were guarding and tending the animals. Job in anguish tore his clothes and collapsed to the earth in tears.

Job's wife consoled her husband, "Cursed be God! How could He have done such wickedness to you—you, who have always been so upright and devout?"

Job would have none of his wife's negativity. "Naked came I out of my mother's womb. I had nothing. All that I had came from God, so why should I detest Him if He should decide to take it all back. No! I still praise and worship God; the Lord giveth and the Lord taketh away." Despite the tragedy, Job was still sinless and perfect.

A few days later, God and the sons of God were again basking in glory when Satan stopped by for another visit. God had a big smile on his face. "Hey, Luci! See, I told you! Job is great, isn't he? Look at what you did to him, and still he worships me."

Satan was not pleased with having lost the first bet, and he decided to up the stakes a bit. "Well, of course he still loves you—you wouldn't let me touch him directly. Give him cancer, hemorrhoids and bad breath, and then he will curse you to your face!"

God took this bet, too. "Do your worst ... but just don't kill him. You'll see!"

Job, bereft of sons, daughters and all belongings, now fell sick. Satan, in the presence of God who watched everything, inflicted painful boils over Job's whole body. He was in agony and his body wasted away. His wife again spoke out against God, but Job shut her up: "What?

Should we only receive good from the Lord?" Throughout his whole ordeal, Job never once sinned or spoke against God.

Now, Job had many friends, and some of them came to him in his time of suffering to comfort him. As they sat around commiserating over Job's turn of fortune, they made several astute observations. "Boy, you sure must have pissed God off! What sin did you commit to be punished so severely?"

Job resented their insinuations. "No! I have not sinned. I have always been righteous and loved God."

"No way! God only punishes the wicked. Evil never befalls the just. You have been punished; therefore, you must be wicked!"

"Not so! I have only ever been good. God knows that I have always treated people fairly: I have looked after the poor and the widowed; I have given sage counsel to kings and princes; I have treated my slaves and animals kindly; I have spoken ill of no man or of God; I have not deserved this fate, but now that this fate is upon me, I wish that I had never been born."

Job's comforters were not convinced. "How can puny little you know the mind of God? He is the greatest mystery of all. You say you have not sinned, but God is ever fair and righteous and knows your sins, even if you do not admit to them. You are sinning now by saying that He was wrong to have punished you. How dare you say such a thing!"

Job argued with his comforters, whom he called friends no longer since they would not see his point of view. They were equally obstinate in insisting on the fact that he must have been guilty of something for God to treat him so harshly. In frustration, Job called on God Himself to be witness to his innocence; and in a whirlwind, the Lord appeared before Job.

Now, did God say "Hey, Job, you've been just great! You know the devil and I, we made this bet, you see, and you helped me win"? No. Did God try to explain himself and rationalize his actions? No.

Instead, God said unto Job, "Who do you think you are? You are trying to understand me? Did you create the heavens and the earth? Do you cause the sun to rise every morning? Can you speak in a voice of thunder? Could you catch the Leviathan on a hook or fill his head with harpoons? I can! I did all these things, not you. Who are you to even pretend to understand My ways?"

Job fell to the earth and cried, "I know that you can do everything and no thoughts can be hidden from you. I have heard You with my ears, and now I see You with my eyes, and I am ashamed. I despise myself and will cover myself with ashes."

"That's better," said God, "I will restore you!"

And God did. Unto Job was given seven new sons, three more daughters, twice as many animals and belongings as before, and he lived to see four generations of grandchildren. Job, that perfect man, eventually died of very old age.

⊰ ⊱

Joseph Campbell often referred to this story as a key example of the Levantine view of man's relationship to God.[3] Like Arjuna, Job was humbled by God and learned to accept the will of the most powerful being in the universe. Is it fair and just what God did to poor old Job? That is not a consideration! It is not up to Job, or Arjuna, to wonder about whether the situation they find themselves in is fair or just. Their role is to act regardless of their personal desire. This is the key teaching of the East: You're put here on this earth to *obey*! The creator of the universe has set down the rules of life and of society, and who are you to quibble with them? Dharma trumps kama and artha. If you wish to find pleasure or

214

achievement, you must find them within the fulfillment of the great plan of life. Give yourself up to God, king and country, and you will be rewarded—not in this life perhaps, but in the time to come beyond this existence.

＊ ＊ ＊

PROMETHEUS BOUND

The philosophy of doing your duty and bowing down to gods even when they are not just is not the philosophy of the early Westerners. Northern Europe 2,000 years ago was mostly a hunting-based economy; the prowess of the individual remained important to the survival of the tribe. Not everyone can hunt successfully. Not everyone can protect the tribe in battle from raiders and warring neighbors. Individual accomplishment was required and highly valued in the nonagrarian lifestyle of early Europe. This tendency toward honoring the individual is reflected in the Greek myths. From Achilles in the *Iliad* to Odysseus in the *Odyssey*, the Greek heroes followed their own path. It was not dharma that tugged the Greeks this way and that, but the Fates. The story of Prometheus is a good illustration of the Western drive of the individual that is missing in the East.

☙ ❧

Prometheus, he who foresees the future and knows the Fates, takes earth and water and fashions a new race of man, but man will not stand without something more. So Prometheus adds his own tears and bids the goddess Athena to breathe life and soul into the creatures. The latest race of man replaces the earlier race that Zeus, in his displeasure, swept away with a gigantic flood.

This was not the first time Prometheus showed favor to men. When Zeus sat down with the earliest race of man to determine the allotment of sacrifice, it was given to Prometheus to apportion the sacrificed animals. The cunning Prometheus hid the bones and sinews beneath an attractive layer of fat, and within the hide, horns and hoofs he hid the choicest flesh and healthy organs. Was Zeus deceived by the trick, or did he know he had to choose that which looked most pleasing despite the inedible bones hidden within? In either case, the choice was made, and forevermore the gods were to be given the lesser parts, while men kept to themselves the meat of the sacrifice. For this deception the gods hated Prometheus, and Zeus, in particular, was greatly angered.

To punish mankind, though they played no role in the lie and were blameless, Zeus withdrew fire from their presence. Prometheus would not let man suffer, so he crept to the forge of Hephaestus and stole a faggot of flame, thereby restoring holy fire to mankind once more. This was not all Prometheus gave to man. He found them witless and gave them wit. It was he who gave them knowledge. He taught men how to read the stars, to count and write, to domesticate cattle and yoke the horse to a chariot, to build and sail ships upon the seas, to drag from the earth ores and to refine them into metals, to know the ways of omens and to cure ill health. Prometheus also gave to mankind his greatest gift: civilization.

Farseeing Prometheus knew that Zeus planned revenge. He warned his brother, Epimetheus, the master of hindsight, to never accept any gift from Zeus. But Zeus was cunning, and he ordered Hephaestus to fashion from clay and water a woman—the very first woman. The gods showered the first human woman with seductive gifts, so she was named Pandora, the all-giving. Athena gave her clothes, grace and skills in weaving and other crafts. Aphrodite gave her irresistible beauty, but also cares and worries along with a cruel longing. Hermes gave her a deceitful nature and put lies in Pandora's mouth. Completed, Zeus sent Pandora to Epimetheus, who, despite his brother's warning, could not refuse the enchantress.

To ensure that mankind would be forever troubled and never live in peace, Zeus sent along with the beautiful evil a little something extra. In his palace he kept two jars: One wherein all good things were found, and another wherein all evil was kept. In prior times Zeus would decide when to let out a little grief and when to release a little relief. The first jar, a second womb, he gave to Pandora without telling her what was inside. All he would tell her was to never open the jar. However, the curiosity of a woman is insatiable and dangerous; so of course, Pandora opened her new womb. All the ills that bedevil mankind flowed forth: death, sickness, old age, pain, poverty, toil and troubles ... all these were inflicted on us, thanks to a woman, thanks to the first woman. While Pandora sat and watched these troubles flow out of her jar, she did nothing. Finally, she stirred and sealed the jar with but one final thing remaining inside: hope. Only hope remained within the jar. Is this a kindness at last by Pandora? Or did she withhold from us the one thing that would make all suffering bearable? Where is hope?

Hope is not something Prometheus needs, for he knows what the future holds. He knew full well that in helping mankind become smarter, stronger and civilized, he would personally pay a price. Zeus bade Hephaestus to fashion unbreakable chains and nail Prometheus, for his punishment, to a mountain far from the civilized world. No man would ever visit poor Prometheus, bound upon the bones of a remote mountain. Each day Zeus sent his heavenly bird to feast upon Prometheus' liver. Each night Prometheus' liver grew back so that the eagle could feast anew the next day.

A chorus of friends came to comfort Prometheus. Prometheus cried out against the injustice of Zeus, but justice is a human virtue. The gods are not bound to be just. Power serves its own ends. Hermes, the mouthpiece of Zeus, also visited and tried to reason with Prometheus: "If you wish to be free, just tell Zeus that you are sorry!

He will let you go. He wants to let you go—just admit to your guilt, and you will be released."

Defiantly, Prometheus replied, "I care less than nothing for Zeus! Let him do as he likes."

Prometheus would not bow down to the will of an unjust tyrant. Prometheus knew that Zeus will have need of him one day. The gods are not so powerful that they can exist without others. Freedom will come in time.

꒰ ꒱

Prometheus was a Titan, a god. Unlike his fellow Titans, he did not go to war with Zeus, and thus was spared when the regime changed. While he was not mortal like us, Prometheus came to represent the spirit of mankind. His defiance of the most powerful god in the universe is a model for the Western man. We are not here to merely obey the powers that be; we can challenge them! We can act on our own, for our own reasons. But we must be very careful!

The myth of Prometheus has many versions, some quite contradictory, but there is much we can extract from it. The depiction of women through the rendering of Pandora we will leave for now, but we will return to it later. The trick that Prometheus plays on Zeus with the division of the sacrifice can be seen as aetiology for the practice of sacrifice. Some scholars believe that we developed sacrifice as a way to ameliorate our guilt for killing another living creature. Of course, it would not help us survive if we burnt the best part of the animal, so we needed a good story to explain why we give to the gods the worst parts.[4] It is also interesting to investigate why the myth shows that mankind's progress and movement toward civilization should be against the express wishes of the gods. Why does Zeus oppose our self-improvements? It is clear that the gods and man are not in sync here.

In Greece, around the 5th century B.C.E., philosophers like Socrates and Plato were rethinking the relationship of man to the world around them. Did we have to live in thrall to the powers that manifest in the universe, or could man himself take control over his own fate? This was a time of tyrants ruling over the great Greek city-states, and most of these powerful rulers were not kind to their subjects. Their behavior was cruel; their reigns illegitimate. The myth of Prometheus, especially in the hands of the poet, Aeschylus, was a seditious teaching and showed that man does not have to yield to those in power. Power could and should be opposed when it was unjust.

We can't just leave poor Prometheus hanging; we need to finish the story. Prometheus, eventually, was freed from his suffering by none other than Zeus' son Heracles (or Hercules, as he was called by the Romans and more commonly known in the West). Heracles just happened to pass by while on his way to complete some of his fabled 12 labors, and he severed Prometheus' chains. Zeus permitted this because he really did need Prometheus. Prometheus, who could see the future, had a secret: He knew what would destroy Zeus. Zeus really wanted to hear this secret, but.Prometheus refused to tell while he was bound. Zeus tried to wait him out but eventually had to ask, "What do you know?" Once freed, Prometheus told Zeus that a nymph named Thetis would bear a son greater than his father. This was good for Zeus to know because he had been lusting after Thetis, but knowing this prediction, he restrained himself. Thetis eventually married Peleus, and her son was the famed Achilles, the great hero of the *Iliad*. Achilles indeed was greater than his father, Peleus, and again we see the difference between men and gods: men want their sons to be better than them; the gods fear this.

❋ ❋ ❋

THE HERO

There are many examples in Greek and Roman mythology of men challenging the gods and oft times succeeding. Jason had killed his girlfriend's brother, annoying Zeus so much that he tried to blow Jason's boat, the Argo, off course. When this happened, the boat itself gave Jason directions. Odysseus safely returned home again despite run-ins with Poseidon and the sun god, Helios. Theseus slew a demigod, the Minotaur, living at the heart of King Minos' labyrinth. Heracles got the best of the god Atlas when he tricked Atlas into taking back the sky and bearing it on his own shoulders. For the ladies, Psyche defied Aphrodite and married her son, Eros. In Europe, individual initiative was valued; these heroes used guile, trickery, bravery and assistance from other gods to accomplish their great deeds. No Indian or Hebrew would even consider standing up to their gods in this way.

The fact that heroes exist at all is remarkable and very European. There are very few examples of a true human hero in the East. In the West, a hero was defined in many ways: He could be the offspring of a god and a mortal woman (or occasionally from the joining of a goddess and a mortal man); the hero could be a revered dead person to whom sacrifices were offered; a hero could be the savior of a city; a hero could be someone who may have lived in the remote past and participated in some great event, such as the Trojan War. A hero was someone who resisted the way of the world and succeeded in his quest. To the Greeks, and this is a bit unusual for our modern sensibilities, the hero was not always a great moral person; even Heracles, the greatest hero of all time, was a scoundrel and severely flawed. Heracles killed all his children by his first wife, Megara, and some stories claimed he killed her, too. These mortal heroes possessed the best and the worst traits of mankind; they had dark shadows in their unconscious landscapes and flaws that help us relate to them.

Thomas Mann wrote that what makes someone lovable are their faults.[5] A perfect man is boring: We can't relate to him. The hero must have his weaknesses or there is no story. Imagine Superman without his weakness to kryptonite or Batman without his dark side—uninteresting! The Greek heroes had huge unconscious shadows; they were brutish and violent, yet noble and caring. Reading their stories makes one want to reach into the pages and give them a shake, to rattle some common sense into them. But, they are precisely like us, with all of our inherent contradictions, shadow and light. We do not grow so frustrated and fascinated with characters found in the Eastern myths, because they are not like us, and it is difficult for Westerners to relate to them or to care about them. The heroes of the Greeks, Celts and Germans reverberate through Western culture to the present day, but there are very few instances in the Near East or Far East of stories that exalt mankind. Most stories there talk of the works of gods, not men.

We love our heroes, and their flaws make them even more lovable. Supermarket tabloids thrive on the human mistakes made by celebrities—what kind of love is this? When Tiger Woods was on top of the world, people adored his talent and achievements, but when he fell from grace, did people love him less? It would seem so on the surface, but people still love to talk about fallen heroes, thus the attraction is still there. One measure of love is the amount of energy one pours out toward another. This is illustrated in a surprising little story:

⊰ ⊱

The man was crazy, a lunatic possessed by a single thought. He spent his nights in the forest, but during the day he would wander through the village yelling about how bad and evil Shiva was. He absolutely loathed Shiva with every fiber of his being, and if anyone made any eye contact with the madman, they were soon sorry. The maniac would regale the unfortunate soul with all the reasons why everyone should hate Shiva. At first, the most senior Brahmin of the village tried to reason with the deluded derelict. He eventually gave up: The man was consumed by hatred and would not talk about anything else but Shiva. Everyone learned to ignore him, and in time he died alone in the forest.

It came to pass one day that the village Brahmin also left this world, and it was with great surprise that he found, there in heaven, sitting right beside Shiva, the crazy man from the forest. "Why?" he asked Shiva, "Why is that man here? He hated you so much when he was alive! How does he merit such honor now in death?"

Shiva replied, "This man thought of me constantly. I was always in his mind. Very few of my followers have so devoted their lives to me that they can think of nothing but me, as this man did. He truly earned his place beside me."

ॐ

Hating someone requires that you enter into a relationship with that person. If you are driven to read all about the weaknesses and mistakes of another person, perhaps a celebrity caught in a scandal, you are in love with that person. Those who claimed to be horrified by Tiger Wood's actions but still consumed avariciously all the stories of his misdeed were in love! Pick any celebrated hero who fell and revealed himself to be human, and you will find people still interested in hearing more about him. They crave the sordid details. This investment of energy is an aspect of love. Wherever your energy goes, whatever you are passionate about—that is what you love.

✳ ✳ ✳

Gods, in the European mindset, were to be handled with great care, were to be propitiated and cajoled into being helpful, but they were not worshipped as examples of great morality. While Zeus and Athena were the gods responsible for justice, this was not justice between man and the gods, only justice between men. The gods were free to treat mankind as unjustly as they wished, just as the Old Testament God had treated Job. Remember, the Babylonian god Marduk created men to be servants of the gods, and the God of Genesis likewise created Adam to tend his garden. Men were here solely to serve the gods.

When the early Christians came into Europe, they brought with them the Levantine ideals of surrender to God, of "Obey!" With the early Christian philosophy taking root in the West, a new way was being foisted upon the Western psyche: total submission to God despite any injustice that may be inflicted by God's church or by God Himself. A dissonance was created in the mind of Europeans that never occurred in the East. A choice had to be made: Do you live in God's world or man's world? Whom do you serve? For almost a thousand years, the Church of Christ sought to bury the Greek and Roman urge for independent thought and action. By the 10th century, the Church overcame the Germanic and Celtic lands as well, again subduing the individualism that was native to those cultures. These have been called the dark ages; the science and philosophy of the Greeks and Romans were lost to Europe, and along with them their myths. At the end of the fourth century, the Roman Emperor Theodosius I (347–395 C.E.) encouraged Christians to smash and desecrate all temples and sanctuaries dedicated to the old gods, in exactly the same way that the Taliban destroyed the symbols of Buddhism in Afghanistan in the 20th century.

While Europe was slipping into darkness, the Islamic empire was discovering the scientific and philosophic legacies of Greece and Rome. It was from Moslem Spain and Sicily that the teachings of the Greeks came back into Europe. This was happening in the 11th and 12th centuries and coincided with the rise of the courtly knight-errant, who, seeking to elevate the noblest part of man, rebelled against the proscribed forms of life dictated by society and the church. The knights were the re-incarnation of the earlier European ideal of the individual acting out of his own center: Heroes were riding once again.

✳ ✳ ✳

When you are told what to think, whom to marry, what you must profess as your beliefs; when you are given a job you haven't earned simply because you were born into a certain family, you are leading an inauthentic life. The whole world becomes one vast wasteland, reflecting the inner sterility of your own psychic landscape. This is the state of life and land in the time of Parzival and the knights of King Arthur. It is now time to check in and see what has been happening to Parzival. When we last left him, he had just gotten married, but his was not a marriage sanctioned by the Church.

⊰ ⊱

Parzival was tired and discomforted; there was nowhere to stop for the night. He dropped the reins and allowed the horse to decide where to go. He was taken to a small lake. A man in a boat was quietly fishing. Parzival hailed the fisher and enquired where he might find lodging.

The man first replied, "There is nothing for you around here." But then the man looked more closely at Parzival and corrected himself. "Well, if you follow the trail just a little bit more, cross the bridge and turn left, you will come to a castle. There you will find what you seek."

Parzival had spent two lovely years with his new bride, Condwiramurs, and she had given him two sons. Parzival had met and passed the trials of youth, but the secular bliss he had found could not fill the spiritual hole that now yawned: He got to wondering about his mother. Obtaining Condwiramurs' permission, he returned home, only to discover that his mother had passed away on the day he had left her. In a daze he began wandering, which always leads to adventure, and which led in due course to the lake with the fisherman.

Doing as bid, Parzival followed the trail and took the left-hand path. He found the castle and was warmly greeted. At dinner he witnessed a very strange procession: In the place of honor was the fisherman, but he was the king, and he was borne upon a litter. He was dressed regally but sighed continuously; he could find no comfort sitting, standing or lying down. The Fisher King's name was Anfortas—the one without fortitude or favor, the weakened one. Parzival was not to hear Anfortas' story until much later in life. If only he had asked now! Oh, how the moans of the king stirred him to compassion, but he was a trained knight, a perfect knight, and a knight must never ask questions—that is what his teacher Gurnemanz had taught him. Good soldiers hold their peace and speak only through action.

The procession of sorrow had at its heart a source of great joy, if only it could be released. Twenty-four beautiful maidens came forth, set up the dinner tables, and set wonderful lights at each station. Next came a young man holding a bloodstained lance; following him came the most beautiful and chaste woman Parzival had ever seen, the virgin Queen Repanse de Schoye. In her hands she bore paradise, both root and branch: the Grail that the whole company of Arthur's knights was seeking. Everyone who beheld the Grail was healed and made whole—everyone, save the queen's brother who was the Fisher King. Anfortas could gain no comfort from the Grail, and out of the stricken king's sickness, the whole kingdom was laid barren and bereft of joy.

Parzival held his peace and asked no questions that night. The king, seeing greatness in the young knight but saddened that he would not ask the saving question, gave Parzival a sword: a beautiful but flawed blade that would fail Parzival at a critical moment. Despite their disappointment, all the guests of the banquet treated Parzival courteously, as well-bred lords and ladies do, and in due course he was shown to his bed. When he awoke the next morning, there was no one around; he had to dress himself and make his own way out of the castle. The drawbridge snapped shut as he left, clipping the rear hoofs of his horse. A hidden page who was lowering the bridge shouted at Parzival as he left, "May the sun hate you for what you haven't done. You are a goose!"

Without realization or intent, Parzival had found the Grail Castle, had beheld the Grail itself, but because he was moved to follow proper social customs, to ask no questions, the grace shown to him was withdrawn. He could have healed the king and brought life back to the land with but one soul-felt question, but he failed. He was humiliated and humbled. Whenever he related this tale, he was met with scorn and derision. He came to hate God for the cruel treatment meted out to him, but he continued his spiritual quest. For five years he wandered, trying to find the castle once more.

One day he came to a hermitage where he was kindly greeted, at first. The hermit asked his quest and Parzival related his sad story. The hermit set him straight: None may find the castle twice! The hermit was Anfortas' brother, who had turned away from a life of privilege to seek his own salvation in the woods. He told Parzival how the Fisher King came by his wound. When he was young, not yet having proved himself worthy to be king and rule, he brashly went forth on adventures. On this particular day, however, he met a pagan knight from the East. Without a word the two began to joust, as is the manner of knights. Anfortas unhorsed and killed the Saracen but in turn was struck in the creative organ and emasculated. A piece of the lance still remained in the thigh of the castrated king. He lives now in great agony; the only peace he finds is when he is fishing. He waits in his Castle of the Grail for a hero to come and free him from his suffering: All the hero need ask is the question, "What ails you?" Part of the Fisher King's curse is that he cannot prompt any visitor to ask the question; it has to come spontaneously from a pure heart. Parzival had his chance but failed. The hermit cursed and sent Parzival away. Before leaving, Parzival vowed to find the castle again and right his wrong, despite the prophecy that no one gets a second chance.

Of course Parzival was still a great knight! The greatest in the land. His service to King Arthur gained him high standing. One day there was a grand feast commissioned by Arthur, where many knights and maidens were to be joined in marriage. It was the social event of the century. Parzival was reminded of his own good wife, Condwiramurs, whom he had not seen in many years. He could not bear to be in the presence of such joy and love without her, and with a heavy heart left the celebration. Riding away from the pavilions, he came across a knight with strange, unknown banners. Seeing each other they immediately began to fight.

Unknown to each other, the two knights were brothers! Parzival's father, while journeying to the East, had won a queen and with her sired a son: Feirefez, now the king of Zazamanc. Here fought two men, the Christian who doubted and cursed God and the Muslim who had come in search of his earthly father. You could say they were two fighting, but they had the same father and were actually one. In ignorance of their true nature, they were doing each other grievous harm. At the telling moment of the battle, Parzival had an opening; he brought his beautiful blade down on Feirefez' head, but the blade failed and shattered. Parzival was now at the disadvantage and had no weapon. Noble Feirefez could not strike an unarmed knight, so he bade Parzival to pause. They sat down to talk, and in sharing their stories they discovered their common blood. With Feirefez' helmet off, Parzival noticed his brother's unique complexion: His skin was mottled with patches of both black and white.

"There is a great party happening just over that hill," mentioned Parzival, "and I suspect you have a bit of an eye for the ladies. You won't be disappointed, and neither shall they, I venture. Are you up for some celebrating?"

"It is a day of great joy—I have found my brother. Let's go drink and perhaps take a look at these ladies you speak of."

The brothers joined the party, where Feirefez, as Parzival suspected, was the center of attraction. Ladies were not the only ones interested in him: The knight's demeanor and skill also impressed King Arthur. In the midst of the celebration, a herald of the Grail Castle came up to Parzival and invited him and his brother to visit the Fisher King once more. Feirefez eagerly agreed, mostly because of Parzival's description of the beauty of the Grail maidens. Feirefez was not disappointed. When the brothers came to the castle, the same procession that Parzival had witnessed earlier was re-enacted: Grail maidens with lights, the squire with the lance, and then the Grail Queen. When the virgin arrived, Feirefez was lost in love.

Parzival, eager for redemption, asked the question, "Dear king, what ails you?" Immediately Anfortas was healed— no answer was necessary.

Anfortas' brother, the hermit, was in attendance and admitted to Parzival, "This is indeed amazing! Through your own strength of will, loyalty and compassion, you have changed God's law."

With his health restored, Anfortas awarded his crown and his kingdom to Parzival. Condwiramurs joined him, and together they reigned over the Grail Castle and raised a noble family in a now prosperous land.

But what of Feirefez? He alone of the hosts that day could not see the Grail in the hands of his beloved, for he was a heathen. The remedy was clear: Before he could see the Grail, and, more importantly, before he could wed Repanse de Schoye, he had to be baptized. His cooperation was easily attained. He simply asked, "Is that her god? Then, He will be my god, too!"

By the grace of the Grail, he was baptized, wed to the virgin queen, and they returned to reign over his kingdom in India.

⚜ ⚜

This version of the Grail legend was written by an actual knight, the knight we mentioned earlier: Wolfram von Eschenbach. His view of what was happening to European society in the 13th century was quite different than the views of the monks who wrote their own versions of the quest for the Grail. Cistercian monks also documented the myth of the Grail and described it as being the cup of the last supper, brought to Britain by Joseph Arimathea. For them the great hero of the quest was not Parzival but Galahad, which in Hebrew is Gilead, which means pure or noble—a perfect name for a Christian hero. In von Eschenbach's hands, however, the Grail was not a cup, but a stone brought from heaven to earth by the neutral angels. Who are the neutral angels? That is another story, this time one from von Eschenbach's greatly admired pagans.[6]

⚜ ⚜

Satan's great sin was not that he didn't love God, but that he loved God too much. When God created the angels, he commanded them to love Him with all their being, and none loved God more than Satan. Later God created man and felt man to be the best thing he had ever made. He

229

commanded the angels now to bow down and serve man as well. This Satan could not do; his love for God was so powerful, he could find no room in his heart for anything else. For this disobedience God banished Satan from his sight. Satan was thrown out of heaven, and he landed in a place where there could be no sight of his beloved. This is hell, the place where there is no hope of ever seeing that which you love above all else.

In the struggle that culminated in Satan's expulsion, many angels fought on the side of God, and other angels fought for Satan, but there were some angels that refused to take sides. These were the neutral angels, and they were the ones who brought to earth the Grail made of stone. This wonderful stone, shining green, was shaped like a shallow bowl and was heavier than gold and yet lighter than a feather.Whatever one wished for, the Grail could grant. For the neutral angels, their one lack was humility, and this the Grail gave them. Once cured by the grace of the Grail, they were called back to heaven, leaving the precious stone behind, in the hands of a noble family.

⊰ ⊱

Like the neutral angels, it was humility that Parzival needed to learn. Once he could accept that his pride would never reopen the path to the Grail castle, once he accepted defeat at the hand of his elder brother, he was eligible to be summoned back to the castle. But von Eschenbach's use of the story of the neutral angels is telling on another level: The story of Parzival and the Fisher King is filled with opposites colliding. Parzival's own name speaks of finding the middle path: *perce à val* means "piercing the valley," going through the pairs of opposites.

In Parzival's story we find the theme of the Christian world colliding with the pagan Islamic world rendered twice: first, when Anfortas killed a Saracen and was terribly wounded in the battle—this, quite obviously, is not the way!—then second, when Parzival fought his own brother, Feirefez. As von Eschenbach explains, they were two sons of one father, just as Christianity and Islam are two sons of one father religion: Judaism. Feirefez' own complexion displayed this dual nature; his skin was black and white, showing he was a pagan but the son of a Christian king, and he eventually became baptized so he could marry a Christian queen. Once married, he headed back to rule his pagan land of India. Baptism did not remove the darkness of his skin. The duality remains.

Recall that it was Feirefez who called the truce that led to peace, but only after Parzival's blade broke. What a lesson we have here for us today! It is not by contending that peace is won; in the procession of the Grail at the Grail Castle, there was the lance, bloodied at the tip, and there was also the Grail carried by a pure virgin. Yielding to nature is the key action here. Letting go of the reins of the horse and trusting to the deepest layers of our unconscious mind to get us where we need to go. It is to our deepest nature that the story of Parzival is speaking.

Society and religion both dictate what we should do in life. Parzival went against church doctrine. He refused the traditional arranged marriage and married for love. This is the cry of the knight: "Amor not Roma!" (Through a telling quirk of language, these words are exact opposites in spelling, and to the knights, in meaning.) Parzival expressed his own individuality here, but he was still trapped by society's rules, and he could not bring himself to drop the duty of the knight when the occasion demanded. He was still young; we can see this happening today, as well. In our youth we go out and slay many dragons, which helps us win a maiden, and we settle into a comfortable, secular life. But the spiritual battles still await us. In middle age, the spiritual crisis comes upon us, and we are off again to face new battles, battles that cannot be won with the weapons of our youth. With the wisdom of age, we learn to drop the belief that we must do what society expects us to do, and we learn to act out of our own center. We act with humility, but also as Anfortas' brother, the hermit, said, "With tenacity and compassion, we are healed; and now—we may heal others."

Parzival journeys into the darkness of the psyche. At critical times we find the symbols of the unconscious guiding him: the waters of the lake, his horse deciding which direction to follow, turning left on the path to find the Grail Castle. Becoming whole is not something that we can do consciously, it requires both consciousness and the darkness within us. It requires fusing together the black and the white, like the meeting of the two brothers, one pagan and one Christian. Note an important point in the story: The question need only be asked, not answered! That is another function of the unconscious: The unconscious asks the questions; it is the conscious mind that attempts to answer. Don't worry about the answers—just allow the question to be asked! Life is not a puzzle to be solved, but lived.

It is also telling that the Grail Castle is not a church; there are no priests presiding over the procession. There is the lance, very masculine and dangerous, and there is the virgin, very feminine and alluring. We find ritual here, but there are no Brahmins or clergy doing the work for us. We have to choose to act in order to receive the benefit. When you allow others to act for you, when the rituals are watched and not performed, you are living in the wasteland. The life you are living is not your life.

Does it really make sense, the myth that people in that time were living under, and many live under today? You are born guilty of a sin that someone else committed; you are saved by the action of someone else, as well. Adam condemns us by his disobedience to the Boss; Jesus redeems us through his sacrifice on the cross. What is your role in any of this? To quietly acquiesce and just watch it all unfold? This is simply doing as you are told and believing what you are told. This is dharma, not moksha. This is not the European spirit of the Greeks, Celts and Germans. This is what Parzival's story exposes to us: To live an authentic life, we have to go out and live that life ourselves.

✳ ✳ ✳

While mythologist Joseph Campbell loved to tell the story, Parzival's story is literature, not myth; but the sources von Eschenbach drew from did come from old myths. The themes found in all the King Arthur legends and the various quests for the Holy Grail are from ancient Celtic myths and hearken back to the earlier days of European culture, before the influence of Christianity.[7]

The symbol of Parzival as a hero acting out of his own uniqueness is a continuation of a powerful Western meme. We have seen it in the ancient Greek myths, and we have now seen its attempt to flower in medieval Europe. The rights of the individual versus the rights of the state and church was a struggle that continues right up to the present day. As a reaction to the outbreak of thinking exhibited by Wolfram von Eschenbach and other radicals of the day, the Catholic Church created the most feared instrument of repression ever seen: the Inquisition. The heresy of the knights-errant was wiped out, along with the whole idea that one could marry for love.

Carl Jung has noted that what we resist persists. The ideal of the individual would not be suppressed for all time; it kept resurfacing in other guises. The rugged individualist ran out of room in Europe, so he went to the high seas and new continents; the great captain explorers were masters of their own fate. In the New World, they became the scouts of new lands, rivers and mountains. In the American West, they were personified as the cowboys who herded cattle across the plains. In the 1950s they were the beats; in the 60s, the Hippie. Countercultural, against "the man," raging against the machine—they are Prometheus, the spirit of the ancient Greek hero who did not meekly accept the will of church, state or even God himself.

Prometheus is still alive and well today; in fact, he is honored as a cultural icon. Jack Kerouac, James Dean, Martin Luther King Junior, Abby Hoffman, Rosie Parks ... the list can go on for a long, long time. The 1960s were filled with this lunge toward individual freedom and civil rights. In America, young people refused to go to Vietnam, not out of cowardice, but because it was unjust to do so. They were publicly saying, "No! I won't lay down my life for my country, because my country is wrong!" The heroes of the '60s were real-life people who touched the need deep in our psyche for individual freedom. In the movies, the medium where many of our modern myths now are presented, we watched Rick Deckard in *Blade Runner* and Jason Bourne in *The Bourne Conspiracy* fighting for their right to be free from the machinery of society. This is exactly what Luke Skywalker is fighting for in *Star Wars*. Movie producers show this to us time and again because this is what we resonate with: It is what sells. Dire Straits' song, "Skateaway", touches this meme from the feminine point of view and with exactly the same theme of individual freedom.

This individualism swelled into the 1970s when the counterreaction set in. All societies are inherently conservative, and they all have their version of the Inquisition to keep things in order. Dharma has been served under many names, from the FBI to the Gestapo, as societies create organizations that ensure the status remains quo. Do you remember the movie *Easy Rider*? Here again are our mythic heroes striving for individual freedom, but here also is shown the machine fighting back and winning. The story describes two bikers travelling through the southern United States, living life large and on the road. Those who have to stay at home do not appreciate the freedom the heroes have taken hold of, and at the end of the movie, the heroes are shot off their bikes and killed. Society will still react to protect itself if the pursuit of freedom goes too far. The Empire does strike back. It is fine to resonate with characters in a movie or read a myth of freedom, but don't try to actually become truly free. That is too much. Remember, not everyone can head to the forest: Society would collapse.

Once again, recall President John F. Kennedy's inaugural address in 1961: "Ask not what your country can do for you, ask what you can do for your country." This is exactly what society and church have been asking of you since the dawn of civilization. Without this cooperation from the members of society, society would collapse. Freedom—yes, but never total freedom. Better to think you are free but act as society requires. So, in our Western society today, we have the myth of freedom, the spirit of individuality, but not the absolute fact of freedom. It can never be that we are both absolutely free and still a functioning member of society. To be totally free, as reflected in the Eastern concept of moksha, one must leave society altogether.

This is our choice and our dilemma in the West today: Do we live in God's city, the state's city or man's city? For many, we have diminished the religious imperative to only one hour every Sunday, if even that, but there are still the tremendous obligations of society to meet. We must be productive, consume, think for ourselves, but we shouldn't go overboard and think that we are truly free. Many of our great movie myths show us this compromise. James Bond can flout all the rules, but in the end he still works for Mother and, in his own way, serves justice, Queen and country. Hans Solo gave up his selfishness and independence and fought for the common cause. It is not easy to stay outside of society, and at the end of the day, is that what you really want?

The modern Western myths, being a fusion of European and Middle Eastern symbols, present a confusing image. It is good to be an individual and decide what you want to do with your life, who you will marry, what job you will have. This level of freedom has never existed before. Advertisers play on this by telling us to buy a certain product or service so that we can be unique. We love to be unique and have our own style. But how can one million people buying the same deodorant be unique? It is a pretense, and it works, to a degree. Jung points out that we don't need to be a unique individual in society, but we do need to be individuated—we need to be whole people, not part people. Joseph Campbell suggested that we determine where our bliss is and follow it; that path may well be solidly inside society, as Indra's guru, Brihaspati, insisted. Early Buddhism taught that one had to leave the household and shake off its dust. The later Mahayana Buddhist teachings, however, allowed us to stay inside secular life and still seek enlightenment. We have several maps we could choose today, but the primary maps still lead us back to society. Time again for our question: Which map is leading you?

Chapter 12: Myths for Women

Gone to Greece! Back in two weeks. — Shirley Valentine

※ ❧

"That man! He is just infuriating and never listens. I am ashamed to call him my father. Why did I ever choose him?" Sati turned to the fire and hid her face from the party. She is embarrassed now to be here: Shiva was right. It was a mistake. It has all been a mistake. The fire, though … the fire can wipe clean everything. It is a holy fire after all—the mouth of the gods, the doorway to the next world and to a new life.

The day began idyllically; Shiva and Sati had just ended their yearlong embrace. She felt fulfilled and warm lying beside her god, recalling the years she spent trying to win his heart. It was not easy getting Shiva's attention. Life was now perfect, almost.

Daksha was the great creator of life. Shiva had been asked to populate the new earth, but he elected to go meditate, instead. In Shiva's absence, Brahma turned to the high priest of the gods, and the job of procreation was given to Daksha. Life comes from women, so Daksha chose to create daughters—lots of daughters, dozens of them. The youngest was beautiful Sati.

Daksha's daughters were given to various gods: Dharma took a baker's dozen; 27 were given to Chandra, the moon; others went to sages and yogis; and to Agni, the holy fire, was given Swaha. Sati (why is the youngest one always so difficult?) would accept no husband save Shiva. He alone she worshipped, and he alone her father despised.

Shiva finally ended his meditation, ready to fulfill the request to populate the universe, but he was surprised to

237

see that Daksha had beaten him to it. Feeling a bit miffed, he decided to retreat back into meditation. Sati, however, had other plans. It is not easy to woo the greatest god in the universe: First she had to get him to notice her. If Shiva was the greatest ascetic and meditator, then she would outdo him. She left the palace and the life of luxury and headed to the forest.

Sati spent her years in increasing mortifications. She wore only rags and renounced food, surviving solely on one small leaf of a stone apple tree each day; then she stopped eating entirely. Finally Shiva noticed, took Sati as his bride, and brought her to his palace on Kailash, the holy mountain high in the Tibetan Himalayas. Here she spent her days in bliss with her husband, and life would have been perfect, if only she didn't have to visit her family every once in a while.

Later that afternoon Sati noticed many people walking by their palace, all dressed up for a party. She asked Shiva, "Where is everyone going?"

Shiva, of course, knew, because he knew everything. "Your father is conducting a great sacrifice tonight. Everyone was invited."

"I was not invited! How can you say everyone was invited, but we weren't?" said Sati.

"It OK; you know your father and I don't get along," came the reply. "And it's just as well. It will be nice to just stay home tonight and watch the stars."

"It's not OK. I am his daughter, and I am offended that he didn't at least invite me. I am going to go to the party and tell him so!"

"Don't go!" warned Shiva. "You know what a temper you have; you'll just get angry and nothing good can come of it."

"You can't talk me out of it. I am just as stubborn as you. I am going."

Shiva had misgivings but had to relent. "OK, but if you are going, take Nandi with you."

This Sati was agreeable to. She mounted Nandi, Shiva's great white bull, and together they headed to the party. But she arrived late, and the sacrifice had already begun. Her father was talking, and his speech was not kind.

Daksha never liked Shiva for good reason: Shiva never acknowledged Daksha. He never gave him any credit for all this work; for his gift of daughters; for looking after the *yajna* sacrifice that was so critical to the survival of all the gods. One time, just before a grand yajna, Shiva arrived before Daksha. All the gods stood up as Shiva entered the hall in reverence and honor. A short time later Daksha arrived, and again all the gods stood, all except Shiva. Shiva thought, "If I stand up, Daksha will be embarrassed because I am the greater god. It would be best for me to remain sitting." Of course, Daksha was not impressed. He thought, "Who does Shiva think he is? He shows no respect to anyone. I am his father-in-law, yet he ignores me."

Daksha's hatred for Shiva was on display, and he didn't notice when Sati arrived. He cursed Shiva. He complained about Shiva's attire of rags of animal skins and snakes. His hair was matted and filled with debris. He did no work; he just wasted his time dancing in the forest or stoned out of his head, pretending to meditate. Shiva was a disgrace to all the gods.

Shiva was right about Sati: She had a temper. She was her father's equal in verbal abuse, and she let him have it. "How can you talk that way about my husband? He is the greatest god in the universe. Time and again he has saved us all. You are nothing compared to him. I am ashamed to call myself your daughter." Her words ran down, but her fury was not spent. She turned her back to her father, who was still reeling from his daughter's sudden appearance and outburst.

The fire beckoned; life was impossible. Sati knew in her heart it was not Shiva's fault that Daksha bore him such hatred. She knew it was because she disobeyed her father and married Shiva without permission. Daksha had picked out many suitors for Sati, but she rejected them all and chose the one her father would never sanction. She was to blame for all this. The fire would make it all better, and she stepped forward.

Daksha was caught off guard, and no one had time to move. They all watched in horror as Sati offered herself to the flames. Their horror paled compared to the pain Shiva experienced. Watching from Kailash, he rose in anguish and tore a hair from his locks and dashed it to the ground. Behind a puff of pyrotechnics, there arose a great warrior, Virabhadra. Shiva directed Virabhadra to take his army, go to the hall, and wreak revenge on all there. This he did: Everyone present was ground down under the attack until all that was left was a red smear on the marble floor.

This act of violence did not go unnoticed—Vishnu was also watching. He appeared to Shiva and took him to the hall. "You've gone too far again, Shiva," said Vishnu. "Now bring them all back and apologize."

Shiva protested, but Vishnu was firm. "Your anger will destroy the whole universe one day if you are not careful. Now bring them back!"

Shiva did, but not quite all. He refused to bring Daksha back to life. "Even Daksha!" said Vishnu.

"No! He is the cause of Sati's death," said Shiva.

"You know that is not true. Sati made her own noble choice. Do not dishonor her with your anger."

Shiva relented and brought back Daksha, but to teach him a lesson, he incarnated Daksha with the head of a goat, a permanent reminder of just who was the greater god. Daksha never again spoke ill of Shiva.

Shiva turned to the fire and gently took Sati's burning body in his hands. He flew back to Kailash with the greatest sorrow anyone could ever experience. As he flew, her body disintegrated, and 108 pieces of Sati fell to the earth. Wherever a morsel of Sati landed, the spot became sacred, and temples were raised in her honor. The greatest temple was built at the site of Sati's fallen vagina. It is to this temple women come who have difficulty conceiving children.

There was nothing left for Shiva; he was alone again. In his loneliness, he returned to his mediation.

⌁ ⌇

There are many mysteries raised in Sati's story. Why did Shiva refuse to populate the universe, leaving the job to Daksha? What is the secret cause of the enmity between the great Brahmin priest of the gods and the even greater Shiva? Why does Shiva, who knows all, allow his wife to go to the party? And most puzzling of all, if Shiva can bring back to life everyone else, why not Sati, too? We will leave these questions unanswered, allowing them to float in your mind. Instead, we will look at two other mysteries: What is the meaning of Sati's self-immolation and her body breaking into pieces and falling to earth? What does this story tell us about the view of women in these ancient times?

* * *

Remember that the invading, conquering proto-Indo-Europeans who overran Northern India were fiercely patriarchal. While their culture eventually merged with the native Dravidian planting culture, which was matriarchal, the patriarchal themes replaced the matriarchal. In planting communities, the god who was usually dismembered and planted was male. Recall the Polynesian story of the god who became the coconut tree, the Ojibwa myth of the god who was killed and planted and became corn, and the Egyptian story of Osiris who was murdered by his brother Seth, torn apart, and also buried. In all these stories, it was a man who was divided and, like seeds, planted in the womb of Mother Earth; the earth goddess brought forth life from the seed of a god. Not so in India. Here the roles are reversed. In the story of Sati, we see that it is a woman who dies and is broken and planted. This is an important preview of what's in store for women in this culture and in all the cultures where the patriarchal viewpoint prevails.

In nomadic communities there is no sacred ground; when you are always moving around, of what use are temples or graves? The sky and its inhabitants are your constant companions. To bury dead bodies is to leave them behind; cremation is the way to return the spirit to the sky. It is evil to bury a body. Recall that it was Angra Mainyu, the Persian devil, who invented burials. This is not the way to treat your dearly departed. In the story of Sati, we see that the sacrificial fire is the door to the realms of the gods and to the next life. Agni, the mouth of the gods, is the only one who can release the spirit trapped in the body. Fire is the path that leads beyond.

Sati's dharma is to destroy herself. Her duty to her father and her husband demands it, for she was the one who caused the strife in her family. This duty of the wife to throw herself into the fire became known as *suttee*, a variation of Sati's name. The word *sat* means "truth" or "being." Sati is the feminine version of sat and means "the true wife."[1] The practice of suttee is meant to be performed after the death of a husband. This is spelled out clearly in the Institutes of Vishnu: "A wife after the death of her husband must preserve her chastity or ascend the pile after him."[2] We find this repeated in the Vedas: "A real woman dies with her husband on the pyre so that she may receive the privilege of serving him again in the next world."[3]

Suttee is highly symbolic and extremely cruel. In the skies of the patriarchal priests, there was a celestial dance that occurred regularly. Venus, as the beautiful evening star, would lead the dying moon into the fires of the sun, and then a few months later, as the brilliant morning star, she would lead the moon back out of the sun for a new round of existence. As in heaven so on earth: It was the proper role of the queen to die with her king so she could guide him through death's door and lead him to rebirth in their next life together. If the king went alone into that fire, he would be lost forever. His wife must accompany him, for life always comes through a woman. This is true physically, but it is also true spiritually. We saw this practice in the tombs of Ur uncovered by Sir Leonard Woolley. We see this practice in India even today.

What a cruel role to inflict upon women! In modern India the practice of suttee is outlawed, but it is still performed, and often against the wife's wishes. The rarity of the practice today does not diminish the fact that it still happens, which means the underlying mythos is still operating in the minds of many people.

* * *

The mystery of women is due in part to the fact that within every man, there is a feminine quality. It is not always one particular woman that mystifies and terrifies a man, but his own inner mystery. He does not understand these tender feelings, and what we do not understand, we fear. Men don't understand the powerful attraction they feel for these creatures, either; women seem to possess a great magic that can make a man lose himself. The fear of women is one of the biggest sources of psychic energy in the patriarchal cultures. It is present today, and it is important to understand what maps we are following in our society. Around the world women are still subjected to horrific cruelty and discriminations: genital mutilations, sequester and illiteracy, being bought and sold as slaves into prostitution, unequal career opportunities, less pay for equal work, objectification, domination and ridicule.

Why is it that women are considered less than men and treated as we might treat pets? We can look to the ancient patriarchal Greeks to see the source of many of the modern misogynistic tendencies still remaining in society.

⊰ ⊱

Run Medusa! Run! But where? How can a woman outrun a god? Poseidon, powered by his lust for her beautiful body, is gaining. She can't run fast enough; she must hide.

There!

The temple of the virgin Athena, the goddess of justice—run and hide in there. Athena will protect your honor.

Poseidon cares not about temples or other gods; his rutting heat is high. He seeks only relief. Medusa becomes trapped inside her failed sanctuary. Athena will not provide protection, for justice is a human quality, meted out between humans, not between gods and humans.

Poseidon seizes, penetrates, conquers; Medusa is broken and discarded. In blood and pain, Medusa looks up at the statue of Athena. "Why did you not help me?"

An angry Athena answers her. "You allowed yourself to be raped in my temple? How could you lose yourself here? You dishonor me, who prizes virginity above all else: You must be punished!"

Athena curses Medusa, whose luxurious hair becomes writhing snakes and beautiful face becomes twisted and ugly. The mere sight of that face will turn any man into dead stone. Ravishing, ravished Medusa becomes a Gorgon; hated by mortal men and a bane to all. It will be brave Perseus who finally rids the world of this evil. Looking into the mirror of his polished shield, he will cut off her head and declare justice finally served for the sin she committed.

⊰ ⊱

This is a monstrous tale. Greek myths are full of "monstrous females and female monsters."[4] There is nothing fair or just about their treatment. Greek men were terrified of the feminine. Greek women were treated at best as property, at worst as enemies. Greek sexuality found in myth had no flavor of love and tenderness—it was about possession and dominance.

Homosexuality was a part of this mythos; young boys were dominated and penetrated by older men. This was a sympathetic mirroring of the great heroes in battle who would dominate their foes and penetrate them with the sword. It was improper for a grown man to allow himself to be homosexually abused; only young boys (between the age of 12 and the age that they sprouted a full beard) and women were to be dominated in such fashion. Homosexuality between grown men was condemned for another reason: Society needed replacement soldiers. If a man forsook women, as one named Hippolytus did, he was forsaking his duty to reproduce.[5] This, society could never abide; the commandment against grown men knowing each other is universal. Consider the story of Lot's daughters in Genesis:[6]

⊰ ⊱

They were fine-looking men, beautiful to behold. "Angels," thought Lot.

The men of Sodom had other thoughts. Lot invited the angels into his house to allow them to rest and wash. He served them a nice dinner, but while he was cooking inside, mischief was brewing outside.

There came a knock on the door. Lot was suspicious and quickly went outside, shutting the door behind him. The men of Sodom accosted him. "Show us the two men who went into your home. We want to know them!"

"Please," said Lot, "do not dishonor me with such ideas. If you are horny, let me give you my two daughters. They are both virgins, and you can do with them as you will! My guests are sheltered under my roof, and I can't let any harm come to them."

"No," came the reply. "Those two men are prettier than your daughters. Send them to us or ..."

Lot went back inside his house and talked to the angels. They knew the wickedness of the city and warned Lot, "Take your family and leave this place. God knows the evil that these men do, and they will all be killed in punishment. You must not tarry here—leave and do not look back."

The angles were prophetic, for indeed God did destroy the city of the Sodomites.

⊰ ⊱

While Lot offered his daughters to avoid the homosexual rape of the angels, the daughters were lucky: They were not taken. This story is repeated almost identically again in Judges, but with a very different ending.[7]

⊰ ⊱

A Levite priest was travelling with his concubine and came to the town of Gibeah, but he found no place to rest the night. Fortunately, his difficulties were noticed by a kindly farmer who offered food and lodgings. Unfortunately, several men also noticed the priest's arrival. Later that evening they came to the house and called on the farmer to bring out the man, so that they might know him.

The farmer went out to the men and said, "Nay, brothers. This man is a guest under my roof. Do not ask me to give him to you. I have a better idea: I can bring you his concubine and my own young daughter. You can play with them in whatever manner pleases you."

The men were not pleased; they wanted the man, but instead the farmer brought the concubine out. The men took her and abused her throughout the night, and when the first light of dawn appeared, they left her. She crawled to the door of the farmhouse, and with her last breath her hand touched the threshold. There she was found when her master came looking for her.

"Get up," said the priest, "we should be going."

When he received no response, he went to the kitchen and found a large knife. He carved the body of his sacrificed wife into 12 pieces, which he then sent to all regions of the land.

❧ ☙

Sound familiar? Where to begin: Do we look at the devaluation of the women, even Lot's own daughters, in relation to the sexual safety of a stranger? Do we look at the callous cruelty of the Levite priest, who orders his concubine to get up, as if nothing happened? Do we look at the horror with which society reacts to the possibility of homosexuality? Do we look at the faint echo of the goddess being cut up and planted? Again, it is not a male here being dismembered, for in the Old Testament, it is the patriarchal mythos that rules. We could look at this story, not as an actual, historical event, but rather as another re-enactment of the patriarchal herding tribes' conquest of the matriarchal planting communities. Or we could look at the sacrifice itself that guarantees the safety of man: This is another very old theme.

❧ ☙

The fleet is stuck; the wind blows against them. The insult cannot be avenged if Agamemnon cannot sail to Troy. Paris is there with Helen, the daughter of Zeus, who rightfully belongs with Menelaus, Agamemnon's younger brother. Paris was awarded Helen by Aphrodite as a reward for his vote; he had been asked to judge who was the most beautiful goddess, and Aphrodite was pleased with his selection of her. The fact that Helen was already married seemed of little matter to either Paris or Aphrodite. Paris stole Helen away.

Why is the wind blowing against the fleet? Agamemnon's folly. He bragged that he was the greatest hunter, greater even than Artemis, the goddess of swift death.

Agamemnon grows desperate and seeks counsel from his priest, who is aware of Artemis' anger. "If you want favorable winds, you must offer a sacrifice. But Artemis will not be pleased with just any meat; she is demanding your own daughter's body be burnt. Only then will you be allowed to sail to Troy and begin your war."

Agamemnon is torn: He loves his daughter, Iphigenia, more than life itself, but more important than life is honor and duty.

Paris committed no sin in his own mind, since the goddess Aphrodite told him that Helen was his proper wife and he should take what is his. Agamemnon committed no sin in his own mind, since the goddess Artemis ordered him to sacrifice his daughter. Where is the morality in life? It is not found among the gods; theirs is raw power. What the gods command, men must do, but it is to men that the consequences of all action fall. Men will ultimately pay the price for their actions, regardless of their intentions.

Iphigenia consents to the deed and death, and with her willing sacrifice, the winds change and the men sail off to their fate.[8]

⊰ ⊱

Just as the hunting mythos provides psychic balm for men who kill animals, just as the conquests of peaceful planting communities are justified and rationalized by claiming it is all part of God's grand plan, so too are men psychologically excused from their atrocities toward women when they can blame it all on the gods. Sometimes, however, they can only blame themselves and hope the gods understand.

⊰ ⊱

During the time of Abraham, there was a famine that forced him to go to Egypt. While there, he was worried for his own safety because his wife Sarah was so beautiful. He was afraid that other men might desire her so much that they would kill him to get to her. He decided to claim that she was his sister. Sure enough, Sarah did attract attention and was chosen to be a concubine in Pharaoh's harem. Abraham didn't protest; he let her go and gained great favor at court for having provided such a wonderful beauty. But God was not pleased with this arrangement, and so he sent a fierce plague upon the people of Egypt. Pharaoh innocently asked why he was being punished, and only then was Abraham's trick discovered. Pharaoh gave Sarah back and said to Abraham, "Go away!"

᭰ ᭴

Abraham sacrifices Sarah to save his own skin.[9] Now who is punished for this deed? Not Abraham! While God disapproves of the deal, it is Pharaoh, the innocent one, who is punished. Sarah is just a piece of property bandied back and forth. Since he got away with it, Abraham later tries the same trick on the King of Gerar and this time gets rewarded with a thousand pieces of silver![10] Abraham performed these subterfuges out of a sense of self-protection, but one day he is ordered by God to perform a different sacrifice: He is told to kill his own son, Isaac, as a test of loyalty, and again, out of fear, he accedes to the request.[11] There is a big difference here, though: Isaac is male, and the sacrifice is aborted at the last second. Would he have been spared if his name was Isabel or Iphigenia? Consider what happened to the dutiful daughter of Jephthah.[12]

᭰ ᭴

Jephthah was a powerful, strong man, but he was also the son of a whore, so his stepbrothers shunned him. They forced him out of his father's house and into exile. He would not remain unwanted for long.

The Ammonites rose up against the Israelites, and the Israelites sought a hero to lead their men into battle. The elders of Gilead went to Jephthah and begged him to return home and fight their battle for them. Such irony, but Jephthah agreed to take on the job on the condition that, if he was successful, he would be their leader. The deal was sealed.

Jephthah prepared for the battle with a prayer and a commitment to God: If God should favor him with victory, then upon his return to his house he would offer up to God whatever came first out the front door. God agreed.

The war went well, and Jephthah's heart was filled with joy at what God delivered to him, until he came home. The first thing out of his door was his precious daughter, his only child. She was wearing bangles and trinkets, and she danced and sang to her father in praise and celebration of his victory, but Jephthah could only fall to the ground and rend his clothes.

A deal is a deal, but the deal pushed hard upon Jephthah. His daughter discovered the cause of her father's distress and tried to comfort him. "If you have made a promise to God, then I must help you keep your word. Don't worry about me, I will be good."

His daughter did have one request, however: "Please allow me two months so that I may go to the mountains and mourn my virginity."

After two months, the virgin daughter returned, and her father offered her as a burnt sacrifice to God.

⇨ ⇦

These stories are both sociologically and psychologically illustrative. They show how little societies value women, but also they explain the psychic discord that exists today. How many men still sacrifice their families in order to fight their business battles? These myths are old, but they still resonate. Women are not immune to their influence; the primacy of the masculine within each woman's psyche can demand the same sacrifice of their inner feminine.

✳ ✳ ✳

The patriarchal cultures conquered and subsumed the matriarchal myths, but men cannot exist without women—some accord was necessary. The Greeks moaned about the reality of women: You can't live with them and you can't live without them. If only they could! Women were a necessary evil, a necessity and an evil, as the story of Pandora illustrated, but they were only necessary to bring birth to new men. Even then the Greeks believed the woman's role in bringing forth new life to be minimal; what a man deposited into the womb of a woman was a complete, but very tiny, human being. The woman's only job was to provide it space to grow. The woman was the soil, but the seed planted in that soil by the man was complete.[13] In this myth, life comes from the man, not the woman; now we can understand why some patriarchal myths insist that a man created the universe and all its life.

Women were needed, and they were feared. Women controlled the means by which a man continued himself: reproduction and sons. The frequent rape stories in ancient Greece, as horrific as they are, may be a reflection of men's attempt to control the reproductive process. Remember, sex was not about love; it was about domination and control. Women are wild, and a man could never be completely certain whether the children they bore were his children. This is critically important in a patriarchal society—a man must know if his sons are really his sons. It is irrelevant in a matriarchal society, because women always know who their children are. The necessity in the patriarchal cultures is to keep your women close, keep them secret, and keep them away from all other men, especially the males of your own families. It is not your worst enemies one has to watch out for; it is your own brother. Your wicked wife may try to seduce him. Whose child did she just bring forth?

Even the gods had to have their wives; it is singular and strange that the God of the Western religions is a devout bachelor. It is not so anywhere else. Think back to the story of the "Humbling of Indra," where we saw Brahma sitting on the world lotus while Vishnu dreams the dream of the universe. Who was it sitting by Vishnu's feet? His consort, Lakshmi. She was originally sitting on the lotus, not Brahma, and her name was Padma: She *is* the world lotus who gives birth to the whole of creation.[14] It was the patriarchal imperative that displaced her and put a man on the lotus, and again we find a man giving birth! The idea should be inconceivable, but in some Brahmin's mind, the idea took root. Padma was removed and put at the feet of Vishnu, the lowest, meanest part of the body. This symbolic repositioning of Lakshmi at Vishnu's feet, and not beside him at the level of his heart or head, shows quite clearly where a woman's place is. We find the same image in the New Testament when we watch Mary Magdalene washing the feet of Jesus. A woman's role is to serve her lord and master.

And yet without the woman, nothing happens. She is necessary. Lakshmi is stroking Vishnu's feet, and that action stirs the dream, which is the dream of the whole universe. We can see this re-enacted today; the husband, reclining on his couch, holds the remote control in his hand and is flipping through several football matches. His wife comes to him and whispers something sweet in his ear, and he thinks, "That would be nice" and leaves the couch. Every Indian god has his shakti, his feminine power.[15] Shiva does not shine without his Shakti; without her he is but a corpse.[16] Shiva without Shakti has no life, but Shakti without Shiva has no form. These two were originally one' then the original Self swelled up and split into two, creating male and female. It is an illusion that they seem separate, but the illusory nature is hard to look past. The emanation of the feminine from the within the masculine is described in many myths:

⚛ ☙

Mahisha, the buffalo demon, was granted a great gift from Brahma: Now he was invincible. No man or god could kill Mahisha, and with this new power he set off to conquer the universe. Indra fell—the greatest warrior god of the universe was no match for Mahisha.

In defeat Indra runs to the creator Brahma for help, but Brahma cannot undo what he has wrought. Together they go to Shiva. Alas, even Shiva cannot defeat Mahisha, so they all visit Vishnu. Predictably, even Vishnu is no match for this devil. No man or god can slay him, and the great buffalo conquers the heavens and rules over everything.

In a quandary, the three great gods ponder what to do. Individually they are helpless before the evil infesting the universe, but together they may be able to regain the lost balance. They join together, three as one, and from this wondrous yoking, creative energy brings forth the great goddess Durga, the one whose name means "difficult to reach."

The mere sight of Durga could shock a man to death. She is black—blacker than the darkness of the night. Around her neck is a garland of skulls; she is death itself come to suck back the world through bloodied teeth. She wears a skirt of severed arms, with snakes for the sacred thread. In her forehead is the moon, the source of life and death. Her mouth bleeds, and her body is streaked with red stains. For earrings she wears dead babies. Durga sets out on her giant lion, with a mane as bright as the sun, to do battle with the devil.

The boon granted to Mahisha was that no god could destroy him, but here he is not facing a god, but a goddess—the original goddess. Durga is the incarnation of the creative power that brought forth the universe, and that will swallow it up again in time. The devil does not yield willingly, and a great battle begins.

The conflict between good and evil lasts many years. At times the demon seems to be on the ropes, but he is tricky and always finds a way to survive. Finally Durga cuts off his head, and that should be that; but as soon as the blood from the buffalo touches the earth, two more demons rise up. She cuts off their heads, but once more when their blood touches the earth, more demons arise. Soon Durga is facing a murderous herd of demonic buffalos. She backs off to consider this new dilemma.

Durga enters a deep meditation and calls forth her creativity. From her ebony body springs another goddess, Kali. She looks a lot like her mother; Kali has a long, blood-red tongue, many arms with many swords and a bowl made from a skull. Together they rejoin the battle.

Durga chops and Kali catches. Before the devil's blood can find the earth, Kali scoops it out of the air and holds it in her bowl. Mahisha protests, "But this is not fair. I am fighting two goddesses, not one!"

Durga responds, "But we are just one. It is your ignorance that causes you to perceive that which is not real." The goddess prevails; evil is defeated. Men and gods are safe once more.

⊰ ⊱

It is up to a woman to do what three great gods cannot! But here again we see the idea of men bringing forth women. This is the Greek idea once more of men injecting little homunculi into women's bodies. It is also the biblical story: Eve came from Adam, not the other way around. This defies common sense and common experience. Can man, even three men together, really be a source of life?

We find this theme in the three Western religions. Yahweh, male, brought forth all existence. He and Jesus are bachelors; they have no need of a woman to bring forth physical or spiritual life. (Fortunately, Mohammed is allowed a wife, and Mohammed's wife, Khadija, plays a very important role in his life.[17] But Mohammed is not a god and so does not figure in this reckoning.) God, the highest being in the universe, is a man: If you really believe that, what does it tell you about women? To quote one professor of biblical studies, "To be a man is to be like God."[18] If so, then to be a woman is to be ... well, not like God, at the very least.

God without a mate is a rewriting of history. Originally Yahweh did have a wife: Her name was Asherah, and the early Hebrews worshiped her as a fertility goddess. Her idols have been found in thousands of early Israeli homes. Asherah is a variation of the names of other great fertility goddesses in the Near East: Astarte, Inanna and Ishtar. (Venus and Aphrodite are the European manifestations.) Asherah is also the wife of El (pronounced "ale"), the Canaanite high god which many scholars believe was also the earliest Israeli high god; his name is found in many passages of the Bible and is found in the name of the Jewish homeland, Isra*el*. During the Jewish Babylonian exile of the sixth century B.C.E., as the idea of monotheism grew in importance, Yahweh was forced to divorce his beloved and go it alone—there could be only one![19] From that time onward, there would be found no more statues of Asherah in Jewish homes.

※ ※ ※

There are other ways to look at the story of Durga, as is true with any good myth. We will defer the mystical import of the myth to the next section. Forget the biological implausibility of a man giving birth to a woman, what does it mean psychologically for men to bring forth the feminine from their own depths? Carl Jung has proposed the concept of the anima, the feminine energies that all men possess, but which are repressed. These ignored energies do not go away, they go underground into our psyche, where they are still active, but active in ways not apparent to our conscious awareness.

The story of Durga begins with a man making a rash promise of power to an archetype of evil, the buffalo demon

Mahisha. The god Brahmin gave the boon to Mahisha: nothing male can kill you! This is masculine arrogance, to think that one can overcome death so easily. Everything must end one day, but it is the hope of ego to continue on in its present form. Wielding his masculine might, Mahisha goes against all the great male gods and defeats them. What the ego has created cannot be defeated by more ego; something different is needed.

The trinity of Hinduism, the three great male gods of Brahma, Vishnu and Shiva, are helpless. Just as we find in the Catholic trinity of the Father, Son and Holy Ghost, something is missing. The number three implies incompleteness; four symbolizes wholeness. What is missing is the feminine aspect of life and power. In the Church this completeness was finally achieved when the cult of the Virgin Mary was allowed to flourish. In the Hindu stories, completeness was achieved with the re-creation of Durga.[20] This bringing forth from the depths of the unconscious psyche that which was repressed for so long is exactly what is needed to solve the masculine problems of the day. Not more macho, and yet, what does Durga do? She goes to war! She employs exactly the same macho tools in her battle with Mahisha that any man would do, but there is a difference.

There was another buffalo story we have looked at, and it, too, required a woman to save her people. In the myth from the Blackfoot tribe of Montana, the chief's daughter learns how to return the blood of the buffalo back to the earth so that the animals can come alive again. The blood must be returned. Kali reverses this: She prevents the buffalo's blood from returning to the earth from whence life could rise again. This removes Mahisha's ability to regenerate. In effect what Durga is doing is withholding her own creative powers from Mahisha, for without women, there can be no life. It was not the years of fighting that defeated the demon. The war was inconclusive. The end came when Durga drew on her inner feminine resources and manifested Kali.

Psychologically, a man who has no connection to his inner feminine will find himself constantly at war, battling demons that he has brought forth out of his own darkness. Fighting harder will not end the struggle, for Brahma has decreed that no man can solve this problem. Only when the feminine, that missing fourth of the trinity, is brought forth and honored, will the devil be subdued.

✳ ✳ ✳

The great goddess is never far from the earth; she is the font of life and creativity, just as the earth is the womb of life. Myths of the goddess are aetiologies of the earth's fecundity, as illustrated by the lovely Persephone:

৺ ৻

Persephone loved the blueness of the anemones waving to the sun in his equally blue home. She sighed happily amid the spring breezes and idly picked the brightest flowers. She did not see the shadow rising behind her; her abduction was swift. She had no chance to call out to her mother, Demeter; she had no chance to tell her what was happening or where she was being taken. Hades rarely left his home in Tartaros, but Zeus had allowed that, on this occasion, he could rise from the underworld and take Persephone as his wife.

Demeter had mated with her brother, Zeus, only the one time; it was his idea, of course. One mating is all it takes for a god to plant his seed. Demeter's daughter grew up as beautiful as the flowers she loved to pick. Apollo and Hermes lusted after her, but Demeter kept her hidden and away from Mount Olympus. She did not want her daughter married: that would have meant she would rarely get to see her.

Hades was also very much in love with the girl and really did need a queen to help him rule the dark land below. He decided to approach Zeus and ask for Persephone directly. Zeus, as the father, agreed to his brother's request but suggested he do the deed discretely, so that Demeter would never find out who took her daughter.

Demeter was distraught—there was no sign of her daughter anywhere. She searched the surface of the whole world, with torches at night and with Apollo's light in the day. Finally, it was Hermes, the only one who could freely visit Hade's realm and return, who told her the story: Zeus had allowed Hades to take Persephone, and she was now the queen of the dead.

Hermes had spilled the beans while Demeter was in a town called Eleusis. She had taken the disguise of an old woman. Here she met four girls who said that their mother was looking for a nanny for their newborn brother, Demophon. Demeter saw an opportunity to even the score with Hades and took the job. Each day she coated Demophon in ambrosia and basted the mortal baby in fire, planning to remove his mortality and make him an immortal. Unfortunately, before she could complete the ritual, she was discovered; Demophon's mother was horrified by the sight of her baby being baked, and she screamed. Demeter, in anger, stopped the ritual and then raged against the mother for denying her son immortality. She tossed the baby aside and left.

What was left for Demeter to do? It was time for a desperate act. In revenge Demeter removed her power from the earth, so that nothing grew. Crops withered, and famine spread upon the earth. When Zeus heard the cries of humanity and realized there would be no more sacrifices to the gods, he called Hades to counsel. Hades knew what was to be asked of him, but he could not bear to be parted from his queen, so he played a trick on her. Before giving Persephone back to her mother, he gave her four pomegranate seeds to eat. The rule of the underworld is that if you eat or drink anything of that land, you must spend the rest of time there. Zeus brokered a settlement: He allowed Persephone to spend eight months of the year above ground with her mother, but she had to return each year and spend four months with her husband.

≈ ≈

The scene in which Demeter prepares Demophon for immortality echo's an earlier Egyptian vignette:

≈ ≈

Isis found that a fragrant tree had grown up around the sarcophagus of her dead husband, Osiris. The tree was so beautiful that the local king had its trunk used as a pillar for his palace. Isis took a job in the palace that allowed her to be near the tree entombing her husband; the job was as nanny for the king's newborn son. As she looked after the baby, she decided it would be a nice gift to make him immortal. Every day she would chant a spell and place the boy into the fire, which would burn away his mortality, leaving behind an immortal body. One day the queen came into the room unexpectedly, found her baby in the fire, and screamed. The spell was broken. Isis quickly had to pull the boy out of the flames, and then she had to explain who she really was. In gratitude for her service, the king allowed Isis to open the tree and take Osiris home again.

≈ ≈

Isis attempted to confer immortality on the baby of the king because she was kind; Demeter's motivation was not so benign. Hades (who later in Greek mythology becomes the somewhat softer Pluto) had stolen her daughter, and Demeter wanted revenge. If Hades would take something away from Demeter, then Demeter would take something away from Hades. By attempting to make Demophon immortal, Demeter would be stealing a soul away from Tartaros, thus obtaining her revenge. When this plan failed, she cruelly threw the boy to the floor and stomped off. We can see a big difference in these two tales between the Egyptian and Greek views of women. The Egyptians were direct descendants of the earlier planting communities; their myths were not from patriarchal nomadic tribes. Egyptian mythologies were not as paranoid about women as the Greek myths were.

Let's look deeper inside the story of Persephone and Demeter. Demeter is the goddess of agriculture, and her daughter is the goddess of grain. Each spring Persephone is allowed to come to the surface and spend eight months above ground. Then she is cut down and returns to her husband beneath the earth. Here is aetiology for the seasons, and the reason crops can only appear at certain times of the year.

Let's look even deeper. There is an explanation, as well, in this story for the nature of marriage in ancient lands. Zeus gives his daughter Persephone to his brother Hades. Zeus does not consult with Persephone; there is no asking of what she would like. He doesn't even consult with the mother. The giving of a bride is totally up to the owner of the girl; she is just property, and the marriage arrangement is simply a contract. Zeus is fully within his rights to do what he did, although it is a bit cruel that he didn't at least let the women know what was in the air—cruel but not uncommon. And why give this young thing to his brother? This was also a common practice.

Ancient Greece, like our modern world, was *patrilocal*. This means that a new wife would go to live with her husband's family. That seems very natural to us, but not all cultures did this; there were some cultures that were *matrilocal*, and the husband would go live with the wife's family. But this is not our case. Today a woman takes on her husband's name; that is part of the patrilocal custom. In Greece, a woman was not allowed to own any property, but if a man should die with no sons, then all his wealth would flow through his daughter to the daughter's husband—the wealth would leave the father's family. That was not acceptable! To prevent that from happening, a man with no sons would marry off his daughters to other family members, usually a brother, to ensure the family jewels stay in the family.

In China, where the culture was also patrilocal and patriarchal, there was another reason for valuing sons more than daughters. The Chinese were ancestor worshippers extraordinaire: Your ancestors were still extant, although in another realm. To help the dearly departed, descendants would give gifts and sacrifices, and without these rituals, existence in the netherworld would be harsh. When a woman married, she completely joined her husband's home and family; she became a descendant of her husband's ancestors and worshipped those ancestors, not her father's ancestors. If a man had only daughters, who would look after him when he departed? Sons were not just nice, they were essential— without them there would be no one to tend to us when we become the ancestors.

＊ ＊ ＊

Of course, the point could be made that not all ancient myths treated women poorly. Eros treats Psyche tenderly, for the most part, and Psyche does outwit Aphrodite, with some magical help, in order to marry her chosen lover. There are many goddesses who are revered for their intelligence and resourcefulness, and not just for their beauty or ability to invoke lust or fear in men. The Greek virgin goddesses, of which there are not many, were powerful women.[21] The virgins Athena and Artemis were not sex symbols, and if any man dared to observe their naked bodies, death would find him quickly.

Artemis (Diana in the Roman world) was the mistress of the hunt, not of the household; she was a wild woman. Untamed and untamable. She was a remnant of an ancient idea that to ensure a good future, you must protect the young—she protected young animals, and she protected young women. (Once they were married, though, women were on their own.) She could also be very cruel, as poor Actaeon found out:

⁂

Actaeon was out with his hounds hunting deer one day. He followed a path that twisted and turned, until he heard splashing and women's laughter. He left his hounds on the trail and crept through the underbrush. Looking through the branches of the bushes, he saw Artemis and her maids bathing naked in a lake.

Artemis was not amused at being caught in the nude. To punish Actaeon for his inadvertence, she turned him into a stag. Actaeon ran away as fast as he could, but his hounds caught his scent. They tracked and attacked their master, never knowing whom it was that they killed.

⁂

The Greeks loved their irony. The Greeks also made a big distinction between nature and culture: Men represent civilization, while women represent the wildness of nature. Artemis is wild; she protected young girls who were not yet civilized, up until the time they were married and tamed by a man. Once a woman allowed herself to be dominated, penetrated by a man, Artemis withdrew from her life, until … childbirth. When a woman is in labor, she reverts back to her animal form; the experience is pure wildness and terrifying for men to behold. Artemis is also associated with sudden, unpredictable death—the heart attack, the swift cut of the sword or the puncture of an arrow, the final stroke of misfortune. It may seem that she is a robust role model for women, but that would be looking with modern eyes at an ancient terror. Artemis is not a positive influence in the Greek world. She terrifies men.

We have already seen how callous Athena can be; recall her treatment of Medusa, whom she turned into a gorgon. The Greek gods and goddesses are complex mixtures of good and evil. That is very apt, because life is a complex mixture of good and evil. It is in the Near Eastern myths that we find the tendency to split these two aspects of reality apart, thus forcing a choice upon us—whose side are you on? If you recognize, as the Greeks did, that we all have both good and evil within us, it is easier to find a place of balance within, rather than trying to change the world without. In the Indian mythologies, there is also the tendency to consider one's hero perfect and without major blemishes, but no one is perfect, not even Rama, the great incarnation of Vishnu:

❈ ❈

King Janaka ceremoniously opened the Earth and prepared her for his seeds. When he looked back at the furrow he just plowed, he discovered a golden-hued, baby girl playing in the dirt. He took his newly born daughter, Sita, from the womb of her mother, the Earth, to the palace and raised her. Sita grew into a wonderful young woman, as pretty as a garden and as honest as a flower.

The bow of Shiva hung in Janaka's armory. The bow was so strong that no man could string it. Janaka promised Sita that he would wed her only to the man who could bend that bow, and in Sita's 14th year that man came. Rama easily lifted the bow, which no other mortal could raise, strung it, pulled back on the string, and cracked the bow in half. Sita, looking down from her tower, fell in love, and the wedding quickly followed.

Sita looked divine, which was fitting for the daughter of the Earth. Rama was divine: He was an avatar of Vishnu

who had come to rid the world of a ravenous demon.
Brahma had been conned again; he granted to Ravana
all that he asked, and now no god could kill this latest
devil. But, of course, Brahma left open one small loophole:
Rama was not a god, he was man. He came to earth, the
son of a king, with one grand intention: to restore dharma.

Ravana spied Rama's wife one day in the forest, and lust
raged within him. He had to have her, but first he had to
get her alone. So he lured Rama away by pretending to be
a stag. Rama fell for the trick and chased the animal. Left
unguarded, Sita was easy pickings; Ravana scooped her
up in his chariot and flew off to his stronghold in Lanka.
Rama went mad with anger and searched up and down
the whole of India, but he could not find his wife. It was
Rama's devoted friend, Hanuman, who made the leap
that uncovered her location; over dozens of miles of water
Hanuman flew, straight to the palace of the devil. There
he found Sita.

Sita was being abused by Ravana's many wives. "Submit!"
they said. "Give yourself to our lord! Why should you be
any different than us? You are his now."

This, Sita could never do, for she was chaste, she was
dutiful, and she was the embodiment of dharma. She
would never willingly do anything that was not proper
and befitting of Rama. In punishment, she was confined
to her cell.

Hanuman was caught by Ravana's soldiers but fought
his way free (which is another story). He left to fetch Rama,
who returned with a great army, crossed the sea by calling
up the floor of the ocean (who gladly obliged by forming
a great land bridge to Lanka), and subdued Ravana. Sita
was returned to his arms, and the world was made safe
for all who honor righteous living.

But!

Whispers ... whispers .... What really happened in the castle of Ravana? Was Sita ever molested or assaulted; did she submit? Did Ravana have her? Rama could not ignore the insinuations of the people, even though the vast majority loved Sita and could not believe anything could despoil her. Still, there were a few crude voices, and Rama could not ignore them. He called Sita to answer the voices.

Sita was hurt by her husband's doubt. If he was stricken by the opinions of others, then she had to assure him of her purity and devotion, and there is only one way to truly purge sins or doubt. She called for the yajna flames to be lit. Into the sacrificial fire, she offered herself to Agni.

Agni knew Sita was innocent of all crimes, so he refused to take her. She chased him, but he danced away, until, finally, he leapt up out of the fire pit altogether, leaving her alone, unscathed and absolved. Rama embraced his wife, and they lived together peacefully for 10,000 years.

It was 12 years before the grand anniversary of Rama's reign; for nearly 10,000 years, he had been a great king. And on this particular day, he looked at Sita and saw a radiance that had not been there before. She was with child, and he could not have been happier. Rama asked his advisors if the whole of his kingdom was as happy as he was; he insisted on the truth. The ministers hedged, so he persisted: Were there any who felt ill-treated?

"There is no need to listen to the babble of coarse and ignorant folk!" said the ministers. But Rama insisted, so finally they answered, "There are a few who say that our king sleeps with a woman who lived with another man. But what do they know? Don't let their foolishness disturb your heart."

Rama was troubled: A king must be above and beyond reproach. He summoned his brother, Lakshmana, and ordered him to take Sita to the forest and to abandon her there to the hermits. Lakshmana reluctantly complied with his brother's wish; all Sita was left with were a few combs, needles and threads, perfumes and a mirror, and, of course, a bulging belly.

"Difficult to understand are the demands of dharma," said Lakshmana as he left. "I am sorry that I have to be the one to carry out such an unjust and cowardly deed."

Rama lived alone. He missed his wife so much that he had a golden replica of her built. The statue stood beside his throne, but it could not fill the hole in his heart.

Sita did her duty. She bore the brunt of unfounded guilt and the distrust of her husband's heart. She gave birth to twin sons. Sita raised her boys with the help of a kindly hermit and his family. Hearing her story, the hermit composed a tale, a great tale—the tale of King Rama. The sons of Rama learned this song by heart, and they recited it at festivals to critical acclaim. So great was their fame that when Rama made plans to celebrate 10,000 years of being king with a great feast of music, dancing and sacrifices, they were chosen to provide the half-time show.

Rama heard the song and knew the singers. He recognized his sons and asked the hermit poet to go fetch his sweet Sita. He forgave her and wanted her home. Returning to the palace and seeing her husband once more filled Sita's heart to overflowing, but she knew there would still be talk. She could do only one thing to make everyone happy.

"Rama," said Sita, "let me prove once and for all my innocent and faithfulness to you."

Rama nodded in agreement. Sita turned in a circle so she could see all the guests, and they could all see her. For someone 10,000 years old, she was looking pretty good; she was still beautiful. She wore her best gown and had her prettiest ribbons and sparkliest bangles. After she had made eye contact with everyone present, she turned her gaze back to her beloved and made her statement:

"Mother! If I have been ever faithful to my husband, please take me home and hide me."

In response the goddess Earth spoke; a heavy rumbling sounded beneath the feet of the guests, and then a loud crack. From a fissure arose four Naga-kings, great snakes of the deep. Between the four was suspended a golden throne upon which sat Mother Earth. She wore flowers and a garland of the waters of the world. She was not angry or sad; she seemed to smile with the patience of time itself. The Earth bears all and feels no burden, but her patience with Rama had run out. She called her daughter to her. Sita climbed onto her mother's lap, nestled close like a devoted daughter, and the pair descended back into the ground from whence they came.

Thus ended the story of Sita.

⊰ ⊱

The connection between Sita and the earth echoes the themes we have explored earlier. Janaka penetrated the earth with his plough, opened her up and begat a child. Sita is the embodiment of the earth goddess and semi-divine. But more than any other woman or goddess, Sita epitomizes the ideal wife. She is the embodiment of chastity, forbearance and total devotion to her lord and master, also known as her husband. She is the ideal role model for all women to emulate.

By today's standards, Rama acted outrageously toward his wife and his soon-to-be-born children. He allowed snide whispers to poison his thoughts about his wife, despite the fact that she had passed the test of fire and was proven virtuous. Caring more about what people thought of him than his own family's happiness, he sent Sita away. His own brother thought he was crazy and cruel, but Rama was the king and totally within his rights to treat his woman any way he felt proper.

We could claim that this attitude toward a wife is archaic and that this myth has no purchase today in the minds of readers, but unfortunately that would be a mistaken claim. This map is still operative in the minds of many people. Joseph Campbell greatly admired Ananda Coomaraswamy (1877-1947), a Sri Lankan philosopher and historian, but he was shocked by Coomaraswamy's view on the proper behavior of the wife toward an abusive husband. Coomaraswamy said that, just because a husband acts inhumanely, it is no excuse for the woman to forfeit her proper role in the marriage.[22] In Joseph Campbell's sojourn to Asia from 1954 to 1955, he heard of an Indian man who created a home for women escaping horrible marriages, and he discovered that these woman were treated as outcastes by society; they were resented because they were not acting like Sita.[23]

✳ ✳ ✳

The view of women as inferior beings, worth less than men, can be found around the world and in most cultures. Even the Buddha refused initially to allow women into his community of followers. It was the Buddha's cousin, Ananda, who finally persuaded the Enlightened One to allow his own stepmother to join the sangha after his father died, but the Buddha predicted, "because I allow this, my teachings will last only 500 years. Women will descend upon the sangha like mildew upon the rice." [24] The Buddha created several rules that nuns had to follow if they were to be admitted to the community:

- A nun must always stand in the presence of a monk;
- Nuns must never spend retreats on their own and must be accompanied by monks;
- Nuns cannot conduct their own ceremonies;
- A nun must never rebuke a monk even though a monk may rebuke her;

• And a nun must never preach to a monk.

Clearly, nuns were inferior to monks. Tellingly, in the Buddha's last days, Ananda asked him how to deal with women.

"Don't look at them," was the unhelpful advice.

Ananda persisted, "But what if we have to look at them?"

The Buddha said, "Then don't talk to them."

Ananda then asked, "What if we have to talk to them?"

The Buddha's final reply was "Then be very mindful."[25]

There is a special place in Pure Land Buddhism, the most commonly practiced form of Buddhism in Asia today, called *Sukhavati*: the land of bliss. This is where the enlightened beings go after death. There, they are reborn as Buddhas sitting on lotuses, and they get to listen to heavenly music and spend eternity in meditation. Akira Sadakata, a professor of Indian philosophy, writes, "The female sex, considered inferior and unfortunate, has no place in Sukhavati." It seems that only men are worthy of being reborn in this heavenly realm. Why is this? Sadakata explains, "... the male priests did not consider womanhood to be a pleasurable state, and thus could only provide for the happiness of women through the conversion to men."[26] Here is the plan: If you are a woman, you are *eligible* for enlightenment. This the Buddha conceded to Ananda when Ananda asked, "If dogs can become enlightened, why can't women?" But although you are eligible, you can't get there while still a woman, so Buddhist priests came up with the idea that, if an enlightened woman dies, she will be reborn in Sukhavati as a man. Problem solved!

Curiously, Jesus is cited as saying much the same thing in the gnostic Gospel of Saint Thomas. The very last line, which some feel was added much later, has Jesus responding to a demand from Simon Peter, who wanted Jesus to order Mary to leave them. Jesus refused Simon, saying,

"I will guide her to make her male, so that she, too, may become a living spirit resembling you males. For every female who makes herself male will enter the kingdom of Heaven."[27]

Although we could, we need not continue to show all the ways that women are portrayed as lesser creatures than men. The causes range from fear and frustration to awe and ignorance, and there are numerous stories found in all ancient cultures that indoctrinate this belief into the psyches of men and women. We might seek some comfort in the idea of an earlier golden age for women, when the goddess reigned, but even then, there is evidence that the top dog was a real bitch. The earth goddess demanded life before she would give life; human sacrifices were the staple diet of these goddesses, and one of the favored meals was young virgins.

For women raised in the European or Asian traditions, it seems that today they are the closest they have ever been to being treated, not as property of men, but as equal participants with men in society. There is much work still to be done; the World Economic Forum's annual gender gap survey shows progress in some key areas, specifically in access to education and health care, at least in the developed world, but the gap between men and women is still large everywhere in the areas of economic opportunities and political empowerment. The Scandinavian countries are leading the way, while the U.S. and Canada are ranked disappointingly low at 17th and 18th respectively.[28] As could be expected, the performances of developing countries lag behind those of the developed world, and while progress is being made, it is slow. There are some notable problem countries that do not have economic excuses for the gender gap, but rather persistent cultural mythologies perpetuate the divide: India is ranked 111th, Saudi Arabia is 131st, and Pakistan is third to last at 133rd. [29]

* * *

What is a woman to do? What stories can she look to for guidance toward developing her full potential, not just as a member of society, but as an individual? There are few myths today that help; many of the stories found in Hollywood, on TV soaps, or in novels are reworkings of Sita's tale—the helpless woman waiting to be rescued, but who is tossed aside if her man finds even the hint of taint around her. The modern stories are not as blatant as the old myths, but too often the heroine can only be healed of her suffering if she can find a man to look after her. Or the stories go completely in the opposite direction and depict a woman being more macho than any man and dominating them: Angelina Jolie as uber-bitch Lara Croft is Durga kicking Mahisha's butt.

Where are the stories where a woman can still be a woman and can find a role in life that fulfills her without submitting to male dominance and society's stereotypes? There are some myths that explain the way things *are*, and there are great myths that explain how things *could be*. The myth of the handless maiden is one of these great myths: it states the problem women face and offers the solution, as well. [30]

⚛ ⚛

A devil's bargain is one where you seem to get something for nothing. It took the miller's wife to see through the deal her husband just struck.

The miller was a hard worker; he ground the grain that kept the whole village fed and happy. When a stranger approached him to congratulate him on his dedication, the miller felt appreciated for the first time in his life. The stranger said, "You deserve to be rewarded!" and offered him many riches.

"What must I give you in return?" asked the miller.

"Oh no—you deserve all the riches I will award you," said the stranger. "But I suppose some payment is in order.

271

How about this: I will come back in the morning and take what you have now in your backyard."

The miller pondered to himself, "All I have in my backyard is that big old apple tree. I suppose I can easily part with it if we get rich in exchange." A handshake formalized the contract.

After the stranger left, the miller's wife walked into the house, and her eyes grew wide. "Where did all these jewels and gold coins come from?" The miller explained the extraordinary conversation he just had and the riches they now possessed.

"No!" said the wife, "You idiot! Just now, what was in our backyard was our daughter Claire. She was picking apples to sell in the market. You would give her up for money?"

"I am sure he meant the apple tree. He'll be back tomorrow and we will ask him. In the meantime, let's eat out tonight. We can afford it!"

The next morning the stranger arrived, and the miller took him to the backyard. "Where is your daughter?" asked the stranger.

"Why do you want to see her?" said the miller. "Here is the apple tree."

"No," said the stranger, "it is your daughter I have come for."

The miller waved to his wife and daughter, who were hiding in the house. "Come out here!'

The daughter had no idea who the stranger was or what was going on, but she could tell that something was amiss. But she trusted her parents and let her mother bring her to the stranger.

"Must you take our girl away?" asked the mother.

"I only want her hands," said the stranger. "You can keep the rest of her. And don't worry, with all the money you have now, you can make life for her very comfortable. You can hire all the servants she will need. She will live a very long, rich life."

The stranger's words soothed the parents' troubled minds. It was true: With their new wealth, they could more than make up for the inconvenience to Claire. The daughter dutifully held out her arms and allowed her hands to be severed. The deed was done; as she cried, her tears healed the wounds and the stumps sealed over.

The parents did hire servants, and Claire wanted for nothing, and yet, as the days passed, she became more and more unhappy. Claire felt cut off from everyone, and there was an overwhelming sense of emptiness. She made the decision one night to slip away; she left behind her parents and servants and ran to the forest.

She spent that night alone, cold and hungry. She could not even feed herself. As she wandered she came to a beautiful garden, in the center of which stood a pear tree with golden fruit. It was obvious this was a special tree, for each pear had a number. She was able to eat a pear as it hung on the branch, and that one pear was sufficient to end her hunger.

Now the garden was owned by the king, and he was especially fond of his golden pears. When he visited the garden later in the day, he noticed that one pear was missing. He asked the royal gardener what had happened, but the gardener knew nothing. They decided to sit in hiding the next day to see what was going on. That is when the king fell in love. He saw Claire eat a pear without using her hands. He was moved with compassion and took her to his palace. It did not take long until she, too, fell in love, and they were soon married.

Claire at first resisted, not because she didn't love the king, but because she felt unworthy. How could she be his queen if she had no hands? The king was resourceful and solved the problem by having his smith fashion silver hands for her. Claire's beauty and her fashionable hands impressed everyone at court. The king really loved Claire and had servants do everything for her. In time, a baby boy arrived, and the servants looked after him, too.

Claire felt sad; she longed to be able to hold and caress her baby, but she could not. The old feelings of emptiness and loneliness came back, and she knew what she had to do: She stole away one night with her baby. What was she thinking? How could she care for herself, let alone her baby, all alone in the forest? But she was not thinking; she was just doing.

She walked long and far that night in complete silence. The stillness of the forest was healing, but by morning she was thirsty. In a stream she bent over to take a drink, and her baby slipped into the water. Claire cried for help, but there were no servants around. She was alone, and in the crisis her intuition took over. She plunged her arms into the water, knocking off those useless silver hands, and— it was a miracle that happened that day, and miracles occur only in times of crises—she drew her baby from the stream, and there at the end of her arms were two real, flesh-and-blood hands.

&

Here we find the sacrifice of Iphigenia and Jephthah's daughter again: The father makes a deal with a god, or the devil, that will provide him with success in his ventures but at a terrible cost for his feminine side. In this folk tale, it is not just the patriarch who agrees to the sacrifice, but also the matriarch. The gods of the nomadic tribes required animal sacrifice, but the planting goddesses require human sacrifice. Claire's mother is a willing participant in her daughter's dismemberment. This is not unusual; women have long been complicit in their own subjugation. The concubines of Ravana harangued Sita to be like them and accept Ravana's domination. Women often form what Clarissa Pinkola Estés calls "ridicule pacts"—groups of women who put down other women by critiquing their hair, their clothes, or their behaviors, their intention being to make everyone just like them.[31]

Like Sita, Claire initially submits to what is happening, to what others expect of her. The masculine logic is that the daughter doesn't have to worry about losing her hands; she can have servants do everything for her. Robert A. Johnson points out in his rendition of this story that the cry of the wounded woman is, "But what can *I* do?" The woman who has everything done *for* her is also the woman who has something grave done *to* her. She can no longer live an authentic life; she must be submissive and take whatever life brings to her.

The daughter's name, Claire, means "clear". She is the only one who sees clearly, and she knows intuitively what she needs to do. Unlike Sita, who goes involuntarily, Claire chooses to leave the masculine, planned world for the wildness of the forest. Claire doesn't kill herself; she kills the inauthentic life she was living. She finds her own path. This is the same move to unconscious wisdom that we witnessed in the story of Parzival, when he let the reins of his horse go slack.

It is in the forest that Claire finds a second important tree. The first tree in the story is an apple tree in the backyard, the same kind of tree found in the mythical Garden of Eden: the tree of good and evil. This is the tree where the first sin occurs. Redemption is found at the second tree—the tree of eternal life, the Holy Rood that Jesus climbed willingly upon. The fruit of the second tree is a pear, feminine in shape and golden in color. Claire is sustained by the feminine side of life, and then she is redeemed by a king, another incarnation of the masculine. Fortunately for Claire, this masculine energy is positive compared to her father's attributes. In tenderness and compassion, the king looks after her, and, for a time, this is enough. But Claire is still trapped in a life where she cannot do for herself. As well-meaning as her inner male is, everything is still at the expense of her femininity. She cannot relate to her own baby in a natural way. The silver hands are beautiful, but they are artificial and cold, and she can't feel her own child. She is again drawn to the forest, to the solitude found within.

The forest represents many things. In the forest you must walk your own path and find your own way. The journey is solitary. Withdrawal into your own deepest, darkest resources is what this story is calling for symbolically. You must leave behind the calculating, thinking, logical world and trust the feeling function found deep within the forest. In the forest we find the gifts of Mother Nature, and they are all free: air, water, food, fresh breezes, clean and wonderful smells. Our masculine nature turns these things into commodities that are bought and sold back to us. At first that devil's bargain seems like a really good deal, until we find out that we have to pay the ultimate price of our freedom.

Who are the handless maidens in the world today? Look around for any woman suffering in a relationship where she has given up her own abilities and freedom in order to serve the masculine imperatives: the daughter of the alcoholic who has to sacrifice her own life to look after her father; the daughter of a mother who demands her girl live the life that the mother couldn't live (and win that beauty pageant that eluded her); any woman who has become the scapegoat for her family or social group and who pays the price for the greater good. These are the women who cry, "I can't do anything about my life!"

This is not to say that we should disregard the benefits of the masculine energies in our lives, but we must not give in to the devil's bargain of something for nothing, either. We must consciously recognize the cost and then pay the price ourselves. The way is not to make someone else pay the price for our gains; we cannot profit if we let the masculine succeed at the expense of the feminine.

Masculine qualities include competitiveness, logic, rationality, creativity with machines, science and engineering. These qualities are possessed by both men and women. Feminine qualities include feelings, compassion, love, relatedness and reconciliation, creativity in the arts, lyrical thinking, dancing and singing. These qualities, too, can be possessed by both men and women. The Greeks tended to look at the feminine negatively and saw deceit, cunning, treachery and trickery, beauty that entrapped, and the power to take over a man's heart and mind and lead him astray. All those are possible, and even likely, if that is the map implanted in women's minds. If you have no other map to follow, then you follow the only map you have. The heroic Greek women and goddesses were either revered for their male qualities or feared for their negative feminine nature. The revered goddesses were virginal and undominated, just as the ideal man should be. They were better than men at hunting or running. They were every bit as ruthless and cunning at getting what they wanted as any male hero, and they didn't care the cost paid by others.

Certainly it is perfectly OK for a woman to exhibit and even excel in masculine ways: Every woman has her inner maleness. But there is a question each woman needs to ask: "Is my inner man enabling my feminine nature or at the expense of my femininity?" Giving up being a woman to become a man is not a solution and will lead to psychic imbalances like depression, loneliness and feelings of inadequacy—all of which will spin the cycle more deeply, with thoughts that "I must be even more masculine so I can feel even more capable."

Which story resonates with you: the uber-bitch or the passive princess? Perhaps there is a time to be Sita and completely submit to the treatment accorded you, and perhaps there is a time to be the alpha-monster, eating men alive and drinking their blood. But realistically these attitudes are not skillful, and they do not serve women well. In fact, few of the ancient stories serve women today. We need new maps to lead women to the roles that are slowly evolving. We need stories of women who can and have changed the world, even if this is just their own inner world, or the small, intimate world of their family or friends, while remaining true women: stories of women who can still manifest the creativity and love that inspires the best in everyone.

In a search for stories that inspire women today and provide positive role models, we find many old myths being rewritten and updated. Old myths, which never did serve women well, are being rewritten in a positive way. One such story that has evolved is the ancient Greek story of Atalanta. Let's first look at the earliest telling of this tale:

☙ ❧

King Schoeneus really wanted a son, but what he got was a baby girl. He was not happy about that, so he abandoned the girl on the side of a mountain and left her to the Fates. A wild she-bear found the baby and suckled her. She grew up with the she-bear until hunters killed the beast. The girl's name was Atalanta.

Atalanta grew up among the hunters and learned their ways. Blessed by Artemis, she became the best hunter in the world. She excelled at all weapons and was fleet of foot. An oracle had warned Atalanta to hold on to her virginity and never let it go, or she would lose herself; so she eschewed men in all ways sensual.

One time Atalanta joined a hunt for a notorious boar. Among the hunters were a couple of centaurs who lusted after her: that was a fatal mistake. She killed them both. She then went on to be the first to strike the boar, and for this she was awarded the hide, much to the annoyance of the other hunters. In later adventures Atalanta joined the crew of the Argos and helped Jason secure the Golden Fleece: she was the only woman aboard the ship, but she was well able to look after herself.

King Schoeneus heard the many stories about his daughter's prowess and decided to reclaim her. He brought her back to the palace, and she became his prized possession. Now that she was a princess, it was only proper that she be married. She resisted: he insisted. Atalanta finally agreed to marriage upon one condition, that she would only marry the man who could outrun her in a foot race. But! There was a condition: If she outran the man, she was allowed to kill him. Many foolish suitors lost their lives in their arrogance. Atalanta was the fastest runner in the world, and all the suitors died at her hand.

Hippomenes was as smart as a horse; he knew that he could not win a foot race with Atalanta without some divine help, so he called on Aphrodite, the goddess of love, to assist him. Aphrodite was not pleased that Atalanta had been ignoring her, so she gave Hippomenes three golden apples to distract and entice Atalanta. He was betting his life that these would do the trick.

The race began and Atalanta quickly took the lead. Hippomenes threw one of the apples ahead of Atalanta, and she said, "Oh look – shiny!" She darted after the apple. This allowed Hippomenes to take the lead, but quickly Atalanta was on him. Twice more she ran ahead and twice more the apples flew. The third apple distracted Atalanta just enough to allow Hippomenes to win the race and win her hand. With the loss of her virginity, Atalanta was tamed and was wild no more.

꒕ ꒖

Atalanta was abandoned by her father because she was a baby girl, not the boy he wanted. We see right there the Greek attitude toward women. She was raised in the wild and was a devotee of Artemis, the goddess of wild animals and wild women, but, remember, only up to the time they lose their virginity. For men, wildness in a woman is frightening. Hurricanes were named after women until the late 1970s when this practice became politically incorrect, because of their unpredictable and destructive capability. Atalanta could out run any man and would submit to none: These are not feminine qualities! These are masculine qualities, which is why the Greeks admired her. She was not a role model for women; she was a sublime fantasy for men, and many of them wanted to marry her; to break her; to dominate her. This finally happened, but only because Aphrodite decided she had had enough of Atalanta's free-spirited, masculine ways. If Atalanta would continue to reject Aphrodite's gift of love, then the goddess of love would force marriage upon her.

In both Hesiod's and Ovid's version of the tale of Atalanta, the story ends with her being turned into a lion. In Ovid's version Aphrodite turns her into a lion because she does not show any appreciation for what Aphrodite has done for her. In Hesiod's earlier version, it is Zeus who turns Atalanta into a lion as punishment for an extramarital affair. The reason both Atalanta and her lover were turned into lions was because it was believed that lions cannot mate with each other, because it was thought that lions reproduced by mating with leopards, thus, in punishments, the lovers would be forever unable to make love. Ironically, that was all that Atalanta originally wanted! To be wild and free and not bothered about all this mating stuff.

Now let's look at the modern version of this tale, in brief:[32]

⊰ ⊱

The king wanted his beautiful daughter to marry, but she had other ideas. Atalanta refused to marry until she decided the time was right. She wanted to see the world first. Her father was persistent, so she finally agreed that she would marry, but only if the suitor could outrun her in a race. Her father readily agreed because, how fast can a mere girl run?

Atalanta prepared for the race day by secretly practicing. She was well motivated, and day by day she ran faster and faster. Soon she knew that no man would ever catch her. However, there was one man who wanted to win the race as much as Atalanta, and he too was secretly practicing. His name was Young John.

The day of the race arrived and all the suitors were lined up at the start: Young John put on his brand new air-cushioned Nikes with a GPS tracker; Atalanta decided to run barefoot. The signal was given, and they were all off. Many inexperienced runners sped out quickly to the front of the pack, but they were soon winded and left behind. As the race neared the end, there were only Atalanta and Young John still running. She could not escape him, but he could not get ahead either; they ended in a photo-finish tie.

The King decided that, since Atalanta had not actually beat Young John, he had earned the right to marry her, but he demurred, saying, "I did not run this race to marry Atalanta; I ran just to earn the chance to meet her and perhaps become her friend."

Atalanta commended the young man, but she also agreed that the time was not ripe for marriage. "I still have to go out and see the world. Perhaps one day we will fall in love and be married, and perhaps not." And so the two became friends, and who knows what the future will hold.

ఆ ఈ

What a change! From Atalanta being a wild woman forced by a goddess to submit to a man, to Atalanta being free to choose her own destiny and to have the man who supposedly won her turn out to only want to be her friend, not her owner; from being a piece of property to being an equal and free. The myth has changed. Myths continue to change. Many of the old faery tales are being rewritten today and offered in movies and books as a new charter for the way young girls should view womanhood. Originally, Little Red Riding Hood and her grandmother were eaten by the wolf and no one saved them.[33] In later versions, a hunter (of course, a man),, comes by and rescues the pair. The message here was that the woods are dangerous, and to stray from the straight and narrow path, determined and dictated by society, will lead a woman to disaster. If this myth were being written today, it would be Little Red kicking the wolf's butt and saving her grandmother *and* the woodsman. In the 2010 Disney movie version of Rapunzel, called *Tangled*, it is not the prince who rescues the maiden in distress: it is the maiden herself. Ten years before this movie, Alix Olsen in Eve's Mouth sang of Rapunzel not being there when the handsome prince hit town:

> All that time alone kinda taught me how to cope, so I shaved my head and I made me a rope![34]

New myths and new stories are coming into being all the time; that is the nature of mythology. One grand myth that may have been created just in the last hundred years is the myth of the great goddess. It is compelling today to think that there was a golden age before the patriarchal warrior tribes invaded and conquered the planting communities; that during the time of the goddess, women were equal to men, and the genders treated each other with respect. We have alluded to this myth several times already, however, there is no direct evidence that this was ever the case. There were

282

definitely planting communities, and, yes, there were many references to a fertility goddess, but this does not mean that women were well treated. Elizabeth Vandiver points out that the Greeks worshiped Athena, but they still sequestered their women and feared them.[35] The stories of a great planting goddess being overcome by the big sky-gods of the proto-Indo-European invaders may simply be an aetiology of the way society treated women. But once more, let's not let the historicity of the stories get in the way of their importance. The stories of the great mother goddess definitely are myths, but they may be modern myths in the same way that the story of Chief Dan Seattle's speech is a modern myth. We love these myths today because they provide a map to where we believe we should be heading. It is not necessary for them to have been ancient stories for them to work.

The newest maps for women are definitely evolving, but they have some way to go yet. Not all women believe that they are equal, free and just as valuable and important as men. While many fortunate young girls may be getting the message, the same cannot be said for all men; the psychic landscape of men is not changing as rapidly, although some progress is being made there, too. There are many men who do have these newer psychological maps within.

It is important to remember that it is not just the inner view of women, by women, that needs changing; a man's inner woman, his anima, also needs honoring. The newer maps that will allow men to embrace their own feminine nature are not so prominent yet. And what about the maps that guide us in the relationships between a man and a woman? We will look at the psychological function of myths as it relates to love next.

Chapter 13: Myths of Love

Romantic love is the single greatest energy system in the Western psyche. — Robert A. Johnson[1]

Love is inadequate: not the emotion, but the word itself. In English we force this one word to carry a vast array of meanings. You love God, you love your country, you love your spouse, you love your lover, you love your children, you love your parents, you love your job, you love chocolate, you love that dress. These forms of love are all very different; we may mean respect, honor, admiration, lust, romantic feelings, commitment, compassion, kindness or any of many other feelings. Robert A. Johnson notes that in Persian there are 80 different words for love. The love of a husband and wife is very different from the love of a man for his father.[2] We have no words in English to describe these nuances. In Sanskrit there are 96 words for love.[3] We are impoverished by the lack of options in European languages.

This is a problem. When a husband says to his wife that he loves her, she may hear that he loves her romantically, like Romeo loved Juliet, but what he may mean to say is that he loves her like a sister or a friend. This is a relationship in trouble! He respects her, wishes her well, but he is not "in love" with her. The problem arises not because he loves her in a different way; the problem is the difference in the expectations of love. There is a tremendous difference between loving someone and being "in love" with someone.

The power of lust was well known to our ancient ancestors; they personified it as a god or goddess. The Greek god Eros embodies sexual energy and the pure zeal of the organs for each other. As we have all experienced, this is quite powerful but very impersonal. It doesn't matter who the other person is, lust compels you to merge physically, and after the merger is over, you go on your way. Remember, Eros was one of the oldest of the gods; he was there at the very beginning, according to Hesiod, along with Chaos, Gaia and Tartaros. Without sex, how could anything be begotten? Lust is a fundamental requirement of life. Later stories tell that Eros was the offspring of the goddess Aphrodite. But who is Aphrodite? As is often the case with Greek gods, we have two stories about her, too. Aphrodite is often called the goddess of love, but this is again where our word *love* is inadequate. It would be better to understand Aphrodite as the Lady of Lust: She embodies pure sexual energy, not devoted affection or a commitment to share life's travails with another.

The earliest story of Aphrodite, the important one from our perspective, also comes from Hesiod. Aphrodite was born of the sea; she rose from the foam that formed around Ouranos' severed genitals. Recall that it was Ouranos' own son Chronos who had assaulted and castrated him. Aphrodite is the result of that passion and conquest, and the combination of the generative organ and the deep waters. She is portrayed as irresistibly beautiful, eternally young, and the cause of lust so strong that even Zeus cannot resist it. Her effect is not long lasting or permanent; lust's power arises suddenly like a spring squall, its energies quickly spent, and it fades away again.

Another form of love was called *agape*. This is common Christian charity or the love Jesus required of us when he commanded, "Love your neighbor as you love yourself."[4] This is the power of the Buddhist bodhisattva who expresses immeasurable compassion for all beings. Agape is just as impersonal as lust, because it doesn't matter who your neighbor is—you are to love him or her. Romantic love, however, is very personal, and very specifically tied to that one person. No one else will do; there are no substitutes who can replace the one you are in love with. Romantic love, the power of being "in love," is a much more recent mass phenomenon than the impersonal loves of agape or eros.

The earliest Greek myths did not speak much about romantic love, but by the time of Rome it was starting to appear in the Western psyche. The Roman poet Ovid, writing around the time of Jesus, captured an early example of romantic love in his story of two lovers called Pyramus and Thisbe:[5]

⁓ ⁓

Their families kept the two young lovers apart, and the lovers' suffering was intense. They could not bear to be separated, but they were not allowed to be together. One night they arranged a midnight tryst in a graveyard, under a mulberry tree: Thisbe arrived first wearing a scarf, but she was frightened away by a bloodied lioness that had recently killed a cow. When Thisbe fled, she dropped her scarf, which the lion then shredded. Pyramus arrived and saw the lioness walking away, leaving behind the blood-stained veil. Pyramus thought that the lioness had killed and devoured his beloved, so out of deep, black anguish he drew his sword and killed himself. Thisbe regained her courage and came back just in time for Pyramus to die in her arms; in immense grief she impaled herself on the same sword, and their blood mingled as she died.

⁓ ⁓

In the East, marriages are arranged—you are given your partner. There is no room for being "in love" in these societies, but there is room for love. In time the two partners grow to honor and respect each other. In the Indian marriage ritual, a promise is made: "You will be my best friend." It is the power of friendship and the commitment to the relationship that sustains the marriage, not the power of romantic love. While Bollywood films may imply that romantic love is now infesting India, statistics show that 90% of Indian marriages are still arranged marriages, and the divorce rates is a very low 1%.[6]

Romantic love is dangerous, as we just saw in the tragic tale of Pyramus and Thisbe; the power of love can lead us to our doom. While this story was set in Babylon, there is no evidence that this is an Eastern myth. Scholars feel that Ovid may have made this story up, or maybe he just changed the setting to make it appear a little more exotic.[7] In any case, the message is clear: If you attempt to follow your heart, death will surely follow. Stick to the rules of society, and you will be safe. Accept the fate society chooses for you, and forget about this romantic nonsense.

✳ ✳ ✳

What are the safe forms of love? There are four levels of love which society sanctions and tolerates. Joseph Campbell noted that in India these formulations of love allow a worshipper to increase his service to and knowledge of God.[8] The first kind of love is the love of a servant for his master: You are my master and I will honor and respect you and do as you command. This sounds a bit archaic today; most workers would not use the term *love* to describe how they feel about their boss, which again shows how inadequate this word is.

The term *servant* is a slippery one. Most translators of the Bible prefer to use this term rather than the more provocative noun *slave*, but, for the most part, where we read *servant* in the Bible, the person was actually a slave.[9] We can find several occurrences in the Bible of slaves being urged to obey their masters, such as in Paul's letter to the Ephesians: "Slaves, obey your earthly masters with deep respect and fear…as you would Christ.[10] This is a key point: You are to love your master just as you would love God! It is obvious why society sanctioned this first form of love—societies are built upon the edict "Obey!" From a religious point of view, this is also a command to love your god just as you would love and obey a near and dear master. This is the first form of religious love and is the most common form of religious worship: "God, you are my master and thy will be done on earth as it is in heaven."

The second form of love is that of a friend to a friend. This is found in the camaraderie of Jesus and his apostles, and in the friendship between Krishna and the Pandava brothers, especially Arjuna. They would hang out together and debate various theories about life, love and politics; they'd go bowling together or have a few beers after work. Friends share good times and bad. This form of love is deeper than the first, but the object of your affection can again be seen as god. A vow to a friend in arms is stronger than almost anything, and honor is won or lost by how you treat your promises to a friend. Similarly, you can love and commit to your god just as you would love a cherished friend. It is the second level of religious love.

Here we can find another example of the inadequacy of the English word *love*: If a man in the West said that he loved his male buddy, people would look at him in a particular and peculiar light—they'd wonder whether he is gay. We hear *love* and unconsciously think it means a romantic relationship. But that is not the way the guy feels. He doesn't have romantic feelings; he loves his friend in another way. In the East (Near or Far), this would not be a problem; men can walk hand in hand, loving one another in a way we haven't defined in the West, and, again, we are the poorer for it.

A man's inability to tell his father how much he loves him reflects the same blocking of the inner feminine qualities by the masculine self-image. The word *love*, when told to one's father, would imply too much and just doesn't fit, so rather than risk embarrassment, both the father and the son say nothing, because saying nothing is better than saying the wrong thing. The blame for this inability in the West to express these deeply held, but seldom admitted, feelings lies at the feet of our poets, who have failed to give us the vocabulary for expressing what our inner woman is dying to express. The newly coined term *bromance* fails on so many levels, not the least by including the term *romance* in this portmanteau, because it implies a homoeroticism that is not intended. While the word was intended to convey the depths of love between two men, its usage can ridicule those very feelings, this ridicule created by the masculine overlords of our minds, our egos, trying to squash the very idea that men can love men. The only time this emotion can surface is when the friends are huggy-drunk. This is not to say that these feelings aren't felt, only that men in the West still have great difficulty expressing them.

The third form of love is that of a parent for their child. Once more, symbolically, God is involved, and this time God is the child. We see this in the reverence paid every Christmas to the nativity scenes, to Mary and Joseph adoring the baby in the crèche. We also find the same love in all the joyous stories about baby Krishna and the toleration of the mischievous pranks he loved to play when he was a little boy. The parallel here to your love of God is also obvious: Love your god like you would love your only child, and sacrifice your whole life to his benefit. This attachment is higher and stronger than the first two forms of love, but there is one more bond that society encourages.

The fourth form of love is that between spouses. This is the bedrock upon which societies survive. "What God has joined together, let no man put apart."[11] This is the strongest glue between two people. Jesus said, "They shall be one, though they were originally two: one flesh."[12] One flesh is much harder to break apart than two individuals. The glue here is the love of the other "as if" the other were God: of course the other is not God, and you know he or she is not God, but you strive to behave as if she/he were God. This is the love in marriage of two people for each other. This is the love that grows in time between two people who were given in marriage by their families. Reciprocally, you can and should love God just as you would love your spouse. This love is the commitment of a nun who takes the ring of Christ as a sign of her marriage to Him.

These four kinds of love are very different, but in our language we have but one word to describe them all. No wonder we are confused by love! And then there is romantic love, completely different from all the other forms of love. Not recognizing the difference between romantic love, being "in love" and married love is one of the biggest psychological problems Westerners face today.

Romantic love is the fifth level of love, and this kind of love is *not* sanctioned by society. This is the love that leads to death, destruction and the destabilization of society. Jesus felt this love for his Father and it drew him willingly to the cross. This is the love that the ninth-century C.E. Sufi mystic Al-Hallaj suffered for his beloved. Remember, Mansur al-Hallaj repeated the heresy of Jesus, "I and my beloved are one," and was executed for it. He explained his desire for extinction through the parable of "The Moth and The Flame":

୫ ୫

Late that evening, as the sun began to set, the moth started to fly home. Along the way someone lit a lantern; the moth saw the light and was immediately attracted to it. He flew to the golden flame and was entranced. Again and again he tried to get closer to the beloved light, but an invisible barrier prevented him. All he could do was back off and try once more to fly through the glass that separated him from his heart's desire, but each time he was cruelly beaten back. All night long he battled until, come morning when the sun rose above the horizon, someone extinguished the flame. Dazed, beaten and dejected, the moth fluttered home to his friends and family.

"Where were you?" said his family when the moth finally arrived home. "We were worried about you—my God! What happened to you? You look a mess: You are bruised and beaten, and your wings are bent."

The moth explained, "Oh, I saw something wondrous last night, a great, beautiful light that shone red and gold and drew my heart right out of me. I tried to get closer, but I could not find a way. But I must! I will! I will go back every night for the rest of my life until I can be with my beloved."

"No!" said his friends, "you will kill yourself. Let such things be; they are too much for moths. Do not go back there. Promise us!"

The moth would not make that promise—he could not. He could not sleep, he could not rest; all he could think of that day was the vision of his beloved. He vowed to himself to find a way to join with the golden light.

That evening the lantern was lit again, and the moth flew all around the glass enclosure. Desire would not let him rest. He explored every avenue possible, and finally, toward the last hour of the night, he found the hole at the bottom of the lantern, where the match is placed to light the lamp. The moth wiggled through this tiny hole and was consumed by the light.

The moth is the yogi, the one who forsakes everything—family, possessions, even his own life—for the flames of eternal bliss, of union with the beloved.

In the first four kinds of love, we are allowed to act *as if* the object of our love was God: in our spiritual practice we are also told to love God in the same ways we would love a friend, a child or a spouse. In the fifth kind of love, the beloved *is* God. There is no pretense here: Without our beloved we are in hell. Recall that what makes Satan's abode hell is the fact that from there God cannot be seen. The pain of that separation can be described like burning in fire, but that is just a metaphor, a hint of the real pain we feel when we can't be with our beloved. Al-Hallaj remarked that the job of orthodoxy is to provide the means for a saint to be united with God, which is all the saint ever wanted.[13]

* * *

The fifth kind of love must be reserved for God alone, because to allow this psycho-spiritual energy to manifest in any human relationship is to invite destruction. The earlier four kinds of love can be contained within the world and within society. But if you unleash the power of crazy, divine love outside the safe walls of the temple (in whatever sacred form your temple takes), you risk blowing apart your whole life. This crazy love, when it alights on another human being, becomes romantic love. In that other you perceive your god or your goddess. Love becomes more important than life, and death is preferred to life without your lover. Romantic love is the crazy love that two lovers named Tristan and Isolde suffered unto their deaths! This is their mythic story:

⊰ ⊱

Tristan is floating … drifting … to where, he has no idea. He has committed himself to the sea. None of the doctors can heal the poison that is stealing his life away. He knows he has no choices left; he must trust fate to take him where it will. He leaves his sword with his armor and takes only his harp. As he lies in the small skiff, he strums the strings in rhythm with the waves; his charming music floats over the waters.

Tristan—such a sad name for such a brilliant boy, but he was born in such sadness. Branchflower was his mother; she was the beautiful sister of Mark, the king of Cornwall. Her heart was captured by the brave and handsome Rivalin, who came to visit Cornwall after defeating the evil Duke Morgan. Morgan had tried to steal Rivalin's lands, which lay just beyond the English Channel, in Lyonesse. With his home secure, Rivalin was free to travel, to visit the great King Mark in Cornwall, but he did not expect to lose his heart there. Branchflower was irresistible, and the two soon fell in love. Mark approved the union and they were married, and soon a baby was on the way.

Bliss is short-lived and must be appreciated when it comes. Morgan rose up again, taking advantage of Rivalin's absence. Rivalin returned home to defend his honor and country and took Branchflower with him. The duke knew that Rivalin would come, so he set a trap, ensnared, and killed the young king. Branchflower heard the news during her labor and birthed a boy in sorrow. The labor was hard; Branchflower was dying. She named her baby Tristan, because he was born in such sad times, had no father, and soon no mother.

Rual, the faithful steward to King Rivalin, took the baby and hid him among his own sons, so that Morgan would never learn that an heir of Rivalin was alive. He raised Tristan as one of his own and taught him all the ways of knighthood, of battle and of court affairs, but he also taught him music and proper manners. He was the most brilliant of children, and soon the most talented of teens. He mastered several languages, the lute and the harp; his voice was like an angel's, but in battle he was swift and decisive. His skills caught the attention of Norwegian traders, who stole him away from his family and took him to sea.

God did not approve of the kidnapping of noble Tristan; the seas grew rough, and the storm threatened to capsize the ship of the traders. Realizing their wrong, they set Tristan free in a rowboat, just off the shores of Cornwall. Tristan rowed to land and was discovered by hunters of the king, who took him to the castle. All Tristan had were his fine clothes, his harp, his upbringing and wit. These were plenty; Mark, espying the instrument, asked the boy to play and was overcome by the heavenly music. He bade the youth to remain with him and over the coming months grew to appreciate Tristan's companionship and skills.

Raul was frantic over the abduction of his adopted son, and he set out to search for Tristan, a search that would take many years. Eventually he came to Cornwall and heard rumors of a magnificent young man, accomplished in all the arts of war, and who had appeared out of the waters a few years earlier. Rual's heart soared with hope that he was close to finding Tristan. He went to the castle of King Mark, where his years of searching ended. Tristan immediately recognized his father and brought Raul to the king. It was a joyous reunion.

King Mark was curious about Tristan's background, so Rual sat them both down and told the whole story. Tristan was Mark's nephew, and Rual was not Tristan's father. Tristan's joy turned to anger: He had thought he had two fathers—Rual, who raised him, and King Mark, who treated him so kindly—but now he found out he had no father, or rather he had a father who was killed dishonorably by a coward named Morgan. Tristan's heart was set on revenge.

Tristan sailed home to Lyonesse with blessings and weapons from Mark. The people back home were delighted to hear that he had not been killed at birth and that Rivalin's heir was back to save them from Morgan's cruel rule. Tristan raised an army of knights, and along with Rual and his sons, he attacked Duke Morgan and defeated him. Morgan's lands were added to Tristan's rightful kingdom, but his heart was in Cornwall. He put his kingdom into the trusted hands of Rual and his sons and returned to King Mark.

Upon Tristan's return, he found joy but also sorrow. Mark was very happy that Tristan had obtained victory over the evil duke and survived unscathed; the sorrow was caused by an old wound to the kingdom. Decades ago, the king of Ireland sent his champion, Morold, to war against Cornwall, and none could stand in the field against the Irish giant. He could defeat any five great knights in simultaneous combat. Morold was the brother of the witch-queen of Ireland, Isolde. With her magic and his king's men, Morold defeated the Cornish knights and forced tribute from King Mark. Over a repeating four-year cycle, Mark had to send precious gifts to Ireland: in the first year, 300 marks of bronze, then silver in the second year, and in the third year. gold; but in the fourth year, Morold came to take away the 30 best young men to serve the barons of Ireland. King Mark's court feared this fourth year, for the barons had to present their sons to Morold so he could choose the 30. It was on this day, the day of the tribute, that Tristan returned.

To Tristan, the tribute was intolerable and the solution clear: Someone must rise up and defeat Morold. But none were brave enough to try. Tristan spoke to his uncle and volunteered. Morold sneered at the young man but agreed to his challenge, and they set up the ground for battle on a small island. When Tristan rowed ashore, Morold was already waiting. Tristan pushed his boat back out to sea, prompting Morold to ask, "Why?"

Tristan replied, "Only one of us is coming back, so we have no need of two boats. Yours will do me just fine."

From the shore no one could see the battle, but they could hear Morold's shouts. Three times the Irish soldiers cheered when they heard their champion's voice, and they cheered even louder when they saw Morold's boat returning. Their cheers died in their throats when they saw it was Tristan coming ashore. He had left Morold's dead body on the island and told the soldiers to take him back to his sister and king and to tell them that Cornwall's tribute to the island across the sea was ended.

Tristan had been cut by Morold's sword, but he hid the wounds from the Irish. After they left, he collapsed into

Mark's arms, who quickly summoned the doctors. Morold's sword had been dipped in poison, and now that poison was consuming Tristan's life. It was a deadly concoction, brewed by the witch-queen herself, and none in Cornwall knew a cure. After weeks of languishing, Tristan bade his uncle to commit him to the sea in hopes that a cure might be found somewhere across the water, or if not a cure, then death. Mark tearfully said goodbye to his beloved nephew and set him adrift.

Tristan committed to his fate, and it took him across the sea to the western isle. There his music was heard by fishermen, who found him barely alive in his small boat. They knew that only the queen could save him, so they took him to her. The witch-queen saw his lovely face and beautiful harp and decided he was worth saving. She instructed her daughter, Princess Isolde the Fair, to care for the stricken minstrel and nurse him back to health. Isolde gazed frequently upon the handsome young man and did just as her mother bade. Within a few weeks, Tristan was physically healed, and he begged leave to return home, claiming that he had left a loving wife behind. The queen allowed him to leave, with the only price paid being a final song on his harp. Isolde the Fair did not realize that she had saved the life of the man who had killed her dear uncle, Morold.

King Mark's happiness and amazement at Tristan's return surpassed any emotion he had ever felt. The barons of his court were not so impressed. They privately thought that Tristan must be a sorcerer: how else to explain his extraordinary exploits? When Mark started to claim Tristan as his heir, the barons worried even more. "Our king must have a queen," they said to each other, "but, if Mark holds only Tristan as heir to the throne, Mark will never marry. He must marry!"

The barons started to insist on having a queen beside their king, and they pressed Mark heavily to wed. Tristan realized there was great honor in agreeing with the barons, and, furthermore, he knew exactly who the right woman was for his uncle. He shared his plan with his uncle, and Mark reluctantly agreed. Tristan would return to Ireland and bring Isolde the Fair to Cornwall to be Mark's queen.

Tristan had a plan: While recovering in Ireland, he heard about a dragon that had been plaguing the countryside. The Irish king had promised he would wed his daughter Isolde to whoever slew the worm. Tristan returned to the western isle, this time with his sword and armor. He found the dragon's lair and succeeded in slaying the flying snake. The battle was not without cost, however; his horse got fried, and the fumes of the dragon's breath poisoned him. Near death's door again, he was taken to the queen for healing. Again Isolde the Fair looked after him and brought him back to life.

While Tristan recovered from his wounds, Isolde decided to clean his armor, as a dedicated lady does for her loyal knight. She was happy that her minstrel was back and that he was also a great knight. While she cleaned his sword, she noticed a splinter had broken off, and the shape of the notch looked familiar. She went to her drawer, where she kept a shard of the sword that had killed her dear uncle: It had been left in the fatal wound that robbed him of his life. She took the shard to Tristan's sword and discovered it fit: This knight was her deadly enemy! She watched him sleeping, while her mind and heart wrestled. She should kill this devil right now, but he had won her hand by killing the dragon. What should she do? She raised Tristan's own sword to strike him dead, but Tristan woke and spoke calming words to the princess.

"Isolde – wait! Why do you want my death after bringing me back to life?"

"Because you lied to me. You are not a minstrel, you are the demon who killed my uncle, and I must avenge his death."

"No, it is not like that," said Tristan, "I came to you out of love. I knew of your father's promise to wed you to whoever rid your country of the worm. Is it not my right to take you home with me now? I, who risked everything, even my very life, to come here to fight the dragon and save your people?"

Isolde lowered the sword in confusion; she didn't know what to do. She sought counsel from her mother, who took the matter to the king. Isolde's mother and father agreed that they should hear what Tristan had to say on the matter, so he was brought before them.

"My king and dear lady, thank you for your kindness in listening to me. I know you bear ill feelings toward me because of the death of Morold, but you know in your hearts that I was simply fulfilling my duty to my own liege. There was no malice toward your dear brother, and I did allow you to have his body back. But my coming to your island was for good, not ill. I rid you of the dragon, brought peace and safety to your land, and I bring you an offer."

The king's and queen's hearts were heavy with memories of their beloved Morold, but they bade Tristan to continue.

"I come to offer peace between our two lands. My king, Mark, needs a queen, and there is no one in the whole world fairer than your daughter. Let me return with Isolde so that she may marry King Mark; she will be the queen of a great kingdom and will be rich and loved by the whole country. Let this marriage bring peace between us, now and forever."

The king did wish for peace, and the queen did wish for her daughter a marriage that would befit her station, so it was agreed that Tristan would take Isolde to Mark.

Isolde was not asked her opinion, and she was very angry about the whole affair. Tristan had lied about being married and being simply a minstrel. He had killed her uncle and then lied about his reasons for coming to Ireland. He did not love her; he won her for another. Now, because of all Tristan's machinations, Isolde had to leave her family, friends and country to marry some old fart she had never met.

The queen knew her daughter's thoughts, so in kindness she sent along Isolde's cousin and close companion, beautiful Brangane, to be with her in her loneliness. And the queen did one more thing: She brewed a secret love potion out of wine, organic herbs and magic. She instructed Brangane clearly, "See to it that Mark and Isolde drink this only after they have been married, and only when they are alone, for the next person they see after consuming this wine they will fall deeply in love with for the next three years." Brangane took charge of the bottle and kept it hidden on the crossing back to Cornwall.

Isolde sailed on Tristan's ship, but she was cold toward him. He tried to soften her up with tales and songs, but she would have nothing to do with him. For his part, Tristan felt elated; he had accomplished all he had set out to do. However, Isolde felt degraded and thoroughly used. The day was hot, and Tristan asked a maid to fetch something to drink. The maid could find nothing suitable, so she looked more keenly until she found a bottle of wine hidden in the luggage. She brought the wine to Tristan, who poured a glass for himself and Isolde.

Reluctantly, Isolde drank with Tristan, but when the potion had been consumed, they were both arrested. Their gaze found each other's eyes, and they could not look away. Brangane found them in this entranced state, saw the bottle empty beside them, and cried, "What have you done? You have drunk your death!"

Tristan replied, "If this be life or death, the potion has poisoned me most sweetly; this death suits me quite well. And if Isolde is to be my death, then I welcome death completely."

Brangane's folly became her burden. She knew that the two lovers were lost, so she did the best she could to hide their affair. Tristan and Isolde could not contain the powerful feelings that overwhelmed then. They struggled to regain control, to maintain honor and loyalty, but they gave in over and over again to love. He became she, and she he; they could not bear to be separated for even a moment.

They knew that their life had to be a lie on the outside so that they could be true to each other on the inside. Isolde had to marry Mark, but she was no longer a virgin. To hide their deceit, Isolde convinced Brangane to take her place in the nuptial bed. The room was dark and Mark more than tipsy when Brangane traded places with Isolde. Brangane paid with her own maidenhead the price of her folly, and Mark was none the wiser.

Love cannot be disguised, and soon the shared looks of longing between Tristan and Isolde caused suspicion among the barons. They discovered the lovers' secret meeting spot and convinced Mark that he was being duped. One night they set Mark high in the branches of a tree overlooking the meadow where Tristan and Isolde would meet. He was armed with a bow ready to kill them both, if their sin proved to be true. Tristan arrived first; the night was clear and the moon full. Standing beneath the tree, he noticed the shadow of a man hiding in the branches. He understood that he was caught in a trap and prayed that Isolde would also notice the shadow.

When Isolde arrived Tristan remained aloof and did not move toward her. She was immediately suspicious and then saw the same shadow that had alerted Tristan. They began a charade.

"Why have you asked for me to meet you here?" asked Isolde. "You know how tongues will talk if we are discovered. Why did you want to speak to me in private?"

"Tongues do talk and have spread idle gossip, my dear queen," said Tristan. "I asked you here only to seek your intervention with my uncle. Please, you must tell the king that I am ever faithful and loyal and have never given him or anyone cause to doubt me. I have heard the stories that impugned your reputation. Please tell King Mark that I am willing to meet anyone on the field of honor and prove your innocence through combat."

Hearing the conversation below him, Mark put away his bow and his doubts. He blessed the two who were most dear to him and returned to the castle to chastise those meddlesome barons.

For a while Tristan and Isolde took more care, but their love tormented them, and they risked everything in its name. Eventually, even Mark saw the messages in their eyes. He didn't want to know, but he knew. The pain in his heart grew unbearable; he loved Isolde more than life itself, but he couldn't stand the pain of knowing her heart belonged to another. He called them to account in front of his court and then banished them from his lands and his life. They were exiled to a distant forest.

Three years they lived in the forest; they survived not on food, but on love and desire. They were not bothered by being alone. They were not bothered by having no luxuries. In the fourth year of their exile, they heard hunters chasing a stag and feared that Mark might be near. They retired to the cave that had become their home and lay upon a crystal bed, fixed like an altar in the middle of the room. They were tired, but before falling asleep, Tristan took his sword and laid it between them. They slept apart that morning.

Indeed it was Mark and his barons who were hunting that day. One member of the party discovered the cave and the two lovers sleeping, so he quickly fetched Mark and brought him to see the pair. Mark, looking down from a window in the ceiling, saw his nephew and queen. He recalled his great love for Isolde and his love for Tristan, and he wondered about the meaning of the sword placed between them. Surely this was the sign of chastity, not lust. In Mark's heart it was clear now that he had misjudged them. He quietly stole away, leaving them to rest in peace, but he also, later, sent a messenger to recal them to court. Tristan and Isolde gratefully returned to life in the castle.

The meddlesome barons did not love Tristan even half as much as his uncle did; they were not so easily convinced. They demanded that Isolde be proven innocent in the eyes of God. A test of fire was convened, and Isolde readily agreed to the ordeal. She schemed with Tristan, and they came up with a plan that, with the grace of Jesus, would lay to rest any doubts about her virtue.

The ordeal by fire was to be conducted in a sacred grove reached only by boat. Isolde had Tristan attend dressed as an old pilgrim. Before she came ashore, she told her attendants, "I wish to be pure and clean when I face God, so, to save the hem of my gown, please ask that old pilgrim there to carry me ashore. He seems like a righteous sort and will not dishonor me." This they allowed; Isolde was carried by the disguised Tristan toward the holy fire.

Within the fire was a metal rod, glowing red with heat. She was to take the rod in her hand: If she suffered any burns, it meant she was lying about her virtue and love for Mark, but if she was unharmed, it meant her vow was truthful. And this was the vow she took:

"I vow that no man has ever held me close in his arms except my husband, the king, and of course that old pilgrim, whom you all just saw carry me ashore."

Isolde took the iron bar and held it aloft for all to see. She was unharmed; Jesus proved her innocence.

Isolde and Tristan were innocent in their hearts, for they were always true to each other, but they knew they could not live the way they had been living. They knew they had to part. Tristan took his leave of Isolde with the heaviest of hearts and a promise that if she ever needed him, he would come. She mirrored his love and gave him a green jasper ring, saying, "If you ever need me, send me a message with this ring, and, whatever my situation in life, I will abandon it and come to you."

Tristan returned to Lyonesse to discover that Rual had left the world. Rual's sons gave back the throne to Tristan, but he found life flat and boring. He wandered and fought in many wars for other kings, gained much praise and honor, but nothing healed the wound in his heart. One day, he helped a neighboring king lift a siege and save his realm. He became good friends with the king's son, Kaedin. They hunted together and fought side by side. Kaedin realized that Tristan would be a great husband for his sister, Princess Isolde of the White Hands. Tristan watched Isolde as she worked at her weaving and other homely arts, and he was attracted to the princess physically, but her unfortunate name kept reminding him of the Isolde who already owned his heart. He could not bear the thought of being with another woman, let alone another Isolde.

As the days passed and Tristan had more occasion to be with Isolde of the White Hands, he saw in her eyes growing affection and eventually love. He started to wonder if it would be OK for him to be with another. Why couldn't he force himself to love this Isolde just as he loved the earlier Isolde? Queen Isolde had Mark for warmth and pleasure; why was he denying himself the same companionship? Three times Tristan almost proposed to Isolde of the White Hands, but three times his heart drew him away. Finally, on the fourth approach, his mind was resolved: He asked for and won her, and Tristan married Isolde of the White Hands.

As Tristan prepared for bed on the night of his wedding, the green jasper ring fell onto the floor. It brought the image of Queen Isolde sharply back into his mind, and his heart was pierced. He couldn't bring himself to touch his new wife, for she was not his true love. He pretended to have a wound that prevented him from being with her, from consummating the marriage, and she unhappily accepted the situation. One day, she inadvertently let slip this state of affairs to Kaedin, who was incensed that Tristan was so dishonoring his sister. He accosted Tristan and demanded an explanation. It was only then that Tristan let his best friend know the sad story of his life.

Kaedin was a compassionate man and forgave his companion. To ease Tristan's burden, Kaedin found another battle for him to fight in, to lose himself in, but this battle was ill chosen. Tristan was cut with another poisoned blade and suffered greatly. There were no medicines that could save him, not even the kind ministrations of Isolde of the White Hands. Tristan asked his wife to send for Kaedin, so that he could talk to him in private. Tristan entrusted the green jasper ring to his friend and asked him to bring Isolde the Fair to his side. Only she could save his life.

Tristan was near his end, but hope kept him going. He told Kaedin, should he return with the queen, to raise a white flag as he entered the harbor, but if she refused him, to fly a black flag. All the while, Isolde of the White Hands had hidden herself so that she would hear what her husband was speaking to her brother, and thus she learned the truth of why she could never win Tristan's heart. She was angry, she was hurt, and she was vengeful; she was determined to pay Tristan back for the false way he had treated her.

Kaedin was a good and loyal friend; he succeeded in his task and brought Isolde the Fair. As they neared land, he flew the white flag of hope urging Tristan to hold on. But Isolde of the White Hands told her husband that Kaedin's flag was black—this was her revenge. Tristan realized that his Isolde was not coming, that she had given up on him, and that life was no longer worth bearing. He surrendered into death's keep. When Isolde the Fair arrived, she found her love dead. The pain was too great—her heart burst, and she fell into Tristan's arms. Together they lay, he in she, and she in he, now and for all eternity.

⇜ ⇝

For Western man, the story of Tristan is arguably the most important myth we have come across. It is highly illustrative for women, too, although it is written from a man's point of view. Within this story a woman can see how a man can get lost in love, and she can see how she herself may unwittingly encourage the drama that unfolds in a romance.

Robert A. Johnson renders one of the most complete explorations of this myth in his book *We: Understanding the Psychology of Romantic Love*.[14] In the 12th century C.E. the Church was failing to provide the complete spiritual wholeness required by the European soul. Corruption was growing within the Church, and the patriarchal attitude completely suppressed the feminine. However, the human psyche is resilient; when something necessary for balance is discarded, it is brought back in other ways. This applies to individuals as well as to cultures. In the south of France, there arose a new religion called Catharism. *Cathars* means "the pure ones." What is pure is spirit only; everything else is corrupted. This is the old dualistic viewpoint of purusha and prakriti once more—the body is evil and the soul divine. One aspect of the divine is the feminine quality, and the Cathars venerated women and the legends of Mary Magdalene. True love was not something found on earth between a man and a woman, but the worship of a divine lady, a female savior who would mediate between God and man. She was pure light, and her manifestation on earth was the lady that a good knight served. To quote Robert A. Johnson:

... the Cathars practiced an exemplary morality and offered an experience of God that was at once personal, individual and lyrical. They returned the feminine to religion.[15]

Catharism was eventually declared heresy, and a crusade was fought against it. The ideology went underground, but the suppressed spirituality resurfaced in the practice of courtly love: the devotion of a knight for a specific lady. Strict rules of romance were developed. First, the knight and the lady he championed must never engage in sex; theirs was to be a purely spiritual relationship. Second, they must not be married to each other (presumably if they were married, the first rule would be harder to follow). Finally, they must both work to keep the flame of passion between them alive. The passion, the flame of desire, resulted in intense suffering; but, after all, that is what *passion* means: to suffer! Romantic love requires—no, demands!—suffering.

With this background we can begin to understand the tragedy of Tristan and all the other knights who were tried and tested against this high ideal, and who failed. Consider Lancelot's betrayal of King Arthur and his illicit love affair with Guinevere: the same story, and with the same tragic result.

* * *

Tristan has everything a man could want, in a man's world. He is powerful, talented, successful, admired and loved by everyone. But nowhere in his world is there any sign of the feminine. His mother died before he could know her. He lives in King Mark's world, where there is no queen, nor even a princess to balance the masculine energy. He thinks life is great and that all he has to do is go on playing his games, and all will be fine, but the repressed goddess will not be denied. The witch-queen of the mystic western isle demands tribute, and the price of remaining apart from her rises with time. Every four years her champion comes to demand the highest tribute of all: life! [16] The tribute of 30 young men represents the sacrifice of your own independence that must be given up when you deny your inner queen.

Tristan fights the queen's champion and thinks he defeats him; that is the masculine mask deceiving him, for in the fight Tristan is mortally wounded by feminine magic. There is no cure to be found in the world of science, in the world of men; he can only trust now his inner strength. He floats upon the waters that symbolize the great unconscious psyche. He leaves behind his sword and armor, his masculine symbols, and takes only his harp—a symbol of the feminine. At some deep level, Tristan understands his wound and what is needed to heal him: not fighting, but music. This is a key lesson for all men who have cut themselves off from their inner woman. Fate takes him directly to the queen of his underworld. It was the queen, Isolde, who brewed the poison that has Tristan near death, and it is only the queen who can cure him. Any man who ignores his anima will face the same poisoning; their life becomes dark and meaningless, they have no energy to live, and they can only drift until, if lucky, they are given the chance to come face to face with their salvation.

While recovering in Ireland, Tristan meets a younger Isolde, one who, if he would but recognize her, could help him balance his life. But Tristan has no interest in Isolde and, once cured, returns immediately home to his life with the boys. It is interesting that to escape Isolde, Tristan concocts a lie: He claims to be already married, to have a woman, so he is released. But who is he kidding? He doesn't have anything feminine in his life; you know he'll be back.

And he does come back. On the conscious level, Tristan thinks he is returning to Ireland to win more fame for himself; he will be thought of very highly if he brings back the most beautiful woman in the world for his uncle to marry. He combines his masculine strength and courage in defeating the dragon with guile and deception in winning Isolde. She thought he was coming to win her for himself, but he denies her; he only wants her to enhance his esteem in the eyes of the men back home. She is but a trophy. He does not see her as a worthy mate for himself, at least not at the conscious level. Unconsciously, his anima is playing with him far more than he was deceiving Isolde. Tristan is continually suppressing his anima, and he does not know the terrible price he is about to pay.

The word *potion* comes from the same root word as *poison*, and the love potion that Tristan and Isolde unwittingly drink is poison indeed. The queen poisons Tristan for a second time, because he did not learn the lesson of the first poison. With the drinking of the love poison, Tristan's and Isolde's lives, as they knew them, as they planned and expected them to be, are over. The anima within Tristan has come to the surface and now controls him completely. He no longer sees the woman he tricked into marrying his uncle; he sees only a goddess who demands his complete and utter surrender to her. Isolde is similarly lost. This man she both hates and admires, the killer of her uncle, the deceiver who is stealing her away from her friends and family, the man she couldn't help fantasizing about and looking at, is now her god. Honor and loyalty no longer hold any meaning or power; the only thing of importance is love.

What is this love that the romantics revel in? This is the crazy love of the moth for the flame. Brangane spoke the truth when she warned the lovers that they had drunk their deaths when they took the potion. There is no way to follow the social rules when the highest priority in life is love. This is the one kind of love that society will not allow; this is heresy to orthodoxy. Tristan replies with "Then bring on death!" He would rather suffer in this hell than be cured of the poison.

Hell only appears to be hell to those on the outside. One view of hell is—people are right where they want to be. Dante saw famous illicit lovers from history in hell, and he thought they suffered, but since they were together and romantic love is suffering, they were right where they wanted to be. Tristan and Isolde chose their suffering over fitting into society. People in love play by different rules: It was perfectly OK to sacrifice Brangane's virginity, if it means the lovers can stay together. It was perfectly OK to lie and deceive innocent Mark. Even God was on the side of the lovers, which confirms all the more how right they are. Jesus conspired to help Isolde pass the test of fire, just as Agni refused to burn innocent Sita when Rama doubted her. God arranged for the moon to be full and the sky clear on the night the barons set the trap for the lovers. God was always on Tristan's side, right up to the end.

Romantic love destroys the ordinary day-to-day life that lovers had before the flames were lit. This is not the love of a husband for a wife. Tristan and Isolde are not married. Being "in love" is the exact opposite of married love. This is a source of great confusion in the West today. We think we are supposed to fall "in love" and get married, but marriage cannot contain the awful power of romantic love. A love affair is not a commitment to sharing the mundane realities of daily living with another human being: doing the laundry, washing the dishes, paying of bills and changing diapers at four in the morning. A love affair means grasping for intensity and excitement that breaks all the rules and being declared innocent because it is all done out of the passion of being "in love."

We need two very distinct maps for the word *love* because romantic love is so very different than married love. Properly used, romantic love can lead toward married love, but we must never confuse these two for the same thing. Romantic love has the sparks, sounds and brightness of a newly lit fire. When the kindling and the scrunched-up papers are lit underneath a few sticks of wood, the result is quite dramatic and lovely to watch; there are sparks and bright licks of flame, but the show never lasts long. If you are watching the fire carefully, you will know when to add bigger pieces of wood, and if the wood is good, if it is dry and the right size, eventually the fire burns into a dull glow that radiates deep heat. There are no more sparks, no more bright flames; there is only a tremendous heat. Now you are experiencing married love.

Just who are you in love with when you burn with romantic love? The poison flowing through Tristan caused him to look into Isolde's eyes, and he could not move. What did he see there? It was not Isolde; he had been seeing her for days, and she never arrested him before. What he was seeing now was his own queen, the shadow from his psyche, his anima. Tristan began to project his own image of an idealized goddess onto Isolde, and she her inner god onto him. Romantic love is a mutual projection. The other person simply provides the hook upon which you hang your god image. If the right hooks are present, then the projection will stay, for a while, anyway. Eventually the hooks start to slip, and the real person shows through the projection. When the projection fades, as it always does, romantic love withdraws its power until a new screen is found, with the right hooks, for the next projection. One falls "out of love" until the next episode of falling "in love."

The woman is complicit in the game of romance because she willingly accepts the projection. Who doesn't want to be loved as a goddess, to be thought of as something special, heavenly, without fault? Who wouldn't want her man to fight dragons for her, to protect her reputation and honor, to love her no matter what stands in the way? A woman will go out of her way to ensure the projection fits: She will dress just so, talk just right, walk sexy, look sexy, build the allure that fires his desires. This is all pretty heady stuff, but it is all ego inflation. We want to believe the words our lover whispers to us, but they are not real, and we live in fear that one day he will discover he has made a big mistake. This fear is compounded if the woman has projected her inner god onto him: the risk now is not just losing her man, but losing her god.

When Mark can no longer tolerate the deceit and the deep pain Tristan and Isolde have been causing him, he banishes them. Society does not tolerate those who put themselves outside its laws and the bounds of common decency. Tristan and Isolde run away to the forest. Here is their chance to build a normal life for themselves; but they miss the opportunity. They live off love and desire, not companionship. They spend three years together, but their relationship never progresses or develops, and when the potion wears off, as it always does, what do they have to keep them together?

The three years are up, the potion is waning, and the real world is calling them back. On the day they are discovered, before they sleep, Tristan places his sword between himself and Isolde. What does this mean? This is a commonly accepted symbol of chastity, and Mark recognizes the symbol. These two people are not together, they are not married; and indeed, the real Tristan and Isolde are not a couple in the social sense of the word. Tristan unconsciously wants to return to society, to come back to the real world, and leave the faery forest behind.

Our projections do not last; they cannot last, because they are placed upon flesh-and-blood people. It is impossible for another person to be a god or a goddess. For a man, in time, that beautiful goddess you fell in love with turns out to have moods, annoying habits, periods and headaches, family members you don't like and friends you can't stand. For a woman, the god who romanced you in the early days turns into a bore who leaves the toilet seat up, never makes the bed, and leaves his dirty underwear on the floor. Eventually, one partner turns to the other and says, "Whatever happened to you? You are not the person I thought you were!" Of course it is exactly the same person, but the projection you cast has gone, and you are seeing the real person, perhaps for the very first time.

We are addicted to being "in love," and when the projection fails, as it must, we scout around for someone else upon whom we can place it once more. We fall "in love" with another, and our whole world is turned upside down once more. The drama returns, but we don't care because it is all excusable: "I am in love!" No matter that the separation from your previous partner is painful and messy; love is more important than any of that. This is the great Western mythos fueled by Hollywood, novels, songs, tabloids and magazines: Love conquers all! If you are not "in love," your life is meaningless; you have no reason to live. But this is romantic love, not human love, and it can't last, so we are doomed to fall in love, out of love, long for love, despair over lost love, fall in love again, and go through these cycles over and over.

Had Tristan restored Isolde to Mark and honored her as his queen, he may have survived the transition. If only he had followed the knightly formula for romance discussed earlier. A man needs his anima just as a woman needs her animus. It is how we relate to these inner psychic powers that is important. Tristan abandons Isolde and goes away, but he keeps with him a relic, the green jasper ring: This is another trap that binds him to her. He pretends to leave, to find a real life, but he doesn't really leave—he takes her with him. You probably know friends who live just like this: They are in a relationship that suffers through cycles of breakup and makeup until the next breakup. "This time for sure, it is over!" they claim, but surprisingly soon they tell you, "We are back together, but it is different this time. He is really going to change." They are so addicted to the drama that they can't let go, but they can't live with the situation, either. Through friendship with Kaedin, Tristan finds a nice, grounded, earthly woman whom any man would be happy to be with: Isolde of the White Hands. But he can't bring himself to relate to her properly. He almost succeeds—he marries this wonderful woman—but at the critical moment, his ring reminds him of the bliss of crazy love. He cannot project his anima onto Isolde of the White Hands, even if he wanted to. The projection doesn't fit, and so he abandons any hope of a normal life with a real woman who will love him in a human manner.

You cannot force someone to fall "in love" with you. We have all had this experience at least once: You are lost in love with someone, but your beloved does not reciprocate your feelings. Welcome to hell. This is exactly Satan's pain when he remembers God saying, "Be gone!" This is agony—your god has rejected you. This is King Mark's pain, and it is also the pain Isolde of the White Hands suffers. It is also true that you cannot force yourself to fall "in love" with someone else, either, no matter how much you would like to or they would like you to. We are dealing with tremendous elemental powers here that well up from the deep unconscious, and there is no way ego can summon or control these powers. The puny conscious mind may scheme and reason and try all sorts of things to try to control the world below, but it fails miserably. When faced with the inevitable, all we can do is accommodate it.

There is a big price to pay for rejecting Isolde of the White Hands. If a man rejects a normal life with a relationship on a human level with a flesh-and-blood woman, he is rejecting life. He is as good as dead. Tristan is poisoned for a third time, and again only his anima can save him. He sends to his queen to come save him once more, and she comes, but too late. Isolde of the White Hands has had enough of her husband's deception; she causes Tristan to lose hope of ever being cured. With the death of her lover, Isolde the Fair also has no reason to live. She, too, had been living a lie with King Mark; she never entered into a real relationship with him, and now with Tristan gone, there is no point for her to continue living. Their love poison turned out to be exactly what Brangane foretold: their death.

* * *

Mysterious and strange is the idea that we project that which resides deep within us onto the outside world and then mistake that external image for something separate, something other, something we have no responsibility for and no control over. We can see that projections do occur when we catch other people doing it, when we listen to busy-body Betty criticize Christie for being such a gossip, but it is very hard to catch ourselves in the act. When a projection that we have cast is brought to our attention, we deny, refute, fight and argue: It cannot possibly be true, because clearly that person is behaving badly (or wonderfully, depending upon which kind of projection we have made). It is not us; it is them!

An analogy can help us see what we can't perceive consciously, and a good analogy can illuminate multiple points with one image. So let's pick one of the most powerful gods, one of the most ubiquitous gods, found in our modern world. This is a god that everybody bows down to every day; his power is so great that if we ignore him, he will take his revenge swiftly, inflicting severe injuries or even death. The name of this god with the power of life and death, with the power to stop the greatest and the meanest equally is ... the Stop Sign.

OK, maybe your initial reaction is one of deflation: You were expecting something much more profound and transcendent than a stop sign, but this is a great example not only of how we project our internal state of mind onto external objects, but also how our ability to conceptualize, indeed our inability to not conceptualize, affects us every day.

What is a stop sign? When we look at a stop sign, the symbology is impossible to ignore. We cannot *not* see a stop sign, but we do not see what is really there; we see only what is symbolized. If we were to plunk down a San bushman from the South African desert, someone who had never seen a road or a car, at a rural road intersection in Arizona and show him a stop sign, and then we asked him to tell us what he sees, our visitor would give a description of the stop sign that is much closer to the reality than what we would describe. He might say that he sees a stick in the ground with a circular shape like the sun on top, a peculiar red sun with white designs upon its face. He certainly won't say he sees a stop sign. We can train ourselves to see what is really there, too; we can see the red as simply red and the octagonal shape and the four-by-four wooden post, but we will also see the symbolic meaning of this device. So deep has this god crept into our unconsciousness that we can never not see him.

The idea of a stop sign is a concept that originates in our mind; it is a convention our culture has agreed upon, a command to drivers to stop. Such is its power that we all stop when we reach the domain of this god. It is not really a god, nor is it really a stop sign—that is simply what we have all agreed to call it. To our African friend, he might see the post as firewood and the sign itself as a potential serving platter. He won't be bound by our concepts; thus he'll be free to develop other uses for the materials. This is the power of an artist and a genius: to see what everyone else fails to see, even though it is all right in front of us. Our native from the Kalahari will also be mystified by our supplication to this strange object: Why do we bow down to this post with red and white blotches?

We have created a concept that exists solely within our minds, and we have buried this concept so deeply that we need no conscious effort to respond to it. We project this concept from the depths of our psyche onto the object standing before us. We react unconsciously to the stop sign when we are driving: we stop. This is the power of our projections; we believe that the stop sign is actually a stop sign—but it is not! It is simply what it is: a piece of wood with an octagon placed on top with a red background and white painted squiggles. The human mind is a conceptualizing machine that loves to create ideas and then project them outward onto the real world. It assigns agency and meaning to what we see and is blind to the fact that all of this comes from within.

The stop sign analogy is a great example of our conceptualizing nature and our ability to project unconsciously the concepts we hold deep within us. Hopefully, through this simple analogy, we can begin to get a glimpse of what we do when we fall in love. We have the concept buried inside our psychic landscape of our ideal woman or man (the anima or animus, to use Jung's terms), and when we find a suitable screen upon which to project this concept, out it goes. The woman standing before you is not seen for whom she is; you see only the "stop sign"—the image from within—not the reality of this poor gal who is actually standing there, and whom you are assaulting with your idealized notion of the perfect woman. Your friends, who are not seeing what you are seeing, are like the Kalahari native: They more easily see the real woman, and they can only shake their heads when they hear you describe what you think you are seeing. They leave you alone and mumble to each other, "Love is blind." Indeed, romantic love is blind for a time, but eventually the spell wears off, and the poison is gone. It may take three symbolic years, as Tristan discovered, but finally, we see reality starkly revealed, and we recoil from its blandness.

Now that we understand how we project what is inside onto the outside world, we can think about the nature of the three Isoldes: the holy trinity of the anima. There is Isolde the witch-queen, Isolde the lover, and Isolde the woman of hearth and home. These are exactly the three aspects of Maya: the reflecting function, the projecting function and the revealing function.[17] The witch-queen reflects to Tristan his own unbalanced, one-sided masculinity in the form of Morold. Tristan thinks he has conquered this device of the queen, but he is mortally wounded in the battle and has to go to her to be made whole. He lies to the queen and steals back to King Mark and the boys, rejecting the wholeness offered, so we know he will have to come back and face the music again at some point. Isolde the Fair is his internal projection of romantic love, the beatific vision, onto a mortal woman. This is where Tristan becomes arrested and progresses no further. Isolde of the White Hands is the path through Maya to the real world. Tristan refuses this last task and remains blinded by the projection. We have seen this trinity as well in Dante's story: Tristan's queen is Dante's Holy Mother; Isolde the Fair is Dante's beloved Beatrice; and Isolde of the White Hands is the everyday woman, Dante's wife, also symbolized by Saint Lucy.

Trinities are incomplete, as we have discovered, and require a fourth; in this case, Tristan is the fourth. All three Isoldes are part of him, and he completes them the same way Mother Mary completes the Holy Trinity of the three Christian males. Tristan's first task is to come into a proper relationship with the three inner women and then to realize his identity with them—they are him. These are again the two great spiritual paths: the Western path of relationship with the divine and the Eastern path of identity with the divine; they are both available. The doorways to them are the sixth and seventh chakra, as we will discover in the next section.

* * *

What is really going on in the story of Tristan and Isolde? Why is romantic love so important to us that we can't live without it, yet we can't seem to live with it? This is the tragedy of losing God. The spiritual side of life in our Western culture has been downgraded to such a degree that we have no place for any gods. This is exactly what caused the Catharism revolution, the rise of the troubadours in France and the minnesingers in Germany in the 12th and 13th centuries C.E. The Church was failing in its role of providing spiritual sustenance, so people started looking elsewhere. The feminine anima was taken out of the depths of the psyche and placed up in heaven, where she belongs. When the conservative backlash from the Church was over, when tens of thousands of people had been killed for believing the Cathars heresy, the poets removed the anima from the Mother of God and placed her upon the grand ladies of the court. The anima was displaced from the heavenly realm to the earthly world, but still the woman holding a man's projection was remote and ideally unobtainable. Remember the three rules of courtly love that would have saved Tristan! The sin occurs when, like Tristan or Lancelot, a man tries to possess his goddess physically instead of worshipping her at a distance.

Romantic love is not a recent phenomenon. We learned from Ovid via his story of Pyramus and Thisbe that it has been around for thousands of years. It has appeared in other cultures, but only in the West has it become the mass phenomenon that it is today. We have inherited the sins of Tristan and Isolde, Guinevere and Lancelot, and we suffer without being aware that there could possibly be another way. But good myths not only explain why things are the way they are, good myths also offer a solution. There is a reason why Hindus do not have the problems we have today in the West: their myths teach them a different way to deal with the power of romantic love. This is their story:

⚘ ⚘

The sound of the flute is irresistible. Krishna stands on one foot, legs crossed at the ankles, like the Planter's Peanut character. His eyes are closed as he sweetly plays his instrument. The music floats on the evening air out of the glade to the homes of the gopis, the cowgirls and milkmaids, who are resting in their beds. They stir in their sleep; their dreams wake them up.

Radha was hoping to hear Krishna's music again—she waits for it every night. She sneaks out of bed, her sleeping husband snoring contentedly without her. Donning her most alluring clothes but holding her bangles in her hand so that she makes no noise, she slips out of the house. Only then does she put on her jewelry and make her way to the forest of Vrindavan.

She is not alone: Thousands of other women also long to dance with Krishna. They are all beautiful and young, dressed in their finest saris and garlands, fragrant with musk and saffron. The sounds of bangles on thousands of ankles create a symphony moving toward Krishna.

Krishna awaits them in his meadow. He continues his music as the host of women descends upon him, but his eyes are looking keenly for the one jewel that shines the brightest: Radha, his beloved. When he sees her, he finally stops playing. He takes her by the hand and leads her to the bower he had prepared.

Among sacred sal trees, white flowers make up their bed. Krishna gazes into Radha's eyes, and she is lost in his. They would have stayed that way for eternity, but finally Radha launches her attack. Her lips devour his, her hand pulls his hair and forces his head back so she can attack his throat. Krishna seizes her in reply, his arms enfolding her tightly. The battle begins. She boldly opens her sari and forces his head to the luxury of her breasts. Their legs intertwine, and she offers her treasure to him. Radha becomes Krishna's slayer. She rocks with the rhythm of love, feeling his trembling joy. Her lips are covered with his dew, and throughout the night they perfect the eight practices of love, including the forbidden and the profane.

The other gopis are not ignored. Krishna multiplies his perfect body many thousand fold and dances with each woman. The sweetness of the night ends with the faint hint of the sun; Krishna restores to every woman her virtue so there are no signs of the night's lovemaking. Before the sun is fully above the horizon, the women are back in their beds, and their husbands are none the wiser.

⚜ ❦

It is interesting to note that the stories of Krishna and his human lover Radha are from exactly the same time as the stories of courtly love in Europe: the 12th and 13th centuries C.E. The romantic poet Jayadeva compiled the story of Radha's hunger for her god Krishna and the great god's love for this mortal woman. The poem is called the "Gita Govinda" or the "Song of the Cowherd". The tale tells of agony and bliss, rejection and mistakes, corrections and consummation.[18]

The Hindus solved the problem of ecstatic, crazy, romantic love by ensuring it remained projected onto a god. Just as we find in the West, romantic love, this crazy love, the moth's desire for the flame, cannot be contained in normal, everyday life. Radha is a married woman, living a normal life with her husband by day, but by night her life is given up to a god himself. She does not expect her husband to be the god of love; he is to be her best friend. She is to honor, respect and obey him in all things, but her spiritual lover is Krishna.

The 19th-century Indian saint, Ramakrishna, was a modern master of crazy love. He employed the "Gita Govinda" as a vehicle, a way to be with God. The scriptures of Vishnu advise that to see Krishna, one must first approach Radha. This is the same equation we find used by Jesus in the Catholic philosophy: Christ through his humanity is related to us and through his divinity relates us to God. In the Indian story, it is Radha who is human and related to us, and through her love of the god, Krishna and Krishna's love of her, she brings us to him. Of course, this seeming separation is all an illusion, for the basic idea in the East is that we are a god. This is what Ramakrishna finally experienced, but first he had to woo Radha. He described his first vision of her:

"It is impossible to describe the heavenly beauty and sweetness of Radha. Her very appearance showed that she had completely forgotten herself in her passionate love for Krishna. Her complexion was a light yellow."[19]

It is the rapture of divine love, of crazy love, that transports us to the transcendent. After experiencing Radha, the door was open to Krishna, and soon Ramakrishna became Krishna. In this merging of his own small identity with the source of the universe, Ramakrishna experienced immortality and transcendent bliss. That is the path that is open to the Hindu.

✳ ✳ ✳

Christians, Jews and Muslims are not Hindus; the myths that work for one culture will not work in another. They cannot adopt the Hindu way of life, but other cultures can look for clues and ideas within the Hindu stories and incorporate these ideas into their own stories. We can look at the solution that Wolfram von Eschenbach offered in the story of Parzival, and the time is right to revisit the lessons found there.

In Europe in the 12th century C.E., a person's life was proscribed: He went to church to participate in the spiritual mystery embodied in Jesus Christ. There, a priest did all the work; a person simply had to ingest a wafer to participate in the mystery. This ritual minimized one's own initiative and involvement. Wolfram's story of the quest for the Holy Grail showed another way. Parzival did not take a wife that was given to him; he earned his wife, loved her, and married her without any sanction of society or clergy. Parzival did not fall "in love" with Condwiramurs, but he loved her deeply and honored her when they were apart. His inability to find joy in the picnics and parties hosted by King Arthur was due to his being away from his wife, but he must be parted, for he had to undertake a spiritual journey: He had to find the Grail. Eventually, he does find the Grail—not in a church, but in a secular castle. There he finds the Grail King, not a pope. And the Grail is being borne by a woman; this is not the communion host being brought forward by a male priest. Wolfram's Parzival is a completely spiritual love story, without religious dogma or societal dharma. It displays the importance of the knight's realization that Amor is the reverse spelling of Roma. He turns the Church's and society's demands around 180 degrees and shows that it is the individual's own effort that will save him and bring him to spiritual and secular fulfillment. Joseph Campbell believed that the story of Parzival, in the hands of Wolfram von Eschenbach, was the greatest love story of the Middle Ages, surpassing the myth of Tristan.[20]

The myth of Tristan also has the solution embedded within it. All Tristan had to do was marry Isolde of the White Hands and leave Isolde the Fair on her throne with King Mark! This is where Tristan fails and Parzival succeeds. It is possible for a man in the West to use the tremendous power of romantic love to honor the feminine within, without projecting her onto another woman who cannot bear the load. This is exactly what Dante did: He married someone other than Beatrice, his one true love, but he did not let marriage prevent his image of Beatrice from being his guide to the beatific vision. Marriage in the West can be a joining together of two human beings, without the burden of asking the other to be a god. We can fan the flames of kindling, but then we must watch and tend the flames with care as they develop into a quiet, deep fire.

Most married people "in love" are not truly married; they have just entered a relationship of mutual convenience. The back door of divorce is always there. However, if a woman vowed to her husband, and a man to his wife,

> "I promise that you will be my best friend even when the illusion of romance has left us; to accept you just as you are, and not try to mold you into someone who will make me happy; to stay with you through thick and thin and all the bad times that life has waiting for us; to put our relationship ahead of your or my own self-interest,"

then they will be truly married, regardless of whether any church or social ceremony was conducted.

Does this mean that we have to give up that buzz that romantic love brings us? Is this exquisite agony forever lost to us if we commit to a human relationship with another person? Not at all. The psycho-spiritual power that moves us to bliss, awe and wonder is still available within every person, and there are ways to manifest and experience it. We do not have to burden our partner with the responsibility for rendering to us the state of bliss; we can find it in ourselves. This is exactly the fourth function of mythology: to put us into accord with the mystical realm of life. This is what we will investigate next.

The Psychological Function of Mythology: Summary

The psychological function of mythology is to create bridges between the small individual and the cosmos in all its grandeur, between the individual and the society in which he has found himself a participant, and between the individual and the mystery that is life itself. There is a lot to do here! Mythologies open us to the world around us and to the world within us. The psychological function of mythology is also the pedagogical function: Myths teach us and guide us through the inevitable stages of our life. Through the stories that resonate within our culture, we learn how we are to deal with life's changes as we grow up, as we grow older, and as we prepare to pass from this world.

The Western myths that created the maps, which direct our initiation into adulthood, walk a fine line. We are directed to achieve great things and seek personal success, while simultaneously told to pare down our individual desires so we can play a proper part within society. This not an easy adjustment, for society demands part people, people who are carved up to fit special niches, but our psyche strives to make us whole. Every person, either consciously or unconsciously, must work out the balance between these two competing imperatives: dharma and duty versus kama and pleasure. If we cannot accommodate these energies, the imbalance manifests as sickness at some level, be it physical, mental or emotional. In the East the cure for this diseased state is called moksha, which is liberation, freedom or enlightenment, and this cure often involves a retreat from the world entirely—retiring to the forest to become a hermit monk or a yogi.

This is not the Western way, and indeed there are also many paths in the East that offer wholeness while remaining within society. Our unconscious need to seek wholeness drives us, but how this drive manifests depends upon our concept of who we are at the level of soul. Our culture provides the myths and maps that answer the basic question, "Who am I?" I am a body that has a soul. Or, perhaps, I am a soul that has put on a body. We act within the world to achieve our ultimate liberation in a manner that depends upon our own internal, unconscious view of our own nature.

The psychological function of myths can be seen as a complement to the sociological function, but these two are also often in competition. At one level the psychological function helps us to accept our roles in society: how to be a good father, a good wife, a good worker. But at another level, we are taught how to become individuals, and by following our own unique path, we are led to psychological wholeness. There are very different maps used in the East and in the West. The Levantine mythologies, based on the idea of men being the servants of the gods and thus servants of society (with our only legitimate role being to "obey!"), came into Europe after the death of Jesus Christ. These stories clashed with the Western instinct of every man to find self-actualization and blaze his own trail through life, despite what the gods may want. These two very different maps are overlapping in the modern Western psyche, and the conflict has not been worked out fully yet.

Are we divine or simply divinely created? Depending upon which story rules in your psychic landscape, your action and reactions to the world of nature and to your fellow beings may be dramatically different. Without being consciously aware of which mythos you are following, you are simply living life on autopilot, following the programming laid down years or even decades ago. This may be perfectly OK, and your life may be flowing wonderfully, in which case you may be well-advised to just leave things alone; or this may be perfectly not OK, and life may suck big time, and you may be well-advised to wake up to why you are living your life the way you are.

Myths are created for a place and time, but when times change, the myths must also. This is true for the psychological function of myth, as well, and is very apparent in the ways the old stories depicted women. The echoes of these ancient memes are still reverberating today; women have come a long way in the last 100 years, but they are not yet treated as equal to men. Throughout history and across cultures East and West, women were feared, misunderstood, dominated and used by men. The mythic stories taught how the perfect woman was to behave: to be always chaste, loyal and devoted to her husband and sons. Women were property, and men were free to dispose of their proper however they saw fit. The myths today are finally catching up to modern society's secular ethics that all people are equal, regardless of gender. The old stories are being rewritten, and young girls today are learning that they can grow up to be free, independent adults who get to choose their own path in life, just like any man; and just as any man, they are free to suffer the challenges inherent in this quest for individuation. For women, the challenge is to be as free as a man but still be a woman, not a pseudo-man. Better myths are still needed.

One of the reasons women are still objectified, rather than seen as real people, is the power that romantic love has gained in our culture. The psychological function of myths guides us in matters of the heart, love and marriage, although not always skillfully. The West today suffers from a misplacement of our spiritual energy. We have lost sight of God and don't know where to look; the older religions have not kept pace with the cosmologies of the day and thus seem quaint. By insisting upon facts that are not true and history that did not happen, religions have lost their mystery. Human nature is such that people are drawn to wonder and awe; the spiritual side of man is part of who he is, and if the myths do not provide the maps showing where this energy can be safely expended, then the spiritual energy doesn't just go away, it goes somewhere else. In the West, it has gone somewhere else—it has become projected onto our romantic partners. This a dangerous place to store such awesome energy: the projections do not hold, and the collapse of the projection can be destructive and agonizing. Fortunately there are some myths that allow for the proper channeling of our spiritual drive, and this brings us to the fourth and foremost function of mythology: the mystical function.

The Mystical Function

The first function of mythology then is to function by showing everything as a metaphor to transcendence.

—Joseph Campbell – *The Hero's Journey*

Chapter 14: The Horror of Life

ॐ ॐ

Even by demon's standards, the monster Rahu was arrogant, proud and greedy. He had some successes, won a few battles, and now he felt he could defeat any god. As the self-proclaimed most powerful being in the cosmos, he deserved—no, demanded!—the most beautiful woman in the world, Parvati, the consort of Shiva. Rahu approached Shiva and presented his demand: Shiva must turn over Parvati, daughter of the great Himalayas, to Rahu!

Shiva contemplated for a brief moment not the request of Rahu, which was patently absurd, but how to teach Rahu an appropriate lesson. Seeing that the demon's greed was insatiable, Shiva decided to show Rahu what true hunger was like. From his third eye came a flash of lightning, which struck the ground beside Rahu, and when the smoke cleared Rahu saw Greed manifest in all its raw power and horror. The new monster was several times larger than Rahu, bore the head of a lion shining brighter than the sun that consumes the stars each morning, and was hungrier than Rahu. Indeed, it had the greatest appetite ever created, and it was poised to eat Rahu in a single swallow. Greed was born to do but one thing: consume.

Rahu was undone and knew that he could not outfight nor outrun Greed, and he knew he had but one course of action available: He turned to Shiva and asked for mercy. The gods must follow certain celestial rules, and one rule is that when someone asks for mercy, mercy must be shown. Shiva ordered Greed to stay its appetite and leave Rahu alone.

Greed obeyed Shiva but spoke on its own behalf. "But what about me? You created me to consume but now stop me from doing what I was born to do. What am I supposed to eat now?"

Shiva knew that, uncontrolled, Greed would devour the whole universe; such was his power and hunger. But then a brilliant idea came to Shiva and he said, "Well, eat yourself!"

This is exactly what Greed started to do. He began with his feet, chewed up his own legs, consumed his own belly and arms, and continued eating until even his lower jaw disappeared. When he was finished, all that was left was a shining face with upper teeth ready to consume anything else that would come within reach.

"How wonderful," exclaimed Shiva, "how marvelous! In honor of your dharma, I shall name you Kirtimukha, the shining face of glory. Your face will be placed over the doorway to all my temples, so that everyone will see what true devotion is."

And so it came to pass that before anyone could come to knowledge of Shiva and Parvati, they first had to pass beneath the visage of the horror of life that consumes life.[1]

Figure 6: Kirtimukha - The Shining Face of Glory

※ ▷

The fourth function of mythology puts us in accord with that tremendous mystery that is life itself. For Joseph Campbell the mystical function reconciles consciousness to the fact of its own existence. This mystery is the Dao that cannot be named; this mystery is the Cloud of Unknowing that can only be experienced. There can be no God here, because to name the experience *God* is to miss what it truly is. We are taught to accept completely the contradictions and horrors that are inherent in life, that all life feeds on life, all life contains much pain and sorrow, and yet all life is ineffably beautiful and wondrous.

The desire to understand the mystery of life is awoken through wonder. We see the stars at night and wonder; a mother suckles her newborn baby and she is arrested in awe; you stand at the top of a mountain, stopped by the beauty of what you behold. In our stillness there are no thoughts, but soon the questioning mind resurfaces and asks, "Why?" The only proper answer is a story, but which story? The mystical function of mythology answers the question "why?" and points to a purpose for life, to life's meaning. But more than purpose or meaning, the great myths take us beyond, to the indescribable *experience* of life.

Up to now, it may seem that we have looked only at the negative aspects of the ancient myths, and with good reason— most no longer serve us. We no longer need myths to instill a cosmic sense of awe anymore; we have scientific models and modern media that do it very well. We don't need myths to tell us how to structure society; we have our secular political sciences, and human ethics and morality, which work far better and much more fairly than the old-time religions. There are still many myths and stories that can help us as we pass through the psychological stages of life, but again, many of the older and even the current stories are not great models for us to follow today. Is it possible that we can find value in the last of the four functions of mythology, the mystical function?

So, finally, we arrive at the mystical aspects of mythology, which Joseph Campbell claimed is actually the first and foremost function. Here we can say that it is our modern secular and scientific models that do not serve us very well, nor do many of the old myths, when they are rendered as history—but when looked at symbolically, they do have a lot to offer us.

We must begin with the recognition that life is sublime.

* * *

When Robert Oppenheimer witnessed the immense destruction he unleashed at the Trinity nuclear test site on July 16, 1945, where mankind ignited the first atomic bomb, he recalled the words of Krishna to Arjuna, *Now I am become Death, the destroyer of worlds.*[2] The vision of the end of the world, which Oppenheimer beheld in the furnace of atomic nuclei tearing each other apart, was sublime. What is sublime is at once horrifying and awesome; it compels one to witness, to worry, to wonder. In its ultimate realization and expression, life is sublime: it is fascinating, totally absorbing and ultimately fatal.

The story of Kirtimukha is mirrored in other myths that recognize the same reality: Life feeds on life. In Greece, the life-eating monster is the snake Ouroboros, whom Plato described as the first living creature.[3] The symbol appeared, perhaps for the first time, in Egypt as two snakes eating each other's tails, symbolic of the gods Ra and Osiris manifesting as the eternal cycle of life and death, and of the contest between the lunar and solar mythologies. In India these snake motifs are common, as well, and the kundalini snake of Tantra and Hatha Yoga is often depicted as coiled up, completing three-and-a-half turns, and with its tail in its mouth. Life feeds on life. We are told to eat up the world, and we have been doing a masterful job of it; there is no place left on this earth that man's appetite has not disturbed.

When we start to investigate the mystery that is life, we are soon perplexed and horrified by what we find. How do we explain the presence and prevalence of suffering in the world? This is a continuing conundrum for religious teachers: If there is a kind and loving God looking over us, how can he let evil loose upon the world? If God created everything, He must have created evil, too—why? Why would He do that? In what way was it a kindness to allow 230,000 people die in a tsunami on Boxing Day, 2004? When something that horrible occurs, we call it an "act of God," but the question remains: Why would God act like that? There seems to be no adequate answer to this question. To say that it is part of God's grand plan that we mere mortals cannot comprehend is not an answer, it is a cop-out, the same cop-out used by the authors of the Book of Job. Perhaps it is a necessary cop-out because, if we can find no other rationale, the alternative is to consider God mad.

How could God allow over 10 million innocent Jews to be murdered in a Holocaust? This was neither an act of nature nor an act of God; it was an act of man and a terrifically evil act of man. How could a personal, loving God stand by and allow this to happen? Life is horrible, yet life is sublime, as well. Where does the overwhelming joy of living, despite the pain, suffering and termination of life, come from? We need stories to explain it all to us, so that we don't go mad with the despair of not knowing why we are and what existence is all about. To acquire the light of understanding, we need to plunge deep into the darkness; we will need to go on a heroic adventure of understanding life through both its horrific and arresting aspects.

‹§ §›

In the most ancient of times, there was no death, and since there was no death, there was also no birth. All that was, was already. But all that was about to change, for one day a murder was committed; balance was lost, and a life left the universe. The universe demands balance, so the body of the one murdered was broken into pieces and planted in the earth, and from its death, new life began. That was the signal: sexual organs, the act of sexual congress, and finally birth arose to balance the loss of life through death. And so it became necessary to seek both death and birth together, for these twins are inseparable.

⚜ ⚜

We have already seen stories of primal cultures where, before two people can marry and beget new life, an existing life must be taken. In the head-hunting cultures of Papua New Guinea, before the husband and wife can marry, the young man has to kill a member of another tribe: He has to get a head, and that head is there at the wedding table; the young child who is to come will have the name of that slain man. [4] The slaying of the buffalo by the American plains natives required the ceremonial returning of the blood to the earth. This is a theme from the ancient planting communities, and it reached its macabre heights in the mythic instruction leveed on India through the rites of Kali, rites of sacrifice that persisted right up to the 19th century, when the British Raj ordered an end to the shedding of human blood in Kali's temples.

Kali goes by many names and incarnations in India. [5] As Shayama-Kali she is a gentle household goddess providing boons and favors. When disaster is upon the land, she is also known as Raksha-Kali and dispels fear when droughts, earthquakes, famine or plague strike. However, in her sublime aspect she is known as Smashana-Kali, the goddess of the cremation grounds, similar in her fierce aspects to Durga-Kali, her mouth dripping with blood, and surrounded by evil female spirits and animals who live on dead bodies. As we discovered in her story told earlier, Durga, the one who is hard to approach, was the source of Kali—conceived to scoop up a demon's blood before it returned to the earth and begat further demons.

Kali is also known as Shakti, the feminine counterpart to Shiva; when Shiva is considered the creator, the source of life, Shakti in her horrific aspect is the source of death. She is often depicted standing astride the corpse of her dead husband: She is the active principle and the activating energy of life; he is the form of life. But if he turns his face away, as shown in the image here, then no energy can flow from her into him, and he is dead; he is *shava*, the corpse, and in this form he has quit the world, just as many yogis do.[6] Shiva in this corpse position is *namarupa*—name and form only; as always in India, it is the feminine that animates.

In the images of Kali, we see the blood red tongue with which Kali licks back the world, the garland of severed skulls, a skirt of arms and hands, from her ears two dead babies dangling as earrings, her blood-soaked sword, and death and destruction all around her. Her very name means "Black Death" and "time", which is the ultimate destroyer of all things, including the universe itself. And yet she raises her right hand, inviting us to not be afraid, and her lower right hand is extended in the boon-bestowing gesture. The symbolic death that she brings is to the sense of ego, the small self, shown here as the severed head held in her lower left hand.

Kali dates back to before the time of the Vedas, before the proto-Indo-Europeans rode their chariots onto the Gangetic plains, back to the earliest planting cultures indigenous to India. She is the most ancient of all the gods, superior even to Shiva, who has succumbed to her. It is Kali that gives life, although, in later stories it is Shiva who gives life purpose. The image of Kali astride her dead husband's body hearkens back to an old story, the story of the horse sacrifice described in the earliest Upanishad.[7] In that story the king's wife, under the cover of a shroud placed over her and the freshly slain

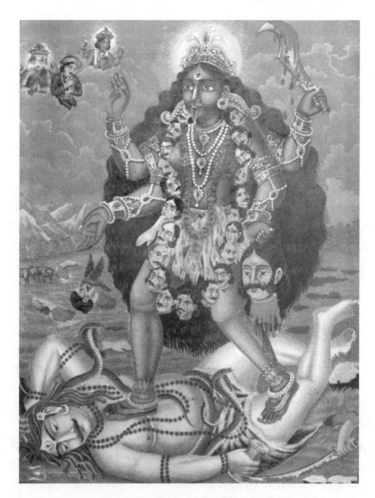

Figure 7: Kali astride her dead husband, Shiva.

prized horse of the king, mimics sexual intercourse with the dead stallion, which in turn echoes an even earlier ritual intercourse of a high-born woman with a sacred bull, all symbolic of the original god fertilizing Mother Earth so that she may bring forth life.

For a community to assure itself of continued food, children and prosperity, for a community to survive and thrive, a price must be paid and sacrifices made. From the writing of

337

Indologists like Zimmer, Eliade and Campbell, and from eyewitnesses who described the events to Frazer, who noted them in his book *The Golden Bough*, we can eavesdrop on an imaginary human sacrifice as practiced by early devotees of Kali before the arrival of the Europeans, in the city that bears her name: Calcutta, now known as Kolkata, the city of Kali:[8]

꩜ ꩜

The *meriah* was a willing participant, a young man of about 15 years, tending toward skinny, with very dark skin and hair as black as Kali. He was chosen weeks before for this singular honor, and honored he was! He was consecrated, given whatever pleasures he asked for, and ultimately he would be rewarded for his sacrifice with many future blessings and a good rebirth. On the few occasions when a meriah was not found, a victim would be stolen; but usually meriahs were simply procured from willing families or bred specifically for this duty. In the days leading up to the ultimate puja, the victim was adorned and anointed with turmeric and oil, then taken door to door through the villages so everyone could touch him, take a smear of oil from his head to dab on their own foreheads, beg a drop of spittle, or pluck a hair.

When the autumn moon had been completely consumed by the sun; when the very small altar was richly clothed within the simple temple nestled against the dense jungle; when a huge black statue of Kali, standing prominently in the center of the temple, was draped in red, orange and white flowers and had her tongue and eyebrows painted blood red, the day of Durga Puja had arrived. In the square in front of the temple, where Kali could see and soak in the ambiance of the festival, were dozens of wooden posts. To each an animal was tied; most were goats, but there were also chickens squawking in protest, adding to the general din of the voices and the shouts of the devotees. The animals' fear was palpable, for they knew their fate: They trembled each time a man came near, and their glassy eyes reflected the red of the torch lamps illuminating the square. In one corner a pit about three feet deep would prove useful soon. Around the perimeter of the square were channels carved in the stone floor to gather and direct the flow of blood to large urns; this blood was to be given back to Kali. In the center of the square was one prominent post larger than the others: This is the post to which the meriah would be tied, but first the animals must be sacrificed.

Naked from the waist up, young men of the lowest castes—for the twice-born can never soil their hands with such tasks—awaited the signal from the Brahmins, and then it began. One man held the hind limbs of the tethered animal, steadying it, while his accomplice neatly, cleanly, and in one deft swing, severed the goat's head. The goat was aimed away from the men so the blood would spurt on the ground, not on them. The severed body jerked continuously for several minutes, while the head was tossed in the waiting pit. The pit filled quickly as pairs of men stalked the braying goats. When still, the body of the headless goat, still oozing life out of its veins, was thrown to eager hands waiting to dismember, cook, and devour the good bits. The heads, bones and bowels would be reduced to ashes that would be spread upon the earth or mixed with the crop seeds to preserve them, but the good meat was to be eaten ceremoniously. When the posts were empty, new animals were brought in; hundreds would be given to Kali this night. The blood filled the gutters, and men began to slip in the red slickness covering the floor. Outside the killing square, the pyre's smoke swirled, at times blinding everyone, and at times rising languidly up into the black, moonless night.

Now at the peak of the whole deliberate business, a new frenzy began. The chosen one, the anointed one, was brought forth—the willing one whose sacrifice would ensure life for everyone else. The devotees shouted louder and waved their torches, but the meriah looked dazed and distant: He had been drugged with opium and would feel nothing. He was blessed; he was lucky—in other cities the meriah had his arms and legs broken so that he could not run away. At those temples, tears were desired, for tears are the symbols of rain; the more tears that the victim was coerced to shed, the greater the rains that would come to water the fields. Here, on this day, Kali only wanted blood.

The Brahmins presiding over the ritual absolved themselves of any wrongdoing with a declaration: "O Kali, we offer this sacrifice to you; give us good crops, seasons, and health." To the meriah they said, "We bought you with a price and did not seize you; now we sacrifice you according to custom, and no sin rests with us."[9]

The meriah was secured to the post, the first cut made, and then the next, and then the waiting mob attacked the victim, each devotee desperate for a piece of flesh. Only the head, the guts and the bones are left for the pyre – all the other flesh was quickly taken to the homes of worshippers in the outlying villages. Running as fast as they could, sometimes in relay teams, the devotees of Kali took their piece of flesh to the Brahmin of their village, who cut the offering in two. One half he offered to the goddess herself and buried it in a communal hole so that the whole village was blessed. Then the priest divided the second lot into as many pieces as there were farmers, and each took his piece home, wrapped it in leaves, and buried it in his land or offered it to the stream that watered his fields.

※ ※

Joseph Campbell reported that one petty monarch in 1830 offered 25 men at Kali's altar in Danteshvari; in the 16th century the King of Cooch Behar offered 150 men in the same temple. [10] In the region of Assam, which is situated just north and a little east of Kali's city, it was customary to offer one victim every year at the Durga Puja. Since the British outlawed this practice in 1835, animals have taken the place of humans, and some sacrifices to this day see slaughtered hundreds of goats, water buffalo, sheep and fowl; blood still flows toward Kali, despite recent efforts to end the killing. Our modern secular society is sickened by the practice, but to the mystics of the old ways, who taught that all life is sorrowful, this is life.

To Ramakrishna and many others, Kali is known as Kali-ma or simply "Ma," the great mother. He saw in her the positive aspect of life, the affirmation of what life could be, not the negation. Paraphrasing Ramakrishna, "If people see Kali as black, it is because they are not close enough to her to see that she is actually colorless."[11] As she was in the beginning, in the planting culture before the arrival in India of the proto-Indo-Europeans, today Kali-ma is once again the chief power, identified by Ramakrishna as the embodiment of Brahman.[12]

Of course, our modern sensibilities recoil at the horror of animal sacrifice. Not even the most ardent Western fundamentalist would revert to the Old Testament practice of personally sacrificing a lamb to God to expiate sin or protect him from calamity. But this doesn't diminish the horrible fact of existence that life still feeds, and must feed, off life. We are remote from the abattoirs today; we do not see our food prepared, killed and dressed for our table—the horror is confined and contained. We don't see what we have done to our planet and nature; the horror we have unleashed upon her is denied, and we try not to see the other modern horrors all around us. Human sacrifice is not lost; it has been sanitized until we no longer recognize it for what it is: We still praise and honor the brave volunteers who willingly go to war on our behalf, these modern meriahs who offer theirs lives so that ours might be better.

There are fundamentalist religious leaders who deliberately evoke the horror of existence in their sermons. They preach of hell-fire and eternal damnation, of retribution both in the here-and-now and in the hereafter. When a catastrophe occurs that moves common people to compassion, these zealots preach that the victims were being justly punished for some imagined sins. Pat Robertson comes to mind: When an earthquake in Haiti in 2010 killed 100,000 people, Robertson said the Haitians were reaping the rewards of a pact with the devil, struck 200 years earlier! [13] When Hurricane Katrina devastated New Orleans in 1995, he implied it was in retribution for abortions.[14] In this view, these victims were sowing what they reaped, in the same way the so-called comforters of Job insisted that, if Job was being punished, he must have done something wrong, because God does not harm the faithful, only the wicked. This is a false view of the reality of life: The reality of life is—"shit happens!" Life is not evil, but it is certainly dangerous.

Darkness is not evil; we mix these terms up in the West and think they are the same. Not so—evil is a human judgment rendered onto darkness: It is an ethical conclusion. In reality darkness is merely dangerous. This is a pragmatic conclusion—you don't know what might lurk in the dark, so you become cautious. A tiger is dangerous, but it is not evil; it is simply living its life in the way tigers live. Do you see the difference? Just because something is dangerous, doesn't make it evil, but even though it is not evil, it doesn't mean you should treat it lightly: It is still dangerous!

※ ※ ※

As we have seen, with the collapse of the cosmological function of religious teaching, which formed the basis for setting social and personal rules for living, the old-time religions started to lose their credibility and their effectiveness.

While the secular social changes have been for the best, since they allow human and humane laws to be enacted and enforced, we lost something vital when the collapse also eviscerated the mystical foundation of life. Our ability to deal with the horror of life has been diminished, and in its place we have turned to placebos, such as mass media and the various drugs of despair, diet and duty to hide the awful fact that life is awe-full. These placebos do work, for a time, but in the end Kali is still waiting, her tongue ready to lick us back into the void: There are horrible monsters all around us.

Our modern fears are not the same as our ancestors'. We do not fear the jungle and its denizens—we never go there. We don't fear that the earth will become barren, because we don't visit nature very often, either, and the shelves of our grocery stores always have food on them. What is out of sight remains out of mind and unfeared. However, if we don't fear God and we don't fear Nature, what do we fear? Today we fear lingering illnesses like Alzheimer's, AIDS and cancer; mass media-generated mania of crime, terrorism and a poor economy; culturally inspired afflictions such as aging, loneliness and separation.

The name of the most dreaded modern monster is "emptiness"—that feeling that your life has no purpose, no meaning, and thus no direction. It is this gnawing emptiness that most people spend their days trying to fill with insubstantial living, for without the mystical power of myths, life can seem empty, and we end up existing in a dull, aching, depressive void of ennui.

Chapter 15: Three Characteristics of Life

At a basic level, the mystical purpose of our myths assuages our guilt over eating life in order to live: even peas and potatoes are living things and we kill them; we take their lives so that our lives can continue. Being conscious of the murder we must commit in order to survive creates guilt that must be accommodated somehow. This is the horror that Joseph Campbell says we wake up to when we become conscious, and it is this horror that our myths help us deal with. To the Buddha, the horror, the simple fact of existence, displays three characteristics, which he named *dukkha, anicca,* and *anatta*. These are known in Sanskrit as the *trilaksana* and in Pali as the *tilakkhana*. It is useful to understand these three primal characteristics of existence before we begin to ponder how to react to the reality, the horror, that is life.

Dukkha

⚜ ⚜

"Once upon a time," began the Buddha, "there was a man who was shot by an arrow, and it struck him in the thigh." The sangha leaned toward the Buddha, eager to hear the story. "Imagine, how must this man have felt?"

While the elder monks, who had heard this all before, sat still, the newest members of the community, who sat closest to the Enlightened One, offered their thoughts:

"Hurt!"

"In pain!"

"Awful!"

"Just so," agreed the Buddha. "Then this poor man was struck by a second arrow ... right in the same spot! Now how did he feel?"

"Worse!"

"In agony!"

"Really upset!" came the replies.

"Correct," said the Buddha. "And do you know the name of this second arrow? It is called 'suffering,' and it is *optional*!"

He paused to allow the meaning of his words to soak in before continuing. "The name of the first arrow is *dukkha*, and that's life! In every life there will come times when pain and sorrow arise; that is the nature of life. But suffering arises out of what we do about dukkha, suffering is always self-inflicted, and to one who lives life mindfully, suffering is always an option that can be dispensed with."

⁂

The most common definition of dukkha is "suffering," but as the Buddha's story shows, this is not a great translation. A better translation would be "unreliability"]or "unsatisfactoriness"]or perhaps "dissatisfaction," and in some cases "sorrow." Looking at the literal definition of dukkha can help our understanding: *ka* means "space," an empty space such as you would find in the middle of a wheel. Imagine a chariot wheel with the hole where the axel rod goes perfectly in the center—the ride would be very smooth and pleasant. This is called *sukha*—the wheel is perfectly centered. Sukha is often translated as "happiness." However, think back to a time when you were riding in a chariot where the center of the wheel was a bit off: Remember how bumpy that ride was and how your bladder almost burst after a few hours? That is dukkha. Another metaphor used to explain dukkha is a potter's wheel: If the wheel is a bit off-centered, the pot being thrown becomes an ashtray.

Have you ever noticed that life does not always work out as you planned or hoped? That is dukkha—that is the nature of existence. You can't count on things. Life is inherently unreliable and unsatisfactory; but that's life. How you choose, whether consciously or not, to react to life is what creates suffering. The Buddha has often been accused of being a pessimist because people quote him as saying, "All life is suffering." But this is a misquote. What he said was "all life contains dukkha," which is quite different. And he didn't mean that all life, all the time, will be tough; rather, if you are alive, there will be times when things won't be the way you'd like them to be.

Dukkha, the Buddha defined, is birth, aging, sickness, death, separation from what we like and want, and getting what we don't like or don't want: All this will befall us at some point in our life.[1] Suffering is the optional part of life; life does not have to include suffering, but we choose to inflict it on ourselves regardless. Some examples are useful to clarify this point. The comedian and psychologist (what a wonderful combination!) David Granirer noted that Christmas is a time when dysfunctional families come together to re-traumatize the hell out of each other. Since all families are dysfunctional to some degree, this observation generally provokes knowing laughter. I can personally recall a time when my older sister and I were reminiscing about our youth and she said, "You broke my Barbie doll when you were six!" To which I replied, "Yes, but you threw my model airplane in the garbage!" Here we were, over four decades later, still reliving an incident that was a very old arrow. Suffering is what we do about and with the pain of dukkha; even after decades, long after the pain has gone, we continue to suffer by revisiting imaginary worlds that no longer exist.

Another incident in my youth taught me the power of the mind to take dukkha and blow it up into something much bigger. A good friend and I were in grade school, around 10 years old, and we had to line up to receive our vaccination shots. My friend was terrified of needles and was ahead of me in the line. He had been freaking out about the shot all day, and when it came his turn, when he got to the front of the line, after he rolled up his sleeve, ready to get the needle—he ran to the back of the line. I got the shot. Yes, the shot hurt (ow!) for a little while, but then the pain was soon gone. For my friend, however, he expanded and multiplied the discomfort a hundredfold—that was totally optional.

What we often perceive as pain and suffering are two distinct realities: pain is simply sensation; it is only what is happening right now, right here in this moment. If you are remembering pain, it is not pain. If you are anticipating pain, it is not pain. Pain can only occur in the here and now. And again, pain is merely sensation. Sure, that sensation can be overwhelming, but if we observe what is actually happening, the raw experience of the moment without adding anything to it, without adding the drama, the self-talk dialogue that we generally inflict upon ourselves, then we are free from suffering and experience only dukkha, the first arrow.

One of the things the Buddha "woke up" to was that dukkha is an *existential* problem while suffering is a *psychological* problem. To work with these, we need very different strategies: the mystical, to help us come into accord with the rawness of existence; and the psychological, to help us with suffering. We see this divide between the existential and the psychological, as well, in the Buddha's second characteristic of existence: *anicca*, known also as impermanence.

* * *

347

ANICCA

⚜ ⚜

"Once upon a time," began the Buddha, "there was a very rich, very old man who had two grown sons. And one night the old father passed away peacefully in his sleep. Now the two sons got along with each other very well, and they amicably divided up their father's estate. The younger son chose to live in the family home with his elder brother and continued to work in the family business."

"One day the younger son started to wonder how he would do if he was on his own. Could he make it without his brother's help? He decided he needed to move out of the family home and start a life of his own. He moved to a faraway city and began a business similar to the family business. It was hard work, but over time he became more and more successful. Finally the day came when the younger brother thought he could afford a vacation, and he decided to pay a visit to his beloved brother.

"The servants were just as excited about the younger son's visit as the family was, and they got busy cleaning up the house, preparing the meals, and making everything just right. One servant was cleaning the old father's den and discovered a secret drawer in the desk. In the drawer was a mysterious box. The servant took the box to the elder brother, who opened it and beheld two rings: one, a plain, ordinary silver ring; the other, an ornate, handsome and obviously very valuable gold ring with many jewels. Upon seeing the golden ring, the elder brother, for the first time, mind you, felt desire. He wanted this ring for himself, so he devised a plan....

"When the younger brother arrived, after all the greetings, a delicious meal, and some sharing of stories, the elder brother brought out their father's box of rings. He explained how the servant had found this box hidden away, so secret that neither son knew about the rings' existence. The elder brother explained, 'I believe that Dad hid these rings away because they were family heirlooms, passed down from eldest son to eldest son, very precious, especially the golden ring ... and I believe that, as the eldest son, Dad would have wanted this golden ring to come to me, so that I can pass it down to my first-born son.' The younger brother simply shrugged and said, 'OK. I will be content with father's simple silver ring. You may have the golden one.'

"The visit of the younger brother was very pleasant, but time moved on, as it does, and soon it was time to leave. On his long journey back to his new city, the younger son got to wondering about his father and the secret box. 'I can understand,' he thought to himself, 'why father hid the golden ring: It is obviously very valuable. But what is so special about the silver ring? It looks so ordinary...' The younger son examined the ring more closely, and there, on the inside of the ring, he discovered a simple inscription of only two words: "Everything changes." He repeated these words to himself over and over again: 'Everything changes ... everything *changes* ... *everything* changes!' This, he realized, must be some special wisdom passed down through the generations, and now this important knowledge had been given to him. Throughout his long journey home, he kept meditating on the wisdom of the ring: 'Everything changes.'

"When the younger brother arrived home, he got right back to work. It was springtime, and business was good, very good—in fact, it had never been better! But while he was tempted to celebrate his great good fortune, he kept remembering the wisdom of the ring: 'Everything changes.' He realized that, as good as times were right now, they would not last. He decided to put away some of his newfound wealth for later and enjoyed what he had while he had it.

"This was wise, for came the winter, the economy collapsed. Times were very bad all around and everyone suffered. Even with the money he had set aside for these bad times, the younger son still faced a very lean period. But again, he remembered the ring's wisdom and realized that, as bad as these days were, they, too, would not last. And so the younger brother lived his life, enjoying good times when they arrived but never getting too high or mighty, and enduring bad times when they arrived while never getting depressed or discouraged; for he knew the secret to happiness: 'Everything changes.'

"Now the elder brother, the one who kept the seemingly precious golden ring, did not know the wisdom of the simple silver ring. Being in the same business as his brother, that spring his business did fabulously well, and he became very rich and lived life high. He threw gorgeous parties, bought many gifts for friends and beautiful clothes for himself. He was manic with delight over his good fortune. But when winter arrived, he lost it all. He became destitute, bankrupt and suicidal. Throughout his life he suffered the joys of good times and the depths of bad times, being blown about emotionally by whatever winds caught him. Unfortunately, the elder brother never learned that everything changes, and that is life."

⊰ ⊱

There is no getting around it: Everything changes. Anicca means "impermanence"; another way of saying this is that everything that has a beginning will one day end. This is the second of the three characteristics of existence, and we need to recognize its reality so we can choose how best to accommodate it. You can choose to see this as another instance of the Buddha being a party pooper. Why does he always have to look at the negative side of life? But change is not a negative, and it is not a positive—it simply is. Consider this scenario:

⊰ ⊱

You are waiting for a good friend to join you for lunch at an outdoor café just off the Champs-Élysées in Paris. You are early and pick a lovely spot on the sidewalk, where you can watch people walking by in their spring clothes, smiling in the sunshine, and nattering in French. You see your friend walking along the street toward you, and you notice she has a flower in her hand. How nice! She is bringing you a single red rose. You greet her with a hug and a kiss on both cheeks, and she hands you the flower. You smell the rose with anticipation and then realize— it's plastic!

⊰ ⊱

What a letdown—your friend just gave you a plastic flower. Now, why are you upset? A real rose will last maybe a week, and then it will become compost. A plastic flower will last forever. What makes the rose precious is its impermanence; we know that it won't last, and so we enjoy it while it is still here. Change, impermanence, is wonderful, if we look with clear eyes. Anyone who has raised a child knows that the diaper stage is not so great; you can't wait until your baby is toilet trained. You look forward to your baby eating solid food, to your baby's first step, to her first day of school, to graduation from high school, to her marriage, to your grandchild's arrival, to … Without impermanence none of this could happen; without impermanence your baby could not even have been born; in fact, *you* could not have been born. Impermanence allows things to happen, and, whether we like the things that happen or not, change is a fact of life. We can choose to embrace it, ignore it, or reject it, but we can't change it.

Impermanence is a Tibetan sand painting. These marvelous meditations produce exquisite works of art, with colored sands forming mandalas of circles and squares, sometimes images and symbols, created by a team of artist monks often placing individual grains of sand one at time in just the right spot. When completed the work is admired for a brief moment and then swept up and forgotten: Such are the works of man, and such is impermanence.

The reality of change is another existential challenge of life; our reaction to change is another psychological challenge in life. There is one more challenge to meet: dukkha and anicca are joined by *anatta*, the third attribute of existence, the reality that there is no 'self.' We met this idea briefly in Chapter Nine: The Soul Question. It is time now to really understand it.

✴ ✴ ✴

Anatta

Let's revisit the sidewalk café in Paris, only in this alternate imaginary universe, we will find that your friend actually did bring you a real red rose:

✌ ✾

The waiter helpfully brings a tall glass filled with water in which you place the flower your friend so kindly brought you. As she talks with the waiter, placing her order for lunch, you take the time to contemplate the rose. Looking closer you see the exquisite shades of dark red on the petals. You notice the shape of the flower and the greenness of the leaves just below the soft petals, and you see that the edge of one leaf is already turning brown. You notice the stems bent by the refraction of the water and the glass. The water ... suddenly you are aware that this wonderful rose grew so lovely because of the water it drank from the ground, water that fell as rain from the sky. You begin to see the rose differently; you see that it is made up of sky!

Realizing there is more to the rose than originally met your eyes, you look even closer. You visualize this single stem growing out of a big rosebush in a lovely garden, and the bush's roots growing deep into the earth. You realize that the rose is made up of earth, too. In your meditation you also see the leaves of the rosebush turning toward the sun

352

for energy and life, and you realize the rose is also made up of sunlight.

Earth, sun and sky all came together to make this rose possible, but there is more. Your friend turns toward you and you smile. Of course, you would not have this pretty flower if not for her; your friend is part of this rose, too, as is the florist who sold it to her, the truck driver who brought it to the store, and the gardener who cared for the flowers and pruned and fertilized the bushes. All of these things are part of the rose, and much more besides: the seed from which the rosebush grew, the previous flowers that created the seed, and the bees that pollinated the flower.

The meal is delightful, and you enjoy talking with your friend, but from time to time you look at the rose, until a broader realization dawns upon you: Just as the rose could not exist without so many conditions being right, your friend and your friendship would not exist without the proper conditions arising. As you listen to your friend talking, you realize that she, too, is made up of earth, sun and sky, and that you are also made up of the same elements. In fact, you now understand that she is a part of you and you are a part of her! Without each other neither of you would be the people you are right now. Without her years of friendship, love and understanding, of being there for you in your times of travail—without all this, you would not be who you are. You "inter-be" with each other, and this understanding brings you great joy.

∪ ∫

Remember, the venerable Vietnamese Zen master Thich Nhat Hanh coined a valuable word: *interbeing*. He hopes that one day it will be in dictionaries. The realization that all things inter-be with other things is liberating; it is an enlightenment realized by the Buddha centuries ago. When you look at anything, a flower or a friend, when you look with awakened eyes, you will see a composite, something made up of many things. Nothing exists of and by itself.

✳ ✳ ✳

DEPENDENT ORIGINATION

We have seen earlier that when someone claims to be liberated, ask him, "liberated from what?" When someone claims to be free, ask her, "free from what?" And when someone claims to be enlightened, ask, "Enlightened about what?" The Buddha is the 'awakened one,' but what did he wake up to? (The Sanskrit word *budh* means 'to awaken.') When asked, the Buddha explained that what he woke up to that night under the tree of awakening[2] was the Law of Dependent Origination:

> I shall teach you the Dhamma: when this exists, that comes to be; with the arising of this, that arises. When this does not exist, that does not come to be; with the cessation of this, that ceases.[3]

This is the essence of the Buddha's realization, and, as Stephen Batchelor coined it, the Buddha's Einsteinian $E=MC^2$ moment is his formula of Dhamma = Dependent Origination.[4] This is also known as conditioned arising. All three of the characteristics of existence are present in this concept: Anicca or impermanence happens out of the nature of arising; anatta or no-self is present because everything that comes into being does so from things that pre-existed; and the fact that this change is sometimes unsatisfactory is dukkha.

Look closely at a flower and find the actual essence, the essential part that makes the flower a flower, or—much more humbling—what makes you "you." When you really look closely, as the Buddha did, you may discover something very perplexing and initially somewhat frightening: You may find … nothing at all! There is no essence to be found. There is no essential "you"—which many people find to be quite scary, for where did "you" go? This topic was discussed amid a series of exchanges between a Buddhist monk named Nagesena and a Greek King called Milinda (also called Menander), who ruled the Bactria kingdom (155–130 B.C.E.) in what today is Afghanistan.[5] The king was very learned, wise and curious and asked Nagesena to explain the assertion that there was no self. Nagesena used the example of a chariot, and he challenged the king to find the part of the chariot that displayed its essence. Is the essential part the wheels, the axel, the sides, the reins, the floor? The king had to admit that none of these component parts was the essence of the chariot; without any one of these pieces, the chariot would not be a chariot. If we can't find the chariot, how do we find ourselves? What is our self?

Here we are stepping onto some very esoteric ground, a ground that has been trod by many philosophers East and West and with very different results. If everything that exists is made up of compound elements, then you and I also are merely an aggregate of such stuff. The Buddha pointed to five aggregates: forms, feeling, perceptions, mental formations and consciousness. Forms include all that is physical, which includes our body made up as it is of earth, sun and sky; feelings include our emotions; perceptions include our five senses; mental formations include the wide expanse of all forms of thinking; and consciousness includes the action of being aware of what we perceive. That is the totality of who and what we are. Where is the self in all this? If you latch onto our consciousness as being the self, be careful—the Buddha was way ahead of you. Consciousness itself is a conditioned thing; it arises when conditions are right. When conditions cease to be right, it goes away again.

The Buddha's concept of consciousness is quite distinct from all the other ideas we have investigated so far. In the Samkhya, Jain or Classical Yoga philosophies, our ultimate and intimate self is pure consciousness: the purusha or jiva. This is the watcher. For example, one yogic meditation involves paying attention to sensations in your body and realizing that you are not your body, you are the watcher of the body's sensations; you are not your thoughts flowing through your mind, you are the watcher of your thoughts; you are not your memories, you are not your personality, you are not your emotions—you are the watcher of all this. Through this realization you dissociate from the material world until all that is left is the watcher. And now the Buddha comes along and says, "there is no watcher either!" There is no self that you can point to or cling to, which is a radical nondualism never before propounded; we have no soul, no little man somewhere deep within running the whole show and who survives when the body dies and is reborn miraculously somehow into a new body.

For the Buddha, there is consciousness, to be sure, but it is not fixed or permanent. When sounds (a form of energy) strike the organs of sound (our ears), the sensation of sound arises, which the Buddha called "ear consciousness." When light (energy) hits the organs of light (our eyes), the sensation of light arises, called "eye consciousness." And so it goes with the energies of taste, smell, touch and even the energy of thoughts, which are perceived by "mind consciousness." Thus the Buddha detected six distinct kinds of consciousness, but each kind is conditional, ever-changing and just as impermanent as anything else: our thoughts can change our consciousness, and at other times we become unconscious; thus clearly we cannot be our consciousness.

Where is our reincarnating monad, our soul, our purusha, our jiva? Is the Buddha saying that we don't have a self? The Tibetan sage Tsongkhapa (1357–1419 C.E.) stated that we could go too far in either direction: in believing that there was a self, in the manner of the Upanishads, some deep subtle soul that exists to experience life; or in believing that there was no self at all.[6] The word anatta in Pali implies exactly that—no self; but what the Buddha was suggesting is more subtle than just the negation of self. What we are is an aggregate of non-self elements that come together to give the illusion of a self; but if there truly is no self, then who is reading these words? Well, you are, of course, but not the "you" that you think you are.

✳ ✳ ✳

BUDDHA NATURE

The radical nondualism where there is no-self flies in the face of common sense; it goes against the stream, as the Buddha loved to declare. Of course I have a self: I perceive, I think, I feel—there is obviously an "I" here somewhere. The idea is so counterintuitive that people in the centuries after the Buddha couldn't help but undermine it, even if inadvertently. Stephen Batchelor has spent a great deal of time and thought investigating what the Buddha originally taught on this topic (and on many other topics) compared to the teachings that were layered on top of his philosophy, or rather his psychotherapies, in the centuries that followed. Batchelor has looked back into the earliest stratums of the Buddhist Dhamma (which means the Buddha's teachings) and found that many of the ideas and concepts common today in Buddhism can't be found there. These later ideas were grafted onto the original teaching and in some cases are quite contradictory to them. One key example is the concept of emptiness, which originally arose as another way to describe anatta, no-self.[7]

To Nagarjuna (150–250 C.E.), an influential Buddhist scholar of the Mahayana philosophy, emptiness is the same thing as contingent arising. To Tsongkhapa, emptiness means that things have no inherent existence. The danger we face when we consider words like *anatta* or *emptiness* is that we begin to think of them as being something, while the intention is to say that there is no-thing. Emptiness is not a place, and it is not a thing; one cannot meditate on emptiness, because that would make emptiness into something, some thing that you can meditate on, but it is not some thing. To try to meditate upon emptiness is an understandable mistake, because we have created a word or a map, and words and maps imply an underlying reality that they refer to. But in this case, the meaning of anatta and emptiness is transcendent; it is beyond meaning, beyond pointing to something. We have to use words to communicate, but when we try to talk about that which can't be described by using words, we fall into a trap caused by the inherent inadequacy of language. This is why, in the Kena Upanishad, the transcendent is described as a place "where words do not go."

Nagarjuna posed a logical analysis, which we can call a *tetralemma*: a dilemma is when two solutions are offered and neither one works, which puts you in the 'dilemma' that whatever you choose is wrong. Imagine this being broadened to four propositions, each of which is unacceptable in some way. You'd have a tetralemma, and this was Nagarjuna's: Things can either 1) exist or 2) not exist or 3) both exist *and* not exist at the same time or 4) neither exist *nor* not exist at the same time. Those are pretty much all the possibilities one can think of, and it puts a hurt in one's head to try to understand them. But let's try. In other words, none of these four possibilities are real, according to Nagarjuna; things are empty of these four possible forms of existence. He said in his book *Fundamental Verses of the Middle Way*, "Nowhere and in no way do any entities exist which originate from themselves, from something, from both themselves and something else, or spontaneously."[8] Or in other words, there is no cause of anything! You may recall the monk we mentioned earlier who once asked the Buddha, "Please tell me whether the universe is eternal or will it one day end, or can it be that it is both eternal and not, or neither eternal or not." You may now understand why he asked the question the way he did, and how these mind-numbing brain-twisters became popular.

Unfortunately, people began to consider emptiness itself as a thing, with all the consequent distortions that arise from this mistake. Nagarjuna observed, "Buddhas say emptiness is relinquishing opinions. Believers in emptiness are incurable."[9] This idea that emptiness was real became a hallmark of teaching found today in Mahayana Buddhism. You may now hear statements such as, "All things arise from emptiness and return to emptiness," as if emptiness was some cosmic void or some power or absolute fact of nature like the Dao; however, that was not the intention of anatta. When the Mahayana teaching reached China, emptiness evolved into the now-famous Buddha Nature. Stephen Batchelor could not discover anywhere in the earliest literature of the Buddha's discourses any mention of Buddha Nature; in fact this concept goes against the stream of the Buddha's original teaching. In modern Buddhist understanding, however, we are all thought to possess this ultimately undefinable quality called Buddha Nature. Even dogs have Buddha Nature, unless and until you ask if a dog has Buddha Nature, in which case you will receive the paradoxical answer, "mu!" which means "no".[10] With the arrival of Buddha Nature, we are now safely back in the dualistic world where there is matter, but there is also this something called Buddha Nature, almost spiritual, which is ultimately "me'"

We are not positing that the idea of Buddha Nature is wrong. Remember, all these ideas are simply models—the proper question would be to ask if these ideas are useful. Certainly the idea that there is a "me" somewhere that survives death and perhaps is reborn can be seen to be useful in many moral ways; there may be any number of evolutionary reasons why this pervasive sense of self arose and continues. Some scholars posit that the idea that we have a soul, which may be subjected to punishment if we misbehave toward others, has helped societies function smoothly; although there are scholars who claim atheists are every bit as moral and self-sacrificing as religious people and often more so![11] But what we are discovering is that, in the original teachings of the Buddha preserved mostly today in the Theravada tradition, the concept of Buddha Nature or emptiness is not what the Buddha meant by anatta. Some philosophers attacked the concept of emptiness because they misunderstood the idea and thought it meant there was nothing. This is also mistaken thinking; emptiness is no-thing but it doesn't mean nothingness or some empty void, which is so often invoked when we think of emptiness. Emptiness is not nothing; it is no thing—get it? If you are still having trouble with this concept, try revisiting the earlier discussion about teapots and mountains.

As Tsongkhapa warned, we can go too far and think that there is no self, or we can get caught up in the idea that we do have some reincarnating monad, or soul, or spark of pure consciousness. These are two extremes, but we don't have to go to extremes. There is a metaphor the Buddha used to explain self in a way that seems to lie in between these two extremes, and one that shows quite definitely that the Buddha did consider our self to be a real thing, just not the thing we thought it was:

Just as a farmer irrigates his field,

Just as a fletcher fashions an arrow,

Just as a carpenter shapes a piece of wood,

So the sage tames the self.[12]

This is more than a simile that likens the person to a field, an arrow or a block of wood; read as a metaphor, we find the Buddha considering the self to be a field that needs irrigation. Channels need to be created, paths for water to flow—in the same way we build habits in the mind through repetitive activities that create neural pathways. The deeper these channels or pathways, the easier certain actions are to repeat, thus becoming habits of mind. The Buddha pointed out that three particularly deep channels that we have carved into our fields are the habits of greed, hatred and confusion. A fletcher is an arrow maker, and the analogy here implies that our self or our mind is also an arrow that flies straight and true, if it is well-made. The arrow is an instrument of sharp discrimination; it is our ability to concentrate and to be totally focused in moving from the bow to the target, from where we are now to our goal. If the arrow is not well-made, it will miss the target, and we will never get where we want to go. The uncarved block of wood is our potential: The wood can become almost anything if the carpenter is skillful. The wood can become a piece of art, beautiful and something to simply gaze upon, or it can become functional like a bowl, if it is carved well. This metaphor can apply to our mind or our body: athletes and gymnasts, dancers and yogis, all mold their bodies into beautiful and useful forms. The wood could represent our potential for self-expression: our work, hobby or passion.

So the sage tames the self. Notice how the Buddha allows us to have a self but a self that is cultivated and always changing, for the self is conditional. What is also telling in this quotation is the emphasis on action. The Buddha did not buy into the varna philosophy that people are born into certain castes; he said, "By action is one a farmer, by action a craftsman …"[13] and by action one is a Brahmin, a priest or a Kshatriya, a warrior or king. A farmer cultivates a field, plants seeds and harvests crops, and by such action he becomes a farmer. A priest conducts rituals, chants secret mystical mantras, invokes powers, and thus becomes a Brahmin.

In this way the sage sees action as it operates,

Seeing conditioned arising, understanding the effects of act.[14]

It is what we do that counts, not our birth. To quote Confucius: "By nature men are similar; by what they do they become different."[15] To quote Stephen Batchelor again: "Rather than dismiss the self as a fiction, [the Buddha] presented it as a project to be realized."[16] We will find many times that the Buddha tries to get us to consider verbs rather than nouns: actions over things. Knowing this, we can look again at the concept of emptiness: not emptiness (the noun) but rather emptying (the verb). Consider this an instruction of something to do rather than something to be or something to experience. Emptying is, as Nagarjuna pointed out, a relinquishing of views, ideas and opinions; a letting go of concepts, rather than a clinging to yet another empty concept called emptiness.

✳ ✳ ✳

You have no doubt had the experience of looking at yourself in a picture taken when you were a child and thinking, "That's me." But the "you" that you were way back then is certainly not the "you" that exists today. Every atom in that child's body has gone and been replaced with new atoms as you grew. Your body has changed, your mind has changed, your personality, your likes and dislikes, your passions and fears—all of these have changed, but still you think that you are still "you." There is something that persists throughout the years that may be impossible to define or detect, but you know you are still "you." However, you are but a wave flowing through the ocean, and waves are but Maya: illusions. Imagine ...

You are standing on shore, looking out over a vast expanse of water, and your eyes come to rest on one particularly large wave. Perhaps it was created by conduction currents deep within the ocean equalizing cold and warmer waters by roiling up to the surface, or by winds far out to sea, or by a big ferryboat plying through the water: no matter. As you watch the wave, it appears to travel toward you; sometimes little white caps form on the crest.

From the scientist's point of view, what you are watching is not one separate volume of water moving toward you but rather a compression wave (also called a gravity wave). The energy of the initial impetus pushes a column of water against a neighboring column of water, compressing the second column of water between the begetting energy and a neighboring third water column that is yet still. Water does not compress easily, so the column of water being pressed becomes narrower and rises up above the normal sea level around it, manifesting as a peak. Gravity doesn't like peaks, so the peak is pushed back down into the ocean, creating another force that compresses the third water column. This pressure repeats what just happened, and a new peak is

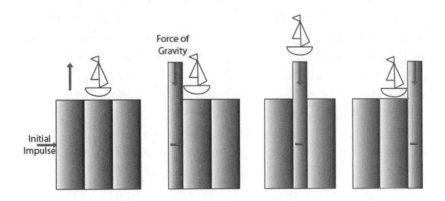

Figure 8: The propogation of gravity waves

formed, rising up and then falling down again. These columns of water are infinitely thin, so we can't perceive the individual peaks; it all appears to us as one single wave, but what we see as a wave is simply water rising and water falling.

Watch as your wave passes a small boat: The boat is lifted up as the wave arrives and then falls down again as the wave passes. There is an illusion of something coming toward you—a wave. But it is not the water that is moving forward; the water just moves up and falls down again. What is moving is energy through the medium of the water.

The child you once were is not "you." We have the illusion of continuity, but every moment there is a new wave of our existence coming into being and falling back again. This is exactly the concept of dependent origination—we *are* due to what has happened. We did not just spring into being one day; when conditions were right, a "you" appeared. When conditions are no longer right, "you" will cease to be. So you see, you both are and are not. The wave passes through the ocean as we pass through life, but there still is something! There is a wave, there is a "you," but when the energy of the wave is dispersed back into the ocean, all that is left is the effect of the wave, analogous to the impact of the life you have led. This is also known as karma, the consequence of our energy as it interacted with the ocean and all the objects found therein. Like a pebble thrown in a pond that creates ripples that touch everything in the pond, become smaller, and seem to disappear, the energy of our lives touches the whole universe and everything and everyone in it. In time our own personal ripples may become too small to detect, but the effect of even one small pebble remains forever. This is immortality—at least, one model for it—and if you find it a particularly useful model, feel free to adopt it.

Chapter 16: Three Attitudes Toward Life

On the surface, the Buddha's three marks of existence don't seem nearly as horrifying as the shining face of Kirtimukha poised to gobble you up in his truncated grin, or the bloodstained statue of Kali ready to consume her sacrificial victims. But upon reflection, the fact that all life contains pain and sorrow (dukkha), and that you *will* grow old and assuredly die (anicca) but you shouldn't worry because you don't actually exist, anyway (anatta)—all this does not move one to rejoice, sit back, smile, and simply enjoy this thing called life. There are terrors and dangers all around us—what are we to do?

There are three attitudes we can take toward these basic facts of existence: We can run away and reject life; we can figure out where it all went wrong and try to fix it up; or we can accept that this is the way life is and come into some sort of accord with it. These are what our religious, philosophical and spiritual myths have to offer us, but as we will see, for us in the West, we have been told there really is only one choice we can make: correction. We must correct the universe. This was not the choice of many of the ancient Indian yogis; they chose rejection.

REJECTION

Two birds, always together and called by the same name, are sitting on a branch of a tree. One bird is eating a piece of fruit, while the other bird sits and watches.[1]

⧰ ⧱

One of these birds has the right idea, but which one? One is engaged in life; the other is remote and aloof from it. According to the ancient Upanishad philosophy, the correct answer is 'B,' the bird that is not caught up in pleasure and activity. The first bird is Arjuna; the second bird is Krishna: One is involved, the other enlightened. This enlightenment is also called moksha, as we have seen, and there are two forms it can take: leaving the world entirely, or realizing one's true nature and staying in the phenomenal world. It is the first choice that Joseph Campbell calls rejection.

If we were to put ourselves in the sandals of an ancient Indian, we also might think that leaving this world of woe far behind was not such a bad idea. We would probably be of the lowest caste, as most people were; we would have no public health care, no pension, no guarantee of our next meal let alone of support to us in our waning years. There would be no public schools, no protection from crime or war, no civil rights to invoke for abuse and discrimination. We would, however, be quite free to get sick, to grow old, or to die without any of the modern miracles that ease our passage. In short, life would suck. Given this backdrop, it does make a kind of sense to say to hell with it all and leave. But there is no point leaving and just killing yourself because … you'll be back! And you'll have to go through this over and over and over again. Where is the joy in that?

The Jain solution of exiting was not an easy one to accomplish. If we cycle back to what we learned about them, you will remember their belief was that any action in the world further tied you to the world. It doesn't matter what your psychological state of mind or intention is—even if you did not mean to step on that ant, if you stepped on it, you accumulated bad karma. If and until you manage to stop acting, which basically means stop living, you will continue to accumulate negative karma—staining your coffee cup as it were—and thus you will have to come back and risk more bad karma. The way out, the way to stop living, was through a strict adoption of non-harming asceticism: not moving, not eating, and eventually not breathing.

The Samkhya and Classical yogis living in the forest had the same basic attitude: They were leaving life behind and getting out. Their purushas, the name they applied to their individual reincarnating monad of pure consciousness, were trapped by the material world of prakriti, and a divorce was necessary in order to be free forever. Just as in the Jain understanding, the world of prakriti, which includes the five non-material mental substances of imagination, memories, dreams, conceptions and misconceptions, was evil and had to be transcended. Most people followed the path of smoke, but these ancient yogis wanted to follow the path of fire: Smoke rises to the moon, where it waits for a time and returns back to earth; fire is the path of the sun, and through that door no one ever returns again. In the epic poem, the "Mahabharata," there is a scene depicting departure through the sun door:

◅ ▻

Bhisma is dying, pierced by so many of Arjuna's arrows that his body cannot even touch the ground; so numerous are the shafts impaling him that there is nowhere left for another arrow to penetrate. Long ago the gods had blessed Prince Bhisma because he had taken a vow to never know the love of a woman, thus allowing his father, King Santanu, to wed again and beget with his new wife another heir to the throne; such was her demand before she'd agree to marry. The boon Bhisma received from the gods was that he could choose the time of his own death, and it was during the great war between the Pandavas and the Kauravas that he decided enough was enough. While he chose to fight on the side of the hundred evil sons of the blind king Dhritarashtra, he also chose to let his nephew Arjuna slay him rather than continue to fight against the five beloved brothers.

Great Bhisma exercised his power and did not go quickly; he lingered until the sun was in an auspicious location, which allowed him time to share his wisdom with the Pandava brothers and other beloved friends. In great sadness and with full attention, the family and friends of Bhisma listened carefully. When the time was finally right, Bhisma began his yoga; he hitched his spirit to the celestial chariot sent to him by the gods, rose bodily into the sky, ascending like a brilliant meteor in reverse, and pierced the disc of the sun. His mourners marveled at the sight of Bhisma's yoga and knew that their uncle had passed through that golden door, never to be incarnated again.

∗ ∗

This was one purpose of yoga in the days of the "Mahabharata," a story told of a mythical time that coincided with Homer's Greek epics. This yoga was a way to yoke the warrior to his spiritual chariot and fly to and through the sun.[2] These yogis were not interested in coming back; they chose the sun door, which meant escaping the rounds of returning.

✳ ✳ ✳

The path of smoke and fire, the path of the moon and the path of the sun are very interesting contrasts. The moon goddess depicted life, death, rebirth and re-death; the cycles of the moon as it casts off its own shadow, reaches maturity and then falls back into darkness mirror the cycles of life on earth. An earthly creature that participated in the moon's mystery was the snake, which casts off its skin of death and is reborn. Shiva, who ultimately represents the moon, rides the sacred white bull that, like the snake, also represents the moon. Against this we have the symbols of the sun, the source of endless light where no shadow or death exists: its animals are the lion, with its golden mane of hair flowing like the rays of the sun, that pounces upon and devours the bull; and the eagle, who flies higher over the land than anything else and who kills snakes, just as the sun consumes the moon each month. In the same epic tale that described the death of Bhisma, the "Mahabharata," we find the story of the birth of the great sunbird, Garuda:

⁂

The great sage Kashyapa, born of a mere thought of Brahman, was married to two sexy sisters, Vinata and Kadru. While sisters in blood, they were rivals competing for the favor of their husband, each believing herself to be the most beautiful. Kadru approached Kashyapa and asked for a thousand sons, strong and brave in battle. She was pleased with the results, for she gave birth to a thousand powerful snakes. Vinata also approached Kashyapa and asked for just two sons, but two sons who would be much more powerful than any of Kadru's offspring. She was not so pleased when she bore two eggs that never seemed to hatch.

Sometimes it feels like gestation will never end, and like many a mother-to-be, Vinata grew impatient. After only 500 years of waiting, she could bear the wait no longer and cracked open one of her two eggs. The unfinished fetus cursed his mother's willfulness and ordered her not to do the same to his brother's egg. So Vinata waited, and after a full 1,000 years of waiting, finally her son, Garuda, was born.

Garuda was a marvelous bird, with feathers brighter and more golden than the sun. He shone like the brightest flame, so bright that he blinded even the gods, who had to ask him to tone it down a bit. Garuda dimmed his brilliance a thousand fold, and everyone sighed in relief.

Kadru and Vinata continued to vie with each other: a snide snipe here and an accidental spill of red wine on a white sari there. One time they made a bet, and the loser agreed to become the slave of the winner. The bet was one Vinata was sure she'd win: What color was Indra's horse? She knew it was all white, but Kadru bet it had a black tail. Kadru knew, of course, that Indra's horse was pure white, but she had a plan: She convinced one of her sons to wrap himself around the tail of the horse. Sure enough, when the sisters went to see Indra, they noticed that his horse's tail was black. Vinata and her son Garuda became slaves to Kadru and the race of snakes. There was one snake, however, who did not appreciate the way his brothers behaved: His name was Ananta, and in protest he left his family and went to the forest to do yoga.

Garuda grew tired of being a slave; he longed to be free to fly wherever he wanted, so he asked his cousins, "How might my mother and I be free from our servitude?" The snakes answered, "Bring us *amrita*, and we will let you go free."

Amrita is the nectar of immortality, found only in heaven and drunk only by the gods. The snakes wanted to become immortals, too, but there was no way they could get the precious liquid by themselves: It was guarded by fire, protected by whirling blades and vicious serpents larger than themselves, and, of course, it was desired by the gods, who would not give it up willingly. But Garuda wanted freedom badly, so he braved all and risked all: He flew to heaven, defeated the gods, outsmarted the machines, and won the nectar.

On his return flight he met Vishnu, who offered him a choice: "Keep going with your crime, or agree to be my steed and I will give you immortality without amrita, and I will let you feed on all the snakes you can stomach."

Garuda chose the latter course, and Vishnu helped him come up with a plan to cheat the snakes waiting below. When Garuda landed, he placed the cauldron of amrita in the midst of the snakes and asked for freedom for his mother and himself. This he received.

The snakes moved toward the cauldron, but Garuda cautioned them, "Before one can receive such power, one must be cleansed! Go clean yourself up and then begin the ritual that will yield everlasting life."

The snakes knew this to be wise advice and so went to bathe, but while they were gone, Indra swooped down and took back the amrita to heaven. All that was left were a few drops, which the snakes tasted with their tongues. That small, sharp taste was enough to split their tongues in two; thus do snakes now have forked tongues and the ability to shed their skin and begin a new life.

In time, Ananta, the snake brother who went to the forest, grew very powerful through his yoga. Brahma noticed and came to him offering a boon: What would Ananta like? Ananta wanted only one thing: to be able to concentrate his mind forever. Brahma agreed but had a favor to ask in return. Would Ananta be so kind as to go to the bottom of the world, spread his cobra hood, and stabilize the whole earth? Things had become a bit rocky lately, and it would be very much appreciated if Ananta would be the foundation upon which everything rested. Ananta agreed, and now the whole world rests upon his mighty head. Vishnu also had a favor to ask: While he was holding up the earth, would Ananta mind terribly coiling up his body so that Vishnu could lie down upon him for a little nap? Again, Ananta agreed: Vishnu now slumbers in Ananta's lap dreaming the dream of the universe.

⇥ ⇤

In other versions of this tale, the enmity between Garuda and Ananta is more personal and far greater. In one story Garuda destroys all of Ananta's eggs, eating all the children before they can hatch. This is a version of an older Babylonian myth where snake and eagle take a vow of peace in front of Shamash, the sun god, but the eagle breaks the truce, earning punishment meted out by the sun. That punishment—to serve

371

man.[3] The motif of heaven's bird against the moon's snake, and of the solar lion against the lunar bull, are common in traditions that claim to transcend the circular rounds of existence. The Buddha, for example, was mythically related to the people of the sun; his clan, the Shakyas, claimed descendancy from the solar race. When he left his father's palace to find the cure for old age, sickness and death, the Buddha-to-be gave out a mighty lion's roar, symbolic of his eventual success in overcoming samsara, the rounds of reincarnation. One of the most popular names for the Buddha today in the East is Amitabha, which means the Buddha of immeasurable (*a-mita*) light (*abha*): a clear solar reference. The myths of the symbols of the sun overcoming the symbols of the moon were presaged thousands of years earlier in Egypt when the mythology of Osiris, the moon god, became superseded by the mythology of Re, the sun god.[4] The way of smoke versus the way of fire is an old theme.

✳ ✳ ✳

Ultimately, the only difference between the rejection of life in this world by the Jains, the Samkhya yogis and the Classical yogis, and the early Buddhists was the methodology, not the intention. In the first three systems of spiritual practice, the tools included nonharming and asceticism. But the Samkhya yogis believed understanding, *viveka*, was also essential, while the Classical yogis believed a state of enstatic absorption, *samadhi*, was required. The Samkhya yogis had to leave the worldly distraction of kama, artha and dharma, head to the forest, disassociate from everything desirable, and combine all this with a clear, visceral understanding of the nature of the universe as explained in their cosmological model.

The Classical yogis also followed the practices of asceticism and retreat to the forest, but their process was a psycho-spiritual one. They had to train their minds to reach a place of no-thought, of no mental movements whatsoever, and then achieve a blissful state of complete introverted aloofness and aloneness, called *kaivalya,* and while in this supreme state of samadhi, die! Only then could they be assured of never having to return. This state of disembodied liberation from life was called *videha-mukti,* and it was not an easy state to achieve. However, there were several possible paths available. One of the most famous paths described in the Yoga Sutra, a compilation of Classical Yoga written somewhere around 200 C.E. by a mythical sage known as Patanjali, has become known as Ashtanga yoga, which literally means the "eight limbs" of yoga.

The first five limbs of Ashtanga yoga include ethical behaviors, called the 1) *yamas* and 2) *niyamas;* 3) finding a solid and comfortable base for prolonged sitting, called *asana;* 4) regulating the flow of energy through the body by freeing the breath, called *pranayama;* and 5) closing the sense doors so that no distractions can disturb the mind, called *pratyahara.* When these limbs are mastered, the inner path opens: 6) concentration, called *dharana;* 7) meditation, called *dhyana;* and finally 8) complete enstatic absorption, *samadhi.* When the sense doors are closed (pratyahara), when nothing of the outside world can touch the mind, then the yogi concentrates (dharana) his awareness on one object, until the seer of the object and the object itself is all that exists (dhyana). Finally, when all is ready (and this final stage can't be forced, in the same way that one cannot force oneself to fall asleep; all we can do is set the stage to allow sleep to manifest), the subject and object disappear, and in their place there is simply consciousness—awareness, but awareness of nothing in particular. Even this state of samadhi has levels within levels, and freedom becomes possible only when the yogi can spontaneous experience the highest level of samadhi, *nirvikalpa* samadhi or samadhi without any content or seed.

Vikalpa means "conceptualization"; *nir* means "to go beyond": so nirvikalpa means "to go beyond any concepts"—the transcendental state of pure consciousness.

✳ ✳ ✳

The Buddha's practices were not as extreme; he offered a middle way between, on the one hand, the goals of kama, artha and dharma found in the household life, and on the other hand, the extreme forest asceticism of the Jains and Classical yogis. He despised the teaching of Mahavira, the great Jain saint, and he had tried and mastered the types of yoga practiced by the pre-Classical and Classical yogis. The Buddha was from Kapilavastu, the city of the mythical founder of Samkhya, Kapila; he knew this philosophy intimately and found it wanting. But make no mistake, the early Buddhist teachings were a rejection—a rejection of the normal ways of life and the rounds of coming back to life. The Buddha taught that two paths lead to dead ends: the path of the mortifying ascetic avoiding all pleasures, and path of the householder who wallows in his addictions toward pleasure. He encouraged men of all castes to leave their worldly lives and head to the forest. In the Sutta Nipata he said, "...dwelling in a house is a constriction, a place of dust, and ... going forth is an open-air life..."[5] A person dedicated to finding release from suffering and achieving nirvana must shake off the dust of the household and go freely from his home and family. All a monk needs is a couple of robes, a begging bowl, shelter during the rainy season and a place to meditate; the monk should seek just enough food, clothing and shelter to meet the minimum conditions of life.

There is another way to look at the Buddha's injunction: "Home" can be seen metaphorically, as a symbol, which by now should not be a surprise. What does home symbolize to you? It is not just four walls, physically, but a place where you may feel safe, secure, and comfortable; thus you become unwilling to risk venturing into unknown territory—and the Buddha is telling us to drop all those feelings and take the risk. Home can also symbolize one's views and opinions— again, mental maps deep within. One may be "at home" with his political view or religious view and feel no need to go outside, to seek new opinions or ideas, to learn about what is going on in other people's homes. This going forth, as the Buddha prescribes, is opening yourself up to the wide world of new places and new ideas.

Nirvana, at the time of the Buddha, was a goal sought by monks practicing a wide variety of philosophical paths; it was a common concept. The word literally means "to be blown out," like a flame extinguished by a breath. A common analogy was that of a burnt string, the idealized state of the monk or yogi: A burnt string still has the appearance of a string, but if you blow on it there is nothing there, it disappears. This was to be the state of the yogi. It looks like there is a man there, but he has extinguished himself. This was the state that the Buddha achieved that night beneath the Bodhi tree when Mara the tempter, the killer, approached him to prevent his awakening. Because there was no one there, the Buddha having achieved this state of nirvana, Mara could not affect him.

It is hard today to imagine the degree of independence that the Buddha recommended for his monks, because we commonly hear of large communities of Buddhists practicing together: monasteries where year-round we can go and find monks and nuns teaching and perfecting the dharma; the diaspora of the greater sangha held together by books, podcasts, local meditation halls, and local retreats; the visits of great teachers such as Thich Nhat Hanh or the Dalai Lama who draw thousands of people together—these all imply that Buddhist practitioners need to lean on each other, to study and practice together under the watchful eyes of elders. But this was not what the Buddha suggested to his followers. The monks only came together during the monsoons, when the rains made the roads impassable. Then, and only then, the monks gathered in communities to hear the teachings, seek shelter and obtain food from the local community of lay practitioners that supported the sangha. When the Buddha lay dying between two sal trees, in a backwater town away from his normal haunts of big cities, he advised his monks to go off on their own: "Let no two [monks] follow the same path."[6] He refused Ananda's request to appoint a successor to lead the community. The value of the community, the sangha, was to help teach monks how to be independent, not to pin them down to an organization. He advised everyone to "be a lamp unto yourself" and if help or guidance was needed, recall the Dhamma, the teachings he had shared with them for 45 years.[7] Moksha is the freedom to create your own path.

This is quite a different viewpoint from what arose very soon after the Buddha died. The emphasis on the individual path and on doing it yourself became subsumed into a focus on the three jewels of Buddhism: the Buddha, his teaching (the Dhamma), and the community (the sangha). This social aspect evolved out of a power struggle between Ananda, the one whose eidetic memory recorded everything that the Buddha ever said and who was the closest to the Buddha, and Kashyapa, the monk who best realized the truth of the Buddha's teachings and understood what Ananda simply remembered. Kashyapa wrested control of the community and put Ananda aside; Ananda retired to the hills and, according to the legends, eventually obtained final nirvana and died at a ripe old age of 120.[8] It was Kashyapa who created the systematization of the Buddha's teaching, which allowed it to be passed down for over a hundred generations. In saving the Dhamma, in creating a lasting sangha, Kashyapa sacrificed the focus on the individual meditating in the forest all by himself, and relying only on his own resources to obtain ultimate enlightenment.[9]

It is ironic that what survived the Buddha was an organization that continued his teaching; elder monks became the authorities, and the Dhamma became the cannon. Adherents were expected to take on faith what they were told, even when they could not experience the truth for themselves. It was all right for a monk to be a "lamp unto himself," but if there was any doubt about the reality of reincarnation and the power of karma, the orthodox opinion must prevail. This was not the way the Buddha had told a group of people called the Kalamas to behave. They were confused by the abundance of gurus, monks and teachers who all claimed to know the truth and who dismissed any other teachings. The Buddha advised the Kalamas to take as truth nothing that they could not verify for themselves: just because someone seems learned, has a long white beard, is teaching from some ancient book, has a certificate from a prestigious university, a fancy title ... this does not mean that they should be believed. The only criteria worth applying is to evaluate the doctrine personally and see if it works, see if it diminishes suffering. If it doesn't work, then drop it.[10]

The Buddha taught a process to minimize suffering, here and now. Ultimately the only way to be completely free from any suffering is to not live any longer; however, except in very rare cases, Buddhism equates suicide as being equal to murder, so just killing yourself is not the solution. Buddhist teaching evolved after the Buddha's day until the solution was to no longer come back for the next life, to reach nirvana where there are no more incarnations. This is an attitude of rejection, when we view it from the religious point of view, but at the secular psychological level, where we can ignore the concept of reincarnation, the rejection of the Buddha was not a rejection of life at all, but rather a rejection of a *way* of life, a leaving behind of the lifestyle and delusions found in the household with all its attachments.

The Buddha rejected the extremes found in the forest yogis of various denominations with their mortifications of the flesh, and the extremes found in the secular life with its desires and fears. The Buddha sounded very much like Jesus who, centuries later, advised his disciples to leave behind their families and jobs and follow him. Jesus urged his followers to reject the normal life and not stop to look back, not even to say goodbye to their families, but to "let the dead bury their own dead."[11] This view can be found in extremis in more modern times in the Puritan ethic of avoiding pleasure, for in pleasure one is tempted into sin. All this displays the attitude of rejection.

✳ ✳ ✳

CORRECTION

The path of the rejection followed by the yogis in extremis, and by Buddhist to a more moderate degree, was a path despised by the Persian prophet, Zoroaster. To him, rejection was a cop-out: our true purpose was to accept the challenge presented by life and correct all that was wrong. It was Zoroaster who first came up with the idea of correcting the universe, and this idea is uniquely Western.

From whence does evil arise? This is an existential problem that all religions must answer, and then depending upon the answer, we order our lives appropriately. In the East, evil is an inseparable part of the warp and woof of life: The Buddha calls it dukkha, and it is inevitable. To the Chinese, within the Dao there are yin aspects and yang aspects; good and evil are necessarily components of the Way, and one can't exist without the other. In the West the problem of good and evil has been explained very differently. There is a fundamental flaw in the universe: Evil exists, but it should not, and our challenge is to fix the flaw. From this Persian postulate, the idea evolved into the biblical point of view prevalent today in the West.

Remember Zoroaster: He is the prophet of Ahura Mazda, the god of light and love; he is the enemy of Angra Mainyu, the source of the "lie." Remember also that the Persians were descendants of the Indo-Europeans, very closely related to the people who went east into India. Their background, stories and languages are very similar; they were masters of the horse and builders of the chariot, herders not farmers, warriors not city folks, and their priests worshipped the sun as the supreme god, not the moon. Where the Indo-Europeans were eventually subsumed by the indigenous planting culture and mythologies of the native Indians, the Persians held firm to their original mythology; not for them was the path of the yogi who sought escape from life.

Creation has been corrupted! That is why evil exists: Angra Mainyu moved against the world, creating everything bad from winter to warts, from murder to menstruation. Angra Mainyu is a principle rather than a person; he is the lie that makes us believe the universe must remain corrupted, so that we can't behold the glorious light and love of god. In this respect Angra Mainyu is equivalent to the Indian idea of Maya, the power of illusion that prevents us from seeing reality as it is. Zoroaster came to earth to set things straight: to remind us of the truth and help us make the right choice; to fight alongside the Sons of Light against the Sons of Darkness; and to restore the universe to its pristine, wholesome state. When the restoration has been completed, at the End of Days, there will be no darkness; no old age, sickness or death; everyone will be brought back to life and given either a 40-year-old body or a 15-year-old body (depending upon how old they were when they died); families will be reunited; and, since there will be no death, there will no longer be any new births. This is why we are here: to restore the universe to its perfect condition, with no hint of evil.

When this mythology is firmly rooted in a culture and its individuals, we can understand the genesis of religious intolerance: in this all-or-nothing battle against evil you are either with me or against me. The idea that we are fighting evil leads to holy wars. These causes of war are not found in the Eastern philosophies, although, unfortunately, sectarian violence does exist, it is just not for ideological reasons. Inherent also in this mythology is the fact that we only get one shot at this thing. Life is not a never-ending circle of death and birth and death; there are no grand moon-like cycles of ages coming and going. We are only given this one chance, and we must take advantage of it.

Remember, the great Persian king, Darius, freed the Jews who were living in exile in Babylon, and many returned home to Israel. Many, however, also remained, and over the next century both Babylonian and Persian ideas infiltrated and informed Jewish philosophy and mythology. It was during this period that the creation myths found in Genesis were compiled and edited, myths that like the Persian myth also saw a fall that contaminated the universe with evil. However, this time the evil did not come from a god but from a man. For the Hebrews, the source of evil fell to Adam, who in turn blamed Eve. This is not a totally satisfactory answer, because it creates new philosophical problems: If evil exists and God created everything that exists, it inexorably follows that God created evil. But! God is inherently good and pure and all loving ... so how could anything evil reside in or come from this loving God? God the creator, goes the Hebrew logic, cannot possibly be the source of evil. Man and his actions must be the source of all evil; both natural evil (the acts of nature) and human evil (the acts of man) stem from this same source.

If this logic makes up your base map psychologically, if you believe that evil befalls people who are evil and thus they deserve what they get regardless of whether the evil comes from an act of nature (an earthquake in Haiti) or an act of man (Al Qaeda bombing the World Trade Center), then you will agree with Pat Robertson that the people in Haiti were reaping the seeds of the evil their ancestors sowed hundreds of years ago, and you would have to also agree that the people killed in New York City on 9-11 deserved to die because they were evil. If they were not evil, God would not have allowed them to be harmed. They were harmed, so … guilty as charged (Remember Job!)!

But there is something not quite right with this logic. God created men, and it is in men that evil has its source, so how is it that God did not create evil, too? To quote Professor Joseph Klausner (1874–1958) of Hebrew University, the Hebrew belief, which informs the Christian and Moslem belief systems, states that

> *Supreme Being of necessity creates evil because of evil persons and for evil persons. Thus, if the evil of evil persons, that is, human evil, should come to an end, all evil would cease, even natural evil in general.*[12]

So, God did create evil, but evil only resides in evil people and not in God himself. Got it? If not, you are not alone. The position is not convincing, but Professor Klausner claims that if we (all mankind) cease our evil, then there will be no more earthquakes, tsunamis, droughts, asteroids, plagues, et al. All of this is our fault. Since it is our fault, it is up to us to correct it.

The Christian idea of correction is a familiar one and was Saint Paul's great realization: Adam sinned, so man was cursed along with Eve, the serpent and the earth itself. Evil arose through the choice of a man, and a correction was needed to set things right. The one appointed and anointed to effect the correction was another man, Jesus to wit. His death upon the tree at Calvary made up for Adam's sin at the tree in Eden. Jesus' reopening of the gates of heaven, which were closed to us by Adam's sin, is a general correction which made it possible for us to enter the Promised Land; but this did not guarantee that each individual person was going to be allowed entrance. There is still a particular correction needed in your life to make you eligible to behold the beatific image: You still have to make your individual choice to serve the Son of God and fight with the Sons of Light to overcome the darkness found in your own unique life. Your personal salvation is still very much up in the air. Where and how do you find your own unique personal salvation?

Remember, in the West the spiritual practice, as we have seen, is not one of identity, as it is in the East; it is one of relationship. In the East the challenge is to recognize that you are it, you are God! In the West, you are not God, but through Jesus you can become related to God. Recall the Catholic formula: We through our humanity are related to Jesus who is born human, but through his divinity Jesus relates us to God. All three of the big Western religions are based upon a relationship of man to God, and the vehicle of this relationship is found in the group.

In Christianity, the group is the Church. *"Extra Ecclesiam nulla salus,"* proclaimed Pope Innocent III (~1160-1216) in 1208. *"There is no salvation except through the Church of Christ."* This was further explained at the Fourth Lateran Council (1215) to mean, f you aren't with us, you are doomed. For Muslims the direction is to follow the *sunnah*: the way to live life and interact with family, friends and your governors as laid down by Mohammed. Those who follow such practices are called Sunni, and they are automatically part of the *ummah*, which is the Nation of Islam or the "one community." For Hebrews, God is not present unless there are at least 10 men convened together, the *minyan*. Without this quorum, God won't bother to show, and you shoudn't try to fool him by disguising a couple of women as men—He knows all![13] The group you relate to, and through which you relate to God, is the "chosen" group: This is the only group in the world that has God's blessing and His mandate to fix things up. By default then, all other groups—gentiles, pagans, heathens, infidels, barbarians—are outsiders; they do not know the truth and just get in the way of the big project. Sometimes they can be ignored, but when they do get in the way, they must be overcome.

Remember, God also gave man dominion over the earth and the animals, the birds and the fishes, and we are to make this garden fruitful so that we can be fruitful and multiply. Nature itself is flawed and cursed by God; it is our job to subdue her, dominate her, and make her serve us. By following the consequences of this mythic belief, we have lorded it over Mother Nature and have drained her wetlands, dammed her rivers, dug deep into her body for precious ores, and dominated all living creatures. We have corrected Mother Nature's wildness so well that all that is left to correct is our own wildness, but for that a different mythos is required, one of acceptance.

✳ ✳ ✳

ACCEPTANCE

> *I think of grass—you know, every two weeks a chap comes out with a lawnmower and cuts it down. Suppose the grass were to say, "Well, for Pete's sake, what's the use if you keep getting cut down this way?" Instead, it keeps on growing.*
>
> — Joseph Campbell *–The Power of Myth*[14]

❧ ❦

"Mother always said that the jungle was dangerous at night; father always warned me that night comes very quickly. I know: I tell my own children the same stories, and yet I find myself now passing through the jungle as the sun is setting. The light is starting to fade and I hear noises. I need to walk more quickly."

Our hero is in a bad place: A loud noise startles him, and he looks back to see a huge tiger come onto the path behind him. He freezes; the tiger is looking the other way. Our hero dares not flinch, because any little noise may alert the cat to his presence. But it's no use—the tiger has the scent of tonight's dinner. It turns its massive head and looks straight at him. Their eyes lock, and our hero turns chicken and runs, just as you would!

With the setting of the sun and the natural darkness of the jungle, the lighting is poor. Our hero stumbles as he runs, but the tiger has no problem and gains quickly. The path swerves alongside a ravine; the man knows he is out of options. He can't outrun a tiger in the jungle, so he takes the only chance he has—he grabs a vine and clambers over the edge of the cliff. A good plan, but it has one fatal flaw: The vine is only 10 feet long, and the ravine is 50 feet high. He is left dangling, peering up at a tiger that is looking down at its prey, sadly just out of reach. In frustration the tiger roars, alerting two more tigers that were lounging at the base of the cliff. They look up and see their dinner dangling at the end of a very short rope.

"Guruji always said to breathe when things were not going well; this is as not well as things get, so I guess I better breathe. What are my options? If I climb up, a tiger eats me; if I jump down, two tigers eat me. What else do I have? Just this vine. Fortunately it looks strong.'"

Unfortunately for our hero, as he is looking at the vine, he notices two mice coming out from a hole in the cliff, and they begin to gnaw on the vine. It is starting to break! He feels the vine begin to give. Soon it will all be over. He breathes.

"What's this? The vine has wild strawberries! And here is a ripe one."

Our hero plucks the berry and slowly places it in his mouth. He smells its sweet scent; he chews and feels the juices flowing in his mouth. It is the most amazing taste he has ever experienced ...

☙ ❧

Well, that's the end of the story ... and like most Zen stories, the denouement is unnecessary.[15] The question left hanging in the air, along with the man, is, why was the taste of a simple strawberry so amazing? The answer is *acceptance*: The man was about to die, knew he was about to die, but while he was still alive, he was still alive and able to live his life to the fullest in that one particular moment, that one particular moment that is actually every moment, if we would but put ourselves in accord with life as it is.

All primal cultures affirm life, accepting it just as it is.[16] This is quite logical: A primal culture could not afford the luxury of members of their society dropping out, living off the food provided by others as alms, and not contributing anything in return. The advent of wandering monks, yogis and teachers that arose starting around the eighth century B.C.E. occurred because societies grew large enough, with enough surpluses, to allow regular people who remained in society to support a number of begging holy men. We find these wanderers along the Gangetic Plains in India, such as Mahavira and the Buddha and their troops, and we saw this arise in Greece where, instead of *sadhus*, there were philosophers wandering about taking jobs as tutors. The same thing happened in China a few centuries later. But for a small primal community, the freedom for individuals to reject or get out of life was just not an option. Neither was the luxury of spending resources to fix or correct life. Primal communities only had one choice, and that was to affirm life positively and with cooperation. These societies accepted life's wild strawberries with gratitude.

We have seen already the fierceness with which primal cultures can put themselves into accord with the reality of life: the ritual sacrifices of headhunters who have to take a life before they can beget a new life; the returning of the buffalo's blood to the earth in order to guarantee the buffalo's return next year; the sacrifice of hundreds of goats and even human beings to the goddess Kali to ensure new life will come. In the Taittiriya Bhramana we find the statement

I am Food.

I feed on Food and on its feeder ...

Food is the exhaling breath

Food is the inhaling breath of life

Food they call death

The same Food they call life.[17]

Food is the source and food is the substance of all living things. There is no point denying it, so embrace it, celebrate it, bow down before it. Participate with joy, with rapture. Life is sublime, it is terrible, it is fascinating; but it is also beyond ethics and morality. Remember, those are human values. Our distaste and shock at the practices of our ancestors are a result of looking at their conditions with modern eyes. If we watch a wildlife documentary that shows a lion chasing, catching, and consuming a gazelle, while we may feel bad for the gazelle, we don't consider the lion to be a murderer. There was no crime committed, even though there certainly was intention: The lion intended to kill the gazelle. There is no sin here; no moral, ethical or religious laws transgressed. As we watch the actions of a great predator without judgment, we must also consider the actions of primal communities, for they are doing the only thing they can do—they are accepting life, in all its horror, as sublime.

✳ ✳ ✳

You may have noticed that both the attitudes of rejection and correction arose in cultures whose primary mythology was dualistic. If you are going to reject something or correct something, that something has to be something other than yourself. However, to accept life you must recognize that life is what you are: food! The Jains, Samkhya and Classical yogis were dualists: They believed that their essence, their soul, was pure consciousness trapped by the material world. Thus, if this is your belief, it makes sense to get out. The main, modern Western religions share this basic belief, but not the conclusion; our souls are embodied, but we are not our bodies, so we have to prepare for the day when our bodies drop off, by fixing up the world so that our souls can go to the right place after life ends. Correction and rejection only make sense in a dualistic world.

Where there are two, a choice must be made. Are you on the side of good or evil? Spirit or matter? But what if there is only one? We come now to the nondualistic philosophies and myths and ask of what ilk are they? Do they offer a way out of life's suffering through a rejection of life or a way *into* life where suffering, although real, is unimportant, a mirage created out of ignorance? Are the myths of the Upanishads, Vedantic Hinduism, Mahayana Buddhism and Tantra life affirming?

Here is the question: Is moksha, the liberation or freedom that is the fourth goal of life, a rejection of life or an affirmation of it? This was the question Brihaspati answered for Indra when he convinced Indra to stay in the palace and rule. That story teaches that moksha is an acceptance of life, but not everyone gives that answer. For many, as we saw with Ananda

Mayi's answer to Joseph Campbell, the question is no longer relevant when true liberation is obtained.

In the Upanishads we learn that all is Brahman, but because of our ignorance, we don't realize this. If we would get rid of ignorance, we would wake up to this wondrous fact. Our own little sense of self is called atman, but atman is Brahman: *tat tvam asi*! You are it! Remember our opening story of the original Self who divided and became all of us. The atman is always free because the atman is always Brahman. Accepting this is accepting life; there is no need to go anywhere because it is all right here. There are many ways of saying and explaining that you are it: teachers have used the metaphor of water, the ocean and waves for centuries to illustrate this point, and so we will add a second theory of waves to our earlier watery metaphor, one that points to a very different conclusion:[18]

❧ ❧

Imagine waves on the ocean, lots of them. Now look at one particular, specific wave. It looks just like many other waves, but it is unique, different, yet still a wave on the ocean. We can see that wave as an individual wave, or we can change our focus slightly and see it as a manifestation of the ocean. This one unique, specific wave is the ocean, but so is that wave over there, and so is that one. Each wave is a unique and different manifestation of the whole ocean.

Now, if *you* were that one particular, unique wave, and you popped up into existence and looked around at all those other waves, it would seem to your little wave mind that those other waves were different from you. Some of the waves are big and scary; some of them are small and puny. You might feel threatened by the bigger waves, but you might also want to poke fun at those tiny waves. You'd feel this way because you have no idea that all of us waves are actually the ocean.

One day, a wave friend of yours tells you that he heard a master wave guru talking about "the ocean," and it sounded really far out. This friend said he was leaving to go off to study with the master to see if he could find the ocean. Now you are intrigued: What is this thing called "the ocean"? You start to ask yourself: Can *I* find the ocean? Maybe! So you search for a teacher and find a wave who teaches something called surf yoga. You sign up.

The surfer yoga dude wave initiates you into a secret knowledge—the ocean is all around us! We are all the ocean, in specific but unique manifestations. As you practice chilling and getting deeper into your yoga meditation, you start to sink into your true nature, until one day … splash! You get it. *You* are the ocean, but so is the surfer yoga dude wave, and so is your friend who is still bobbing all over trying to figure out who he is.

Why didn't you see this before? Ego! Ego is the feeling that you are just a wave, separate from all the other waves, and as long as you feel separate, it makes sense to protect yourself, to erect barriers between you and the other waves. But now that you know your real nature, you realize there is nothing to fear.

From now on, whenever you see a wave, you know in your heart of hearts that, if there is a wave, there has to be an ocean!

⚜ ⚘

The wave failed to recognize its true nature through a trick of Maya. It is Maya that confuses the ego into thinking that it is it. Ego is the small sense of self, and Maya keeps it ignorant of the larger Self that it really is. Recall that Maya has three functions: the obscuring function, the projecting function and the revealing function. Any perception we have of dualism in the world, of ourself being separate from others, of the wave being separate from the ocean, is all just a trick of Maya: It is her obscuring function that hides the truth. It is her projecting function that creates the illusion that the wave is separate from the ocean. This is a false concept, residing only in the mind, not in reality; it is as ridiculous as thinking that heat is separate from fire. Maya projects all of our unconscious symbols and concepts out onto the screen of the real world, where we believe them to actually reside. Maya confuses, Maya projects, but when seen as she is, Maya reveals. The confusion ends, the projection withdraws, and reality is revealed in its true nature, but in a way, remember, that can never be described.

Chapter 17: Aum in Four Syllables

The world appears dual, but this is a projection of the mind. This trick of Maya is also a function of our language; we see everything in terms of subjects and objects. That is the nature of words and thoughts. To go beyond, to transcend this state of duality, we need to go within, and this is the advice of a tiny Upanishad called the "Mandukya." Weighing in at a whole 12 lines, this has to be the most succinct explanation of illusion ever written. In it we learn about *Aum* and about the nature of Brahman.

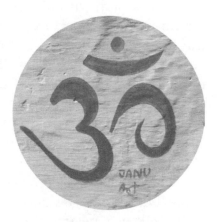

Figure 9: Aum

In the West we often see Aum word written as "Om"—one syllable, two letters. This is a shorthand summary of the sound of the universe. Just as Jesus is God incarnate and the Koran is God in-biblicate, Aum is God in-sonate.[1] "In the beginning was the Word," and it was the Word that created the universe.[2]

੩ ੬

Saul kept us waiting, hanging onto every word. We were waiting in Down Dog, a rather challenging pose when held forever. Saul explained the original discovery by the earliest yogis of the magical word, Aum.

"Aum," said Saul, "was discovered long ago when the very first yogi sat in a hot tub!" Among the modern sweating yogis, there were a few laughs.

"Seriously!" he continued. "And you can rediscover Aum for yourself, the next time you step into a hot bath. The first sound you will make is "ahhhh." After a few minutes soaking in the tub, you will say, "oooo." After about five minutes you will say, "mmmm!" Finally, there will be silence.[3]

⚛ ⚛

Aum has four syllables and four distinct sounds. Starting at the back of the throat is "ahhhh," then the sound moves forward, filling the cavity of the mouth with "ooooo," then the humming vibration occurs when the lips are closed, "mmmmm." Finally, there is the sound of silence. When the modern, Western version of the word is chanted as "Om," some sounds are missed; generally we will hear only two—the "ohhh" extending as long as one's lungs can last, and then a brief "mmmm." Any silence is restricted to the time it takes to refill the lungs and blast out another round of sound.

Aum is the *pranava*, the boat that takes us to the yonder shore, beyond illusion and duality.[4] In the Vedas the word *Aum* itself was never actually revealed; only euphemisms like pranava were used, because Aum is the ultimate power of the universe, and power must be guarded, kept secret.

The four syllables are symbolic: We can consider them as referring to the past (A), to the present (U), to the future (M), and to that place where time cannot flow (the silence)—the place before time began, before God said, "Let there be light" and before the Big Bang. In the Mandukya Upanishad, the four syllables are pointers toward understanding truth. "A" represents the waking state of consciousness, "U" the state of dream consciousness, "M" the state of deep sleep consciousness, and finally, the silence—the place beyond all definitions of consciousness, a place that can't properly be named but must be given a name so that we can converse. So this nameless state is simply called *turiya*, the fourth.

In our Western rational world, governed by Aristotelian logic, we believe that in our waking state we are more conscious of the world than when we are dreaming or in deep asleep. This waking state is the state of duality, and we think it is the highest state. It is in this state that I can say things like "I am holding a water bottle with a Lululemon logo." This is the realm of subjects (I) and objects (my water bottle). But consider this: Imagine I am dreaming, and in my dream, I am holding my water bottle. Now what is subject and where is the object? The dream me is holding a dream bottle; the difference between subject and object is not so distinct, but there is still the dreamer (subject) and the dream (object), so we have not yet transcended duality. Dream consciousness is the level of myths, for myths are from the same source and share the same energies as the dream world. But now we go deeper, into deep dreamless sleep: There is no dream and no dreamer, so we are closer to reality, to having no subject and object, but there is still consciousness, because if someone yelled, "Fire!" we would wake up and run out the door.

Where is your consciousness when you are deeply asleep? It is still there, but it is covered over by darkness, just dimly aware of the world. Go deeper, past sleeping consciousness, to the fourth, the nameless state. To give it a name would be to make it an object; to say it is consciousness is to make it a subject; this state is beyond all words. The goal of Classical Yoga is to go into this deepest state, awake—to remain conscious but not conscious of any thing, because there are no objects to behold and no subject to do the beholding. Similarly, the goal in Vedanta and the teachings of the Upanishads is to be in this ultimate state of yoking your consciousness to reality, where you have transcended duality, and now you rest in Brahman. This is the difference between Classical Yoga's purusha consciousness, which is forever separate from the world of prakriti, and the Vedantic view:

Since you went into this fourth state awake, you are still aware of the illusory world—you are still atman, who is aware that she is Brahman. You have not snuffed yourself out in nirvana, not yet, for you still remain embodied. But with this Vedantic realization, you no longer have to come back and be reborn. Remember, for Vedanta followers, all is Brahman; all is one, and there is no place like Aum.

Chapter 18: Mahayana Buddhism

There have been a few great rulers who were primarily responsible for the success and spread of Buddhism in Asia. The first of these was King Ashoka ([304–232 B.C.E.). Ashoka conquered virtually the whole Indian subcontinent, save for the southernmost tip, but after one particular battle, when he looked out upon 100,000 dead and dying bodies, when he heard the wailing of kin over the loss of loved ones, his pride turned to anguish. Ashoka vowed to give up his warring ways, his fierce governing style, his penchant for burning to death women who insulted him, and he turned to the teachings of the Buddha. As a committed convert, King Ashoka began sending missionaries throughout Asia and into Europe; his missionaries went as far as Egypt and Rome, to Sri Lanka and Indonesia. He built stupas and monasteries, which also helped to spread the Dhamma, the Buddha's teachings. He modeled his government after the Buddha's teachings of compassion. He, more than anyone else, was responsible for the spread of the Buddha's wisdom. In his stupas, the rock monuments, we find the earliest written records of the Buddha's words, and they are of great interest for what they don't say as much as what they do say: They help us disentangle later Buddha thought from the earliest ideas.

One hundred years after Ashoka, the Greeks had reconquered the lands around the Indus River, which were earlier won by Alexander the Great, and created a new kingdom, a new country, called Bactriana by the Greeks and the Greco-Bactrian kingdom by scholars. Here a succession of Greek kings secured the region that today is home to much of Pakistan, Afghanistan, Turkmenistan and a bit of northeastern Iran. Around 155 B.C.E. the king we met earlier, the one who debated with the Buddhist monk Nagesena, took the throne of Bactriana: King Menander. Known as Milinda in India, he became a devoted Buddhist and promoted the spread of the teaching throughout his kingdom. While Menander's impact on the success of Buddhism was not as great as Ashoka's, Menander lived and ruled in a very interesting location: He was on the crossroads between East and West. The Silk Road that connected Rome to China passed through Bactriana; here the European influences of Greece and Rome mingled with the ideas of Persia and Egypt and the philosophies and customs of India, and all of this started to flow into China to the northeast.

This part of the world became very important for Buddhism in the following centuries due to the arrival of the Kushanas. We are not sure where the Kushanas, in China known as the Yuezhi, came from or what language they originally spoke. Were they Indo-Europeans, or Mongols from above the Great Wall of China? Were they forced to relocate by the pressure of other refugees, in turn being pressed ever more westward by the central Chinese, or did they move simply because there were better opportunities down south than what they faced back home? Whatever the case, they were the ones that eventually took over control of the Greco-Bactrian kingdom, and they expanded their domain into northern India and up into western China.

The greatest ruler, Kanishka (~127 C.E.) was reportedly a very cruel monarch who then, like Ashoka, repented and became a Buddhist. The influential Buddhist scholar, monk and poet Ashvaghosha was a member of his court (Ashvaghosha was the one who gave us the story of the Buddha and his three temptations during the night of his illumination), and this causes historians to believe that the rise of the Mahayana form of Buddhism, and certainly its propagation into China, is due to the patronage of Kanishka.[1]

When the Roman emperor Theodosius I built upon Constantine's edict that the only permitted religion of Rome was to be Christianity, refugees began pouring into Kushan. Theodosius sanctioned the destruction of all pagan temples, the burning of their books and the persecution of their priests and philosophers, artisans and scholars. These educated and talented people fled the Roman Christian persecutions and brought their skills and knowledge to the East—to India. It was during this time that the Golden Age of India flourished, thanks to the brain drain from the West. This was a fertile time for Indian mythologies and philosophies, similar in importance to the Islamic flowering of brilliance in the eighth and ninth centuries and the European Renaissance of the 15th and 16th centuries.

Our point in this brief rendering of history is not to take us away from the mystical importance of mythology, but to show that the rise of Mahayana Buddhism, and even Tantra, was not due to purely Indian efforts but rather to a cross-fertilization of ideas and philosophies that took place from about 100 B.C.E. to about 500 C.E. and that infused many Western ideas into the Indian mind. It was the form of Buddhism developed in the far northeast of India, not in her heartland, that went into China. It was over this period and in this place that great vehicle, the large ferryboat of Mahayana Buddhism, was constructed.

᷃ ᷄

Siddhartha Gautama of the Shakya clan, native of Kapilavastu, sat completely still, transformed from a bodhisattva, one destined for awakening, to a full-fledged Buddha. For seven days and nights he did not move from the foot of the Bodhi tree, the tree of illumination. He totally lost track of the time; he was no longer subject to it. Finally he got up, walked a few paces and then turned, stood, and gazed at the spot of illumination for another seven days. He saw that some beings in heaven doubted his illumination, so he constructed a rainbow bridge of jewels that spanned from earth to the heavens, and he walked in meditation back and forth for seven more days. When he finished he sat again at another tree and gazed at the tree of enlightenment for a final seven days. During this last meditation, the realization dawned upon him, "This cannot be taught!"

Brahma, the supreme god in heaven, was attending to the Buddha, watching over him throughout his meditations, eavesdropping on his very thoughts. When he heard the Buddha thinking that there was no point trying to teach what he had awoken to, Brahma thought, "Oh-oh ... I better get down there right away!"

Brahma appeared to the Buddha and said, "Buddha, you gotta teach!"

"If I were to try to teach this Dhamma that I have obtained, it would be tiresome and vexing," explained the Buddha. "Subtle is this knowledge, and no one would understand me. It would be a waste of time."

"Buddha," repeated Brahma, "you gotta teach! Sure, most people won't have a clue what you are talking about, but there are a few people with little dust in their eyes; they will understand. Teach for them."

The Buddha considered. It is true that there were many people suffering in the world, looking for a way to end their pain and trying a host of remedies that were worthless. These poor people did not realize that their simple craving for solace was a cause of their suffering. Perhaps he should try to help, even though very few would benefit and most would misunderstand him. Still, what's the alternative? Just sit here for the next 45 years and do nothing?

"All rright," said the Buddha to Brahma, "as you wish. I will teach ... but they won't understand!"

॰ॐ ॐ॰

Now here is an unusual thing: God comes to earth to plead with a man to help out? Normally it is a man beseeching God for help. This story, of course, is not meant to convey an historical event. As Stephen Batchelor puts it, it is not like Brahma was actually listening up there in heaven, heard the Buddha vacillate, decided to confront the Buddha, appeared in a puff of metaphysical smoke, and said, "Listen, Sunshine, get on with it: teach!"[2] Rather, it is easier to see that this was a metaphor for what likely was going on in the Buddha's own mind: "On the one hand, I really should try to help people out and explain what I have realized, but on the other hand, what I have discovered is hard to follow, and most people won't understand, and that is going to be a royal pain in the butt, but still ... I should give it a try and see what happens."

Why would the Buddha think that this realization was going to be so hard to explain? Recall that what he "woke up" to was the idea of dependent origination: Because that was, this is. It sounds quite simple, and intellectually most people can grasp the idea, but the consequences of this simple idea were earth shaking for the people of the Buddha's time. Dependent origination directly leads to the fact that you have no self, there is no atman within you. And if there is no atman, there can't be any Brahman, either, because everyone knows that atman is Brahman: lose one, and you lose the other. The Buddha has just killed God! Sure, there are still gods, ones like Brahma in the above story, but Brahma is not Brahman, and the gods are just as confused as we are. Plus, if there is no self, there is no death! In fact, *you* were never born, because only things that have an ending can have a beginning, and if you were never born, how can you ever die? The Buddha has freed you from samsara by killing the metaphorical you: You are soulless. This is radical stuff, and very few people would be happy to hear this news. No wonder he hesitated; everything he was going to teach went against the stream of common sense. But this knowledge was necessary in order to stop our suffering.

In the stories of the Buddha's birth, he is shown as arriving in this world, not vaginally in the normal way of newborn babies, but popping out from his mother's side, like Eve budding off from Adam's ribcage. We can now understand the symbology: the Buddha was born at the level of the heart, and his decision to teach, despite his misgivings, shows his awakening to more than knowledge—he awoke to tremendous compassion. This is a crucial component of the bodhisattva, one who, through great compassion, puts off his own entry into nirvana until all beings everywhere are also free. There is a key distinction between this definition of the bodhisattva, so important in the Mahayana tradition, and the Theravada definition, which was cited in the above story: A Theravada bodhisattva is someone who has not yet obtained enlightenment, but who will ultimately succeed. The Mahayana bodhisattva is an already enlightened being who has delayed his entrance to final nirvana, called *parinirvana*, the extinction of death, until everyone else is also enlightened.

YANA

The Sanskrit word *yana* means "vehicle" and is often translated as "ferryboat." The metaphor worked well in ancient India, with its large river systems, seasonal floods and few bridges. Most journeys required traversing water at some point. The Buddha's teaching was the boat that carried you. The Jains also employed the imagery of their great teachers providing a ford, a way to cross the water. But, as we have found with Sanskrit words, there are many possible definitions we could choose. Yana can also mean "a course, a device, a machine, an instrument, a technique, a method, or a means."[3] Skillful means, also known in Sanskrit as *upaya*, is the technique that helps the student achieve the goal. In Buddhism we are offered the choice of two kinds of yana or means: the small ferryboat, known as Hinayana, and the larger boat known as Mahayana.

The Hinayana is the small raft that can ferry only one person across to the yonder shore, but the Mahayana (*maha* means "great") can take a vast number of people and comes with a captain of the ship to guide you, the captain being the bodhisattva. In a one-person raft, you are on your own. Hinayana is a derogatory term; it was coined by the followers of the Mahayana schools. Hinayana literally means "the defective or inferior way." You can see a superior attitude being displayed here, a looking down the nose at the earliest practices. Followers of the earliest Buddhist doctrine called their practice Theravada: the way of the elders, and they feel that they know and follow the original teaching. Followers of Mahayana feel that the Buddha held back his true teaching and offered only the inferior teaching to the early monks, because they would not understand the true doctrine, which was not widely available until long after his departure.

The differences in the two yanas are worthy of investigation: With the rise of Mahayana, a philosophy of salvation appeared in Buddhism. Not by your own efforts are you saved, but through the grace and compassion of a god-like being, the bodhisattva. Some forms of Mahayana belief became very similar to Christianity, in that the follower could only go so far on his own toward the Promised Land—a savior was required to complete the journey.[4] And in the most popular form of Buddhism in Asia today, the Pure Land sect, there is indeed a promised land, Sukhavati, which we will come to shortly.

There are two approaches being offered here: You can work on your own to cross the water to the shore of nirvana, or you can trust someone else to carry you across. In India these are known as the way of the monkey and the way of the kitten: A baby monkey has to cling tightly to his mother as she moves through the trees, or it will fall; a kitten is picked up by the mother and carried by the scruff of the neck and has no choice in the matter. In Japan these two ways are known as *jiriki*, which means "one's own power" and *tariki* or "other power." To rely upon a bodhisattva to save you is tariki; however, to save yourself through your own effort is jiriki. Theravada Buddhism is jiriki, the way of the monkey. Mahayana Buddhism is tariki, the way of the kitten.[5]

This divide is also found in Western thought. A British (or perhaps Celtic) monk named Pelagius in the fourth century C.E. taught that man could achieve heaven without divine intervention, through his own efforts. Saint Augustine disagreed and taught that only through divine grace could one be saved. Augustine's view prevailed, and Pelagius' doctrine was declared a heresy. We in the West still have not worked this out: In politics we have extreme conservatives that believe every man should fend for himself and not rely upon the state for assistance (the way of the monkey or jiriki), while liberals believe that state intervention is necessary to help those who cannot help themselves (the way of the kitten or tariki). Strangely, when the field of debate is switched from politics and economics to religion, the positions are reversed: Conservatives believe that only through God's grace can we be saved and individual effort is not enough, which is the view of Saint Augustine; and of Saint Paul, who taught that God gave us the 10 Commandments knowing we couldn't possibly live up to them, and only by His grace can we be freed from sin.[6] Liberals in the spiritual traditions, on the other hand, believe that following or trusting in someone else to set you free is not the way to go; it is your journey, and you succeed or fail through your own efforts.

Which is the map you follow? Is it by your own power that you achieve your desired goals or is it only, at the end of the day, by the grace of a greater power that you are successful? Do you follow this model consistently, or, like the conservative and liberals above, do you change your view depending upon circumstance?

NIRVANA

The earliest Theravada practice was a solo journey, a retreat, as we have seen, from life. Mahayana Buddhism turned around the emphasis of ascetic retreat to the forest and brought it back into the home. No longer would someone have to be a monk, live a reclusive life, and give up friends and family in order to reach the shores of nirvana. The rise of emphasis on the bodhisattva, the one who deliberately forgoes release from the suffering of the world and instead embraces it, made Buddhism universally accessible and allowed it to take root in China, Korea, Japan and eventually Tibet.

The expansion of the world that contained just one Buddha to a universe that contains innumerable bodhisattvas is one point of departure from Theravada Buddhism to Mahayana Buddhism; another is the reinterpretation of nirvana. Nirvana was all the rage in the Buddha's time. Most of the philosophers and gurus of his day were offering their ways to reach this final extinction, extinction that is from samsara, the rounds of rebirth. When pressed for a comment, the Buddha also offered his way to nirvana, but in his typical style, he turned the common concept on its head. When asked, "Is there such as place as nirvana?" he replied, "Yes! Nirvana is the absence of greed, hatred and confusion." The Buddha named greed, hatred and confusion (some would say "delusion") "the three poisons," and they are the cause of our attachments, and our optional suffering: Drop them, and you dropped suffering; drop them and you instantly transported yourself to nirvana. With this understanding, nirvana was no longer a place to get to, as was commonly taught by other teachers. Nirvana was a psychological state of mind.

In the Mahayana teaching, a more succinct formula was offered: Nirvana *is* samsara! Samsara, remember, was considered to be the rounds of birth, death and rebirth, cycling forever until one achieved nirvana, the complete retreat from the cycles, never having to be reborn again, reaching the so-called yonder shore. Notice how the Buddha changed the emphasis and the intent of nirvana: Nirvana and samsara are the same thing! Heinrich Zimmer offered a story to explain this more clearly for modern readers, which we will paraphrase:[7]

૭ ૬

You have lived your whole life in Vancouver. It's a beautiful city with sunshine, sea, mountains and trees, and occasionally some rain, and occasionally lots of rain. It has dog parks, Starbucks and Lululemon stores on every corner, tall buildings, and everything you need to live a healthy life. But, despite all Vancouver has to offer, life still feels somewhat flat to you; there is something missing, something you can't quite put your finger on. So you go through your days with this vague sense of dissatisfaction, of feeling incomplete.

One day a friend tells you about a special teacher, Guruji Joe, who claims to be able to make anyone blissful. It sounds unbelievable, but you go with your friend to a talk given by Guruji Joe, and you are taken by his presence and power. Guruji explains that there is a better place than Vancouver, a place where everyone can live in total harmony and without suffering, where everyone can live in joyous bliss forever, a mysterious land called … Victoria. That sounds good to you, so you become a follower, quit your job, and join his community, which lives in an apartment building close to Stanley Park, a luscious area in the heart of Vancouver. The days are filled with talks and work, study and cleaning. Joe explains that one day you will all board a magic vehicle, called a Greyhound, and will ride this bus toward the yonder shore, where life will be sublime, where Victoria awaits.

"When?" you keep asking Joe, "when can we go? I am ready now."

"Soon," says Joe. "Work diligently at your studies and don't worry about time."

Finally, after several years of working, studying and living with Joe, the day has arrived. Guru Joe calls all the students together and explains what will happen next. The first stage is to board the bus. Excitedly, everyone clambers aboard the magic Greyhound, and the journey begins.

Joe mentioned that your path would take you over water and under water, a symbolic baptism into the new life ahead, and sure enough the bus goes over the Oak Street Bridge and under the Deas Island Tunnel—you have just passed over and under a mighty river—but then you reach the divine departure point of Tsawwassen Ferry Terminal. Just the name sounds special: Tsawwassen (you never could pronounce it properly). Here you all board the ferryboat, the Queen of Esquimalt. a huge boat with space for hundreds of people. As you stand at the rails of the boat, you can dimly see, off in the distance, the outline of Vancouver, the home of your birth, of your youth, of your friends; and now you are leaving it all behind forever. You mentally say goodbye to all the dog parks, Starbucks, Lululemon stores on every corner, and the tall towers. The ship is sailing.

Life aboard the ferryboat becomes routine: You get used to lining up at the cafeteria for the cardboard hamburgers, and you actually start to enjoy the food, the swaying of the boat under your feet, the view of the Gulf Islands as you glide by, the occasional sightings of dolphins and killer whales. You completely lose track of time, and you no longer remember how long you have been on this journey. But you slowly become aware of a change of energy from your fellow passengers, and you hear their whispers: You are about to arrive at ... Schwartz Bay!

Guru Joe reappears in front of you and guides you back to your Greyhound, but you demur. "But I like it here," you tell Joe. "I want to stay on the ferry and eat more cardboard hamburgers and look at orcas and the pretty islands. Life is very comfortable here."

"You have to leave the boat now," says Joe. "Once you have crossed the water, you no longer need the boat; let it go. Trying to cling to what got you here will prevent you from further growth and advancement. You must let go!"

Reluctantly you join your fellow seekers, far less excited than they. In your seat on the bus, you can't see the dock, but you feel the big bump and sideways yaw of the boat as it greets the land. You have landed, but this is not yet your destination. The bus takes you down south, it is not a long drive, and as you get closer to Victoria, you find your excitement returning. Now, like your friends, you can't wait. Everything that you have been working for over so many years is about to be achieved.

The bus stops. Guru Joe helps everyone climb down, and you finally find yourself standing on the sidewalk in your beloved Victoria. You can feel the calm, the peace, the bliss of the city, as you look all around and see ... look, over there is a man walking his dog in the park, and—oh look ... over there is a Starbucks right across from that Lululemon store, and there are lots of tall buildings. Suddenly you realize! You catch Joe's eyes and they are sparkling, smiling. You realize you are back in Vancouver! Victoria *is* Vancouver; you haven't gone anywhere, but unless you made this journey, you would never have known.

Vancouver is Victoria and nirvana is samsara!

In Asia today the most common form of Buddhism is not Zen Buddhism, not Theravada Buddhism, but a form of Mahayana Buddhism called the Pure Land. In this map people believe that if they but speak out the name of the Buddha of Immeasurable Radiance, Amitabha, or in Japanese Amida, this alone will guarantee them rebirth in the land of Sukhavati, the Pure Land of Bliss (unless of course you are a woman, in which case you can be reborn there, you will just be born as a man). Sukhavati, known in Japan as Jôdo, is a golden realm filled with beautiful lakes, jewels, lotus ponds, heavenly music, delightful birds and flower petals floating down from the sky, which are gathered daily and offered in homage to all the buddhas of all the lands.[8] When you are reborn here, you are born on a lotus, which opens to allow you to take in all the delights. Getting here is an example of tariki, the way of other power, the way of the kitten. In Japan you may hear many monks during a meditation mumbling, "namo Amida butsu" over and over, slurring the words so all you actually hear is "namomidabutznamomidabutznamomidabutz …" This is a mantra of homage to the infinite light of the Buddha. According to legend, the land of the Golden Buddha Realm is located 1,000 miles west of Japan, but this raises the question: is the myth true? Is there really such a place?

A Zen master was once asked by his student, "Where is the Golden Buddha realm?" Now that you know the context of the question, you are ready for the answer: "This world, with all its squalor, with all its poverty, with all its crime and suffering, *this* is the Golden Buddha Realm!"[9] Samsara is nirvana.

Jesus gave a similar answer. In the Gnostic gospel of Saint Thomas, discovered in the town of Nag Hammadi, Egypt, in 1945, Jesus was asked, "When will the kingdom of heaven come?" He replied, "The kingdom of the father is spread out upon the earth, and men do not see it."[10] Samsara is nirvana.

> *Nirvana means extinction, the extinction of all notions and concepts, including the concepts of birth, death, being, nonbeing, coming and going. Nirvana is the ultimate dimension of life, a state of coolness, peace and joy. It is not a state to be attained after you die. You can touch nirvana right now by breathing, walking and drinking your tea in mindfulness. You have been "nirvanized" since the very nonbeginning.*

— Thich Nhat Hanh – *Touching Peace*[11]

* * *

THE FOUR NOBLE TRUTHS & THE EIGHTFOLD PATH

This is it! This Mahayana attitude of acceptance is pretty clear and miles away from the attitude of rejection, of shaking off the dust of the household and heading to the forest, fostered in Theravada Buddhism. But, how to do it, how to practice it? The Jains required fierce asceticism, and Samkhya and Classical yogis required mental gymnastics. But how does one adjust his attitude so that he can live with samsara in all its squalor and pain as if it is nirvana?

When we last left the Buddha, he had just decided to teach, even though he knew it wasn't going to be easy. His very first attempt proved that![12]

੩ ੬

The Buddha pondered: Who should he share his understanding with first? He thought of the two gurus who showed him the path of yoga and deep samadhi in that year after he left his father's palace. "Perhaps, out of gratitude, I should go to them." But a kind spirit informed the Buddha that both of his teachers had recently passed away and would have to come back in another lifetime to hear his teachings. Next, the Buddha thought of his five friends who had hung out with him for the five years he spent in the caves, practicing austerities. Of course! He will share with them his Dhamma. The same friendly spirit informed the Buddha that his friends had moved to Sarnath, a deer park in Isipatana, a suburb of Varanasi. Sarnath was at least a month's walk away, so he better get started. Just as the Buddha began his hike, however, he met a monk of another tradition.

It was common in those days of wandering mendicants for one monk to pass another on the road. They would stop and politely ask each other a standard series of questions: "Hail friend! Who are you? Where are you from? Who is your teacher, and what does he teach?"

The monk whom the Buddha met offered to the Buddha the standard refrain, but with a difference. "Hail friend! You look so peaceful, so calm! Your eyes are bright with knowledge, and your face glows with health. How is this? Who is your teacher, and what does he teach?"

The Buddha had his first chance to teach, to share what he knew. He replied to the inquisitive monk: "I have no teacher, no community. I am self-illumined, enlightened and awake to the knowledge of buddhas from time immemorial. Worlds below me, worlds above me, there is nobody in the world like me."

The monk was surprised and disappointed by the Buddha's obvious conceit. He said, "I wish you well, my friend. Good luck with that!" Giving the Buddha a wide berth, the monk snuck by and hurried down the road.

"Hmmm," said the Buddha to himself, "perhaps that was not the best way to teach. Fortunately I have a long walk ahead of me; it will give me time to come up with a better approach."

❧ ❦

By the time the Buddha met up with his five friends, he had worked out a way to explain his awakening. He decided to model this teaching along the same lines that a doctor uses to investigate the illness of a patient. He called his approach the Four Noble Truths. When you go to a doctor, the first thing the doctor needs to do is to establish if you are sick. This is the Buddha's first truth—suffering exists.[13] Next the doctor will try to find out if there is a cause of your illness. This is the second truth—there is a cause of suffering. Now the doctor will try to see if there exists a cure. This is the third truth—there is a cure for suffering. Finally, knowing that a cure exists, the doctor will give you a prescription. This is the fourth truth—the Eightfold Path.

The Four Noble Truths were so important that the Buddha could not just state them as facts; he had to fully realize them. He had to make sure that everyone knew these conditions were real, that they could be realized and transcended. He said:

> "Such is dukkha. It can be fully known. It has been fully known.
>
> Such is the arising. It can be let go of. It has been let go of.
>
> Such is the ceasing. It can be experienced. It has been experienced.
>
> Such is the path. It can be cultivated. It has been cultivated.
>
> As long as my knowledge and vision were not entirely clear about the 12 aspects of the Four Noble Truths, I did not claim to have had a peerless awakening ... "[14]

"It can be cultivated" is a telling statement. The word in Sanskrit that Buddha used is *bhavana*, "to bring into being, to cultivate." It is cognate with our English word *be*. When we look at the prescription offered by the Buddha to end our suffering, we see that he offers a path, but it is not somebody else's path, it was not his path—it is your path. Remember, this was the guy who said, "Put no head above your own. Check everything out for yourself." Find *your* path. This is exactly what the knights of King Arthur's Roundtable decided when they began their spiritual quest for the Holy Grail: "They thought it would be unfitting for them to enter the forest in a group."[15] They had to find and create their own path, and that is what the Buddha is telling us to do as well.

The Buddha was actually inviting us to begin *pathing*, but we have no such word in our English dictionaries. To understand what he meant, we need to make one more visit to the perplexing problem of subjects and objects, one more visit to teapots, mountains and things. Our English language does not work when there are no subjects and objects; when we say "something" it implies there is a thing, so when we are trying to describe something that is not a thing, it is no wonder that confusion arises.

Consider the word *rain*. We use this term as if there really was a thing called *rain*, like there is a thing called Uncle George. We can say, "Look, Uncle George is running." And when the running has stopped, we can see George huffing and puffing. Obviously there is an Uncle George, but where is the rain after it stops raining? We can't point to the water on the ground and say, "That's rain," because it is not; it is water. We could point to George before he starts running, but we can't point to rain before it starts raining. If you point to a cloud, a cloud is not rain. That cloud may never transform into rain; it may just dissipate or move on. We like to objectify, to *thingify* things, but that gives us an inaccurate view of reality. Where is the wind when it is not windy? We can expand our understanding by focusing less on nouns, as is our wont in the English world, and look to verbs.

The rain does not rain, there is no rain, there is only raining. The wind does not blow, there is no wind, there is only winding (See! We don't even have a proper word for this). Having nouns is a requirement of our language, not a requirement of reality.

When students and scholars of Buddhism hear about the Eightfold Path, they naturally default to thinking about the path as a noun instead of thinking of path as a verb. For this reason, Stephen Batchelor, who penned the above translation of the Buddha's words, deliberately used the verb *cultivate*: the Buddha is not telling us to follow the Eightfold Path, but to take action, to *cultivate* an Eightfold Path and bring it into being in our own life.

Batchelor has provided a more complete statement of the Four Noble Truths:[16]

1. Fully knowing suffering

2. Letting go of craving

3. Experiencing cessation [of suffering]

4. Cultivating an eightfold path

Notice the emphasis on the verbs. Batchelor boiled it all down even more succinctly:[17]

Embrace,

Let go,

Stop:

Act!

This form of Buddhism puts one right in the middle of the third attitude toward life: acceptance. This radical acceptance is another reason that the Buddha thought his Dhamma would be hard to teach and that no one would "get it." The Four Noble Truths ask us to embrace our suffering. This is again counterintuitive and goes against the stream of common sense. When we are suffering, we want to end it or run away from it, not investigate it. But that is exactly what the Buddha is telling us to do. Rather than follow the spiritual practice offered in other traditions, of dissociating our spirit from the phenomenal world, which is the cause of our pain and illusions, we are told to observe the phenomenal world in minute detail. The Buddha's meditations were always on phenomena: the breath, sensations, thoughts and feelings.

* * *

What is this medicine, the Eightfold Path, being offered by the Buddha at the end of the Four Noble Truths, the prescription to end suffering? This analogy to medicine is very fitting because the cure is therapy, probably the first psychotherapy offered in the world. The cure is a way to live life mindfully and skillfully. The Sanskrit word used with each of the eightfold steps is *sama*. Sama means "same," just as it sounds in English, but it can be translated as "equal, sum or whole, right, authentic, skillful or appropriate." It is most often translated as "right," but this can wrong and misses the subtle truth of the path. Right implies that you are living wrong, which is a judgment most people would react to defensively: "What do you mean I am not living right?" But *skillful* or *appropriate* implies that one could live one's life more skillfully, not that you are doing anything wrong. These are the translations we will use. The Eightfold Path then is:

1. Appropriate understanding
2. Appropriate thinking and intention
3. Skillful speech
4. Skillful action
5. Appropriate employment
6. Skillful effort
7. Skillful attention
8. Skillful concentration

Knowing the reality of life, the three marks of existence (dukkha, anicca and anatta: unsatisfactoriness, impermanence and no-self) are the first step on the path, which is appropriate understanding. This does not come easy; to really, viscerally, understand these facts takes some work, some cultivation and some bhavana. And so it goes with each of the steps. Work them. You will discover that these steps, when cultivated, affect every facet of your life: your interactions with others, with the planet and with yourself; your reactions to situations when they are not what you'd like them to be; your ability to enjoy samsara, the world right here, what's happening right now.

Whenever the Buddha was pressed for time and wanted to explain what his teaching was all about, he pulled out his formula: the Eightfold Path. When he lay dying beneath the sal trees and a monk from another tradition wanted to hear the Dhamma, the Buddha said that wherever the Eightfold Path can be found, there you will find awakened beings. Shortly after obtaining his last convert, the Buddha left, and we, too, shall take our leave of him here.

Chapter 19: Tantra Yoga

The Buddha's teaching has aspects of rejection (leaving the household life) and acceptance (accepting the three conditions of existence). Classical Yoga was purely rejection: escaping the rounds of samsara. Mahayana Buddhism was purely acceptance: nirvana is samsara—there is no need to go anywhere. A new form of yoga evolved around the same time Mahayana Buddhism flowered; it was called Tantra Yoga and had the same intention as Mahayana Buddhism—a radical acceptance of this world as it is right now. The main tool employed in Tantra Yoga is the awakening of goddess:

❧ ☙

She is asleep. Her body is wrapped around itself, her head tucked away to block out any distractions, lying in the deepest darkness, hidden from the world and waiting to be awoken when the moment is right. Above her, preparations have begun to bring her back to life; channels long blocked are being reopened, allowing some light to filter through. The path she once travelled in her fall to the depths, a channel long and thoroughly sealed, is being purged, and the way stations opened. However, she will not awaken through expectation or longing, nor through coercion or force; she will awaken only when her song is sung and her lover beckons. Her name is Shakti.

❧ ☙

Shakti is the consort of Shiva. We have met many consorts of Shiva already: Sati the pure, Parvati the determined, Kali the destroyer. There are many maps of Shiva, and many ways to model his role in existence, but in all maps and models he is never far from his shakti. There is shakti the energy that is life itself, and there is Shakti the goddess, the personification of the energy that resides deep within. And where is the home of shakti? For Carl Jung it is in the unconscious landscape of our psyche, but to the Tantrikas, Shakti's home is at the base of the spine, a place known as the root chakra: the *muladhara*. There, as we have just seen, she is coiled up like a small snake, awaiting awakening.

Tantra is a philosophy that evolved during the Golden Age of India, which you will recall began around 300 C.E., but Tantra's roots go way back, into the dim past, beyond the Vedas, into shamanic traditions. Some scholars believe Tantra first arose in Buddhist Mahayana thought and practice and from there seeped into Vedanta Hinduism, creating a completely new school of yoga.[1] The word *tantra* can mean "warp, woof, weave, extension, system, ritual, book or doctrine," but for our purposes, we can understand it to refer to a new worldview, a new way to look at reality.[2] The basic map of Tantra holds that the universe contains one underlying essence, but it manifests in polar opposites, like the Dao that exhibits both yang and yin, like the original Self that swelled up and became two, male and female. Tantra conceives the whole of reality as the interplay, the dance, the embrace, of Shiva and Shakti: the masculine and the feminine, the subjective and the objective, eternity and time. Liberation is available right here, in this body, right now, at this time. All that is required is to experience the unity of Shiva-Shakti, but for that, some work is needed.

Tantra was a radical departure from early Vedanta: It taught that anyone can achieve liberation regardless of caste or gender, or moral development. In this way, Tantra mirrors the Buddha's democratic teachings that everyone can achieve nirvana. Remember that Shankara, the great Vedanta reformer, taught that only Brahmins could become liberated. For this and several other reasons, mostly due to its unorthodox practices, Tantra was looked at by most Brahmins with disdain and disgust. There were right-handed and left-handed schools of Tantra, whose rituals were symbolic of the ecstatic, sexual union of Shiva and Shakti and whose rituals actually enacted the union. But before we can venture into this arena of Tantric practice, let's look at what the model presents; let's look at the subtle nature of nature itself.

＊ ＊ ＊

The Samkhya philosophers created an imaginative ontology that began with the postulate that consciousness (purusha) was completely distinct from creation (prakriti). When purusha comes near, prakriti is activated, and out of this embrace evolves the subtle levels of mind, the energies of sensation, and the gross elements easily discerned by mere mortals. Most spiritual schools considered this model pretty good, save for the beginning dualistic assumption. Tantra fixed this problem by unifying purusha and prakriti: The universe is not dualistic, but it appears this way due to the effects of Maya.

Maya is a complex concept because many philosophers have defined her in different ways. For Shankara, Brahman is the ultimate reality, and this phenomenal world, while it exists, is not real; it is an illusion cast by Maya. In this philosophy Maya stands in distinction to Brahman, which many scholars feel makes Vedanta actually a dualistic philosophy![3] In the eyes of the Tantrikas, however, Maya is a function of Shiva-Shakti, and her illusion is cast over purusha, deluding the mind into believing the universe is dualistic. If the earlier psychonauts had just journeyed a little further, they would have penetrated the five veils of Maya and discovered above her, waiting for acknowledgement, the unity of Shiva-Shakti.[4]

Shiva and Shakti are two sides of the same coin and can appear to be two, depending upon your point of view. But there is only one, as shown in this diagram. If we gaze at the

Shiva aspect of existence, we find the unfolding of subjectiveness, the consciousness of the world. This is equivalent to Brahman or purusha. But Shiva is not alone: If we gaze and meditate upon the Shakti aspect of existence, we find the unfolding of objectiveness—the objects of the world that the subject perceives.

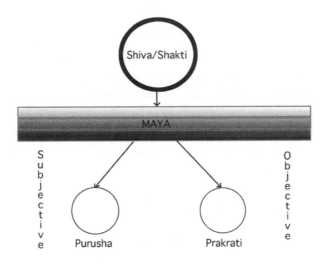

Figure 10: Shiva and Shakti are one

Neither the Buddha nor Shankara thought matter and spirit to be identical. For the Buddha, matter was real and was the cause of suffering, and there was no spirit. For Shankara, only spirit was real, and matter was an illusion. In both philosophies a great refusal was required to break away from the clutches of matter wherein all suffering found it roots. In Tantra, however, matter and spirit are identical, and thus there is no need to dismiss or disregard matter. In fact, it is only by having a body that one can become liberated or enlightened, so maybe this body was not meant to be dissolved or ignored, but honored and cared for. The 20th-century sage, Sri Aurobindo (1872-1950) taught that ego and its desire is the obstacle, not matter or phenomena; if we can disengage or renounce desire, then we will behold the bliss, Ananda, which is the sole cause of existence.

"It is only by this Ananda at once transcendent and universal that man can be free in his soul and yet live in the world..."[5]

We have noted that Shakti is asleep, coiled up in her bed at the base of our spine, awaiting awakening. When she stirs, she will try to rise, but the path is blocked at several centers, called wheels or *chakras*. These are psycho-spiritual vortexes of energy, sometimes called lotuses or *padmas*. Before Shakti can rise up and embrace her lover, who is waiting for her above the crown of our head, the way must be cleared. When she gets there, after our yoga practices have stimulated her awakening and cleared the path, the embrace of Shiva and Shakti will shake our worldview, and we will realize the oneness, the bliss of ananda, which is the basis of everything. We will still be here; there will be no need to die or leave the body. We will still exist physically, but psychically we will no longer be deluded; our body will be transformed into an adamantine body,[6] perfected, and we will possess great, magical powers called siddhis.[7] But these are to be ignored, for they lead back to delusion and desire.

The central channel traversed by the kundalini energy, or the goddess Shakti depending upon your map, is called the *sushumna nadi*, and it is very subtle. The kundalini, you may recall, is another name for the snake that is coiled three-and-a-half turns at the base of the spine. The snake again represents the moon, rebirth, cycles of time, and the goddess, so we can equate kundalini to Shakti; energy is feminine, form is masculine. Nadi means "little river," and some texts claim we have 72,000 of these streams within us flowing with subtle energy, while other texts talk about 300,000 or even 350,000. Again the point isn't whether the maps are real, but are they useful? Of all these little rivers of energy, only 12 are named and only three are described in detail, the main one being the central canal: the *sushumna*. While it is located inside the spinal column, it is not a physical tube; it has not been found in autopsies and is only discernable by the psychonauts in their meditations. Running alongside the sushumna are two collateral nadis: The *ida*, which runs up the left side, is the lunar channel with feminine energies coursing through it, comforting and cooling; and the *pingala*, which runs up the right side, is the solar channel, with masculine energies flowing, activating and heating. When the energies of male and female, sun and moon, are balanced and the channels fully opened, then and only then is it safe to proceed to open the central channel.

The kundalini snake is an old image. The idea of a snake or a pair of snakes rising up a central rod predated, in Mesopotamia, the flowering of Tantra by almost 3,000 years. The libation cup of King Gudea, shown,[8] depicts the snake god Ningishzida; his name in Sumerian means "lord of the good tree." (Now where else have we seen a serpent involved with a good tree?) Ningishzida is an underworld god, just as

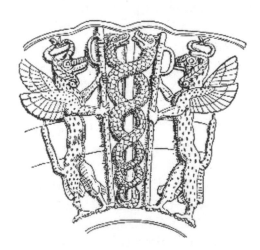

Figure 11: A representation of the image on a libation cup of King Gudea of Lagash showing Ningishzida, the Lord of the Tree. [Circa 2000 B.C.E.]

the Greek Hermes became over a thousand years later. Hermes, too, had as a symbol a staff, his caduceus, with two snakes curving along it. Note the seven points of crossing curve and cross in the same way the ida and pingala do, and everywhere the ida and pingala cross, there is a chakra. The Hindu Tantrikas intuitively detected these seven chakras, mapping nicely to their concept of seven *lokahs*, heavens or worlds. Seven is also the number of moving objects in the sky, the number of days in the week and the number of worlds above us in the heavens. However, not everyone followed the exact same map; Buddhist Tantrikas discerned five energy centers along the sushumna, mapping nicely to their idea of five meditation Buddhas.⁹

✱ ✱ ✱

It is fascinating to accompany Shakti as she rises through each of these energy vortexes and to witness the psycho-spiritual effects as these centers open. We will do so following the map most often used by Joseph Campbell,¹⁰ but, naturally, there are many versions of this concept and many other maps we could follow.

THE MULADHARA CHAKRA — THE ROOT BASE WITH FOUR LOTUS PETALS

Located at the base of the perineum, the lowest part of the torso, between the anus and the genitals, this is the base upon which all rests. Here, there is virtually no psychic awakening; everything is oriented toward mere physical existence. People stuck here are the anal-retentives. We, unfortunately, all know one or two of this type of person—basically, they are the assholes of the world. Joseph Campbell has a nicer word; he calls these people "creeps" and equates this level of existence to the dragon.¹¹ Campbell notes that with advances in modern zoology, we do know a lot these days about the behavior of dragons. Dragons guard things like precious jewels and beautiful virgins, and yet they have not the slightest idea of what to do with either. This is just hanging on for the sake of hanging on.

This chakra is the root because it is the base from which the whole edifice rises, and as such there is no need to deprecate it. The Tantric philosophy sees that which is low and that which is high as equal, the same thing.

Each of the first five chakras symbolizes an element: the root base is equivalent to earth, the grossest, densest and lowest element, and it is associated with our grossest cognitive sense: smell. This is a logical place to erect a structure, having first firmly rooted it into the ground. Here our potential to be who we can be is immanent, awaiting development and growth to the transcendent.

THE SVADHISTHANA CHAKRA — HER FAVORITE RESORT WITH SIX LOTUS PETALS

Located at the level of the sex organs and the bladder, which is the organ pertaining to the element, water. Becoming psychologically active here involves transcending mere behavior and simple existence and rising to the level of sexuality. Life here is Freudian; everything means sex in some overt or sublimated way. Sex is the goal of life, and, if frustrated, this energy goes off and creates something else, such as civilization. Sex is passion; this is Aphrodite and her son Eros, not Amor as sought after and fought for by the knights of King Arthur.

Sva in Sanskrit means "self," and this is the level of the self in terms of desire: "I want for myself these pleasures." Sex is just the base desire. Associated with this chakra is the sense of taste: this is not just the gustatory taste found in our mouth, but all our tastes for particular experiences: again, desire. The six petals symbolize the six negative emotions: anger, lust, greed, confusion, pride and envy, which all arise from the egoic sense of sva—self.

The Manipura Chakra — The City of the Shining Jewel with 10 Lotus Petals

Located at the navel or the solar plexus—our second brain—this is the center of power and wealth. If the second chakra is Freudian, the psychology here is Adlerian: the will to power. We strive to achieve, to overcome our inferiorities imagined and real, to grow, to be secure and safe. This is a fierce energy. This is the element, fire; it is the power to consume and the power to digest, necessary when considering the stomach, but dangerous when out of control in our lives.

Each chakra has a god and goddess presiding, and here is the home of the goddess Lakini. She is not a gentle vegetarian; she loves meat and is often depicted at sacrifices besmeared with blood on her breasts, her mouth drooling and dripping with the fat of the offerings. She symbolizes the ability to destroy but also transform, for fire doesn't just burn, it can also bake. People who are creative in the arts or in the healing professions and people who are successful in business all live out of this center. Sometimes they overextend and become exhausted, depleted, their third chakra "burned out."

The Anahata — The Unstruck Sound with 12 Lotus Petals

At the level of the heart, something transformative occurs: a transition from the purely physical phenomenological level of existence to the spiritual. The psychology here becomes Jungian, [12] and the process toward wholeness begins. This chakra requires a bit more reflection and contemplation.

Here there is an inflection between the dualities of matter and spirit. If we consider the first three chakras forming one line and the last three chakras forming a second line, the fourth chakra is the point joining them, like the bottom vertex of the letter *V*. In the enlightened being, these two arms fold up and merge: the first chakra merging with the seventh, the second with the sixth and the third with the fifth. Whereas the first three chakras relate to raw, animal existence concerned solely with the three aims of life, the last three chakras bring us further into the spiritual realm. Every animal wants to keep on living, to beget the next generation, to be powerful and free from fear; we are no different. Our earliest religions were all barter systems; the purpose of sacrifice was to wrest from the gods health, wealth and kids. "Dear gods, I will give you this if you give me that." The Old Testament contains several such covenants with God, contracts between mankind—or at least a selected subset of mankind—and God, wherein God promises to protect men, make them fruitful, powerful and safe in exchange for certain obligations on men's side. This is asking the gods, or God, through your prayers and sacrifices to serve your animal nature, not your spiritual nature. To be honest, this is where most religious life is still found in the world—people asking God to serve their base needs: "Help me through this difficult time"; "May my team win the Super Bowl"; "Let me win the lottery."

The first three chakras represent the three temptations of the Buddha that night beneath the Bodhi tree: fear, pleasure and duty. Recall that these are the three goals of life: kama, artha and dharma. Moksha, the fourth aim of life, is the spiritual practice that allows us to transcend the base instincts of life, and it begins here at the fourth chakra, at the level of the heart. Even in the earliest Vedas, the heart was considered the bridge from the material life to the spiritual life. Tantrikas are advised to get their mojo rising as fast as possible to this level, so as not to be distracted or trapped in the lower rungs.[13] However, don't think that these bottom three chakras disappear once you reach the higher levels; if you move up to the fourth floor apartment of your building, the lower three levels still exist![14] There is no point in being "holier than thou" and claiming that you no longer need the lower floors—of course you do. Even the Buddha still needed to eat. We learn to assimilate and accommodate these lower energies in a more skillful way, once we have ascended to the heart. And the higher chakras have their dangers, too, if the heart is not awoken first. Awakening the heart involves (and it's no surprise) the qualities and emotions of love, compassion, calmness and acts of kindness. (Note the inclusion of "acts" here: Of what use is compassion if it does not lead to action?)

Here at the fourth chakra, the associated element is air, through which sounds travel. When the heart opens, an inner sound becomes apparent; this subtle sound is called *nada*. Anahata, the name of this chakra, means "unstruck." This is a bit of a puzzle: What is the sound that is not made by two things striking together? What is the unstruck sound? We have heard this one before: It is Aum—the sound of the universe, and the only sound without a cause.

At this level is found the symbol of the yoni, the female organ of creation, and the lingam, the symbol of male sexuality. They are also found at the first chakra, the muladhara, but here at the anahata, they are golden, representing spiritual birth. This is the Virgin Birth—not a physical birth as normally thought, but a spiritual second birth through the inner energies of your own heart. Here we can see that the Virgin Birth, such a common motif in so many mythologies, is not a question of biology, is not "down there" at the level of the sex organs, but up here at the level of the heart; the meaning is symbolic. What does it mean to *you* that you are bringing forth God from inside yourself without any exterior assistance? This is the proper way to use the map being offered when you read about a virgin birth. Like the mantra Aum, it is within you because you are it: *tat tvam asi*.

THE VISHUDDHI – PURGATION WITH 16 PETALS

We are now moving into the realm of transpersonal psychology. The *vishuddhi* is located at the throat, which controls communication and skillful speech; this is also the realm of purification and cleansing. What is pure or being purified here? Some scholars, like Georg Feuerstein, feel that the reference is to the element *akasha*, space, which is perfectly pure, the most subtle of all the elements.[15] Joseph Campbell considers this to be the level of purgation, the *act* of purifying.[16] This is the mirror of the third chakra, but instead of focusing your power outward to control others and the external environment, we bring the power inside to clean up our own act. This is the beginning of the spiritual practice of the yogi: the purification found in extreme asceticism or Hatha Yoga, as well as the daily rituals—going to confession, fasts, and penances—of the more mundane religions..

Purgation has equal symbolic importance in Eastern and Western traditions. We saw how Dante was led by Virgil to the mountain of purgatory, the place where souls who sinned, but not so badly that they warranted hell, were given time to cleanse the stains of their life and prepare themselves for the beatific vision. Campbell points out that this is like being sent to summer school: You didn't quite learn the lessons you should have at regular school, so you are given a second chance by being sent to a place where tough teachers will beat some learning into you.[17] In the East, we don't get sent to summer school; we repeat the whole year! If we aren't ready to go higher, we come back and live another life, and this next life is our chance to purge our karmic stains.

At this chakra we have reached the last of the five elements, and we are about to go beyond the physical realm completely. It is time to behold God.

THE AJNA – THE COMMAND CENTER WITH TWO LOTUS PETALS

Located right between the eyebrows, the third eye position, the subject beholds the object of his devotion. Here you see *your* God, your *ishtadevata*, in whatever form you conceive Him to take. If you understand God to be Yahweh, here he sits; if you conceive God to be Vishnu, here he sleeps. Your ishtadevata refers to your chosen image of God, the one you pray to the most.

Since we are in the realm of subject and object, there are two petals on this lotus: male/female, spirit/matter, right/wrong, God/you. This is the realm of duality, and you are not yet your god. You may not even seek that last step up: like Ramakrishna who loved sugar but did not want to become sugar, you may be content to remain here and just worship your god.

You behold your God as Dante beheld Beatrice, as Tristan beheld Isolde, as the moth beholds the flame. You are held in a state of aesthetic arrest, as defined by James Joyce when he referred to "proper art." [18] Proper art is the art that can stop the mind, like holding a newborn baby or watching a spider's web with dew drops shimmering in the morning light, like listening to a movement of Mozart or contemplating Michelangelo's "Pietà." The mind is still, and you live in the rapture of Presence. This is the spiritual equivalent of the second chakra; where the sexual urge was all about you and your pleasure, here the duality is outward focused, onto the beloved.

Unlike Ramakrishna's urge to resist becoming sugar, the moth wants the flame but is held back, prevented from the final step by the glass of the lantern. This barrier, the last obstacle in the spiritual path of the East, is Maya. Notice, though, there is no last step in the spiritual practices of the orthodox West. Since the base map says we are not God, there is no way to become God. We remain at the sixth chakra, and all we are allowed is to bathe in the vision of the Ultimate. In Gnostic traditions, however, in the Christian mysticism of Meister Eckhart and others, the barrier can be transcended. We can go past Maya to the Ultimate.

Maya—Mary

Maya's obscuring function prevents many from realizing that there is another level above the beatific vision, beyond the bliss of being with God. Her projecting function transmits into the dualistic realms the image of the Ultimate reality, so we think that God is it. Meister Eckhart (1260-1327), the controversial German mystic and theologian, said that the ultimate leaving is to leave God for God; we have to leave behind our concept of God, the limited objective descriptions, for the ineffable experience of God.[19] For this kind of heretical teaching, Eckhart was summoned to Rome to answer for his blasphemy, but he died before he could be tried.[20]

Maya is found between the sixth and the seventh chakra as either a barrier to transcendence or the final curtain to pass through. In the Western philosophy of Christianity, she is exactly where Mother Mary sits: God the Father sits above Mary; his energy of creation, the Holy Spirit, flows through her into the world of objects and subjects, where it incarnates as her son, Jesus. *Ma* means to measure forth, to create, which is the function of all mothers; they bring forth the universe, but in this case the seed is from the Father. In her revealing function, however, Maya allows us into the ultimate, transcendent experience; we *become* sweet sugar.

The Sahasrara — The Thousand-Petal Lotus

We have gone beyond: *gate, gate, paragate, parasamgate, bodhi svaha*—beyond, beyond, far beyond.[21] We are at the peak of the holy mountain, beyond the top of the physical body, at the summit of the sushumna, located a couple of inches above the crown of the head. Here Shakti is now united with her beloved Shiva; all becomes one, and both subjects and objects are transcended. *"Shivoham!"* shouts the yogi. "I am Shiva!" The body can drop off now, or you can choose to remain in the body and descend back to let your consciousness reside in the heart chakra; that is the choice made by the bodhisattvas.

Here the first chakra is complemented and completed; the physical and the spiritual merge, and all of life is an expression, all of existence is an expression, of the one true reality. The journey is complete, and the practices proven productive.

✳ ✳ ✳

Carl Jung showed that through active imagination we can work with the energies of the psyche that are beyond normal conscious or voluntary control, but we need to know how the symbols work. By using our own symbols, discovered through paying attention to significant dreams and other associations that erupt during our daily life, we can reshape them and re-implant them, effectively creating a new map to follow unconsciously, a new map that is more appropriate or skillful in taking us where we need to go, which in Jung's view is to wholeness. The creators of the Roman Catholic Mass were skilled craftsmen of the unconscious landscapes of their followers. They developed over centuries the right full-bodied experiences draped with mystical imagery that awoke the senses on all levels, resulting in resonance between the outer message and the inner experience. In the same way, the Tantric rituals are equally effective and share similar modalities.

What are these Tantric practices? How do we wake the snake, goad her to rise, and prepare the channels? In the West there has arisen an association of Tantra practices with wanton sexuality, which is as ridiculous as associating Catholicism with cannibalism. The comparison is illuminating; in both practices ritual is very important, as Carl Jung notes, and the symbols utilized have similar intentions. For example, both rituals are conducted by a master of ceremonies: the priest or the guru. The Roman Catholic Mass is a masterpiece of psychic manipulations, working skillfully with the symbols of the deep unconscious, through its rituals and mystique, invoking the presence of God, bringing us up to the sixth chakra where we can behold our beloved. (Of course, a Catholic priest would not use the imagery of the sixth chakra; that map is a bit too outré for the Church.) Tantric rituals use similar tools with similar intent, bringing the participants not to the sixth, but to the seventh level, evoking the experience of being God, not merely being in His presence.

A community is required in both traditions. The church itself is the organ through which the relationship to Christ is established; in Tantra, the other practitioners are the vehicles through which the ultimate is experienced. We take in the world through all of our senses, and well-constructed rituals feed us and provide experiences on all perceptible levels. The Roman Catholic parishioner enters the church and is immediately assaulted by the fragrant incense; already he is transported beyond his menial daily experiences, being readied for the transformation ahead. So, too, in the Tantric rituals: incenses fill the room where the ceremony will be performed, the scent sometimes tinged with the sweet smell of marijuana and other spiritual herbs. Kinesthetically, we are actively involved in the Catholic Mass, a baffling series of sitting, standing, kneeling, standing, and sitting—an outsider never quite knows when to do what but shouldn't try to figure it out; just flow. In Tantra, there are movements and postures, as well, which have spilled over into the famous asanas of Hatha Yoga, where they have taken on a life of their own. Tantra employs bodily positions called *mudras*, which manage inner energies and prevent them from leaking out. Our ears are involved as we hear music and sing chants. Originally the Catholic Mass was conducted in Aramaic, then Greek and finally Latin, which added to its power and mystique, something that was lost when the Mass switched from Latin to the vulgar languages (something that Pope Benedict XVI wanted to undo). The chanting of mantras is a key part of Tantra, as well: From the universal sound of Aum to your personally assigned mantra, the sounds create presence and awareness, altering the normal mode of consciousness to one of extreme, focused attention. At times our eyes are closed to enhance the effects on our other senses, but at times we look deliberately; the crucifix, the statues of Mary and the saints, the light through the stained-glass windows all serve the same function as the mandalas, yantras and statues of Shiva and Shakti in ecstatic embrace. Visualization is a powerful practice in Tantra; it brings focus to one object; it provides a template through which the ultimate image can radiate. Finally, the last of our five senses: Even our taste buds are involved ritualistically. Through the mysterious transubstantiation of the Mass, bread and wine become the body and blood of the Savior and are consumed, tasted. In Tantra, normally proscribed foods are consumed: meat, fish and wine. For conservative Hindus these foods and all intoxicants are off limits, but in Tantra they are ritualistically employed to alter the normal state of consciousness and broaden awareness,to realize that everything is divine. There is nothing defiled when everything is God.

The embrace of Shiva and Shakti in sexual rapture is found also in the Vajrayana Tantra of Mahayana Buddhism, especially in the Tibetan traditions. Here the image is of *Yab-Yum*: the male and female energies copulating to bring forth all of creation. Yab represents the supreme Buddha, beyond all incarnated Buddhas, and his consort Yum represents the *prajna-paramita*, the Wisdom of the Yonder Shore.[22] This meditation on both the male and female realities of existence elevates women from the evil things we find in earlier religious symbology—pestilent Pandora, cursed Eve, the scourges of men's souls—to equal and necessary aspects of reality itself. Men are to meditate upon the partner they have, that they are gazing upon, as Shakti herself, and not this particular embodied woman; women are to meditate upon the partner they are with as Shiva, not that particular man.

The union in Tantra is symbolic in the same way that consuming the body and blood of Jesus in the Catholic Mass is symbolic; one does not actually consume the flesh of another human being, because that would be cannibalism. Catholics are *symbolic* cannibals, symbolically partaking of the willingly offered body of Christ. In the same way, Tantrikas do not actually engage in sex with a partner; they visualize the experience intensely as if it were real, visualizing not so much the sex act, but the union with their god or goddess. Remember, this is the value of a good myth: We act *as if* it were real. However, there have been throughout history a few so-called "left-handed" schools of Tantra whose followers did believe that the symbology had to be enacted in full, living color. This was very rare, but these stories have colored Western views of Tantra to the point where many modern "neo-Tantra" teachers leverage the sexual practices, claiming to be able to liberate people in their own bedrooms. For the most part, these left-handed practices were frowned upon by the right-handed schools in the same way that orthodox Catholics frowned upon the parody of their rituals found in Satanic masses.

Just as not every Catholic needs to wait to go to Mass on Sunday to practice his faith, not every Tantrika needs to join a group to practice Tantra. Solo practice can be done utilizing the tools mentioned: murmuring mantras and taming the vital breath, making mudras and visualizing yantras, or meditating upon the goddess. However, to advance in the practice, a guru is an absolute necessity to guide you and keep you on the path and to help you avoid the dark patches where many have fallen and lost their way or physically, and even psychically, hurt themselves. A premature kundalini awakening can blow out the nadis and destroy the chakras in the same way that connecting your garden hose to a fire hydrant can cause an explosion. One must take care in preparing the body and the mind before turning on the full flow of energy. When done properly, the experience of Shakti rising and finally meeting Shiva is sheer bliss. Ramakrishna was often asked by his followers what it felt like to have the kundalini awaken. He said that sometimes it would feel like a little ant was creeping up the spine, sometimes like a snake zigzagging her way up, sometimes like a bird hopping or a fish swimming, and at other times it was like a monkey leaping from branch to branch, sometimes going straight from the second chakra right up to the top in one mighty leap.[23] When he tried to describe the top chakra, Ramakrishna would always pass into an ecstatic trance and could speak no more.

✳ ✳ ✳

THE ATTITUDE OF ACCEPTANCE — REPRISED

It is tempting to think that the attitude of acceptance is the "right" attitude and that we should all adopt this approach, as shown in the compassion of Mahayana Buddhism that works toward eliminating the suffering of all beings; the oneness of Tantra where both the phenomenal world and the spiritual world are equally valued; the Gnostic Christian traditions that see Christ everywhere and in everything—"Split a piece of wood; I am there. Lift up the stone, and you will find me there."[24] But that is missing the point. There is no "right" map; there are only more useful or less useful maps. Affirmation is not "right"—it is one way to deal with the reality of life, but not the only way, as we have seen.

What appears to be acceptance can be a veneer laid on top of rejection; the Eastern wild card of reincarnation is always in the back pocket, ready to be played if things get too sticky. Reincarnation is a rejection; it slides us back into a dualism between life as it is and as it is supposed to be. If one admits to reincarnation, one must also admit to something that gets reincarnated, and thus we have the age-old split between substance (our body and the phenomenal world) and spirit (the reincarnating monad in all its guises). Buddhists have been critiqued from the beginning for wanting to have their cake and eat it too; if there is no self, what is it that gets reincarnated? No solid answer exists, but many metaphysical theories are posited, none of which can be proven and thus must be taken on faith, going against the Buddha's own prescription to test everything to make sure it works.[25]

Thich Nhat Hanh offers a very Buddha-like way out of this dilemma by replacing the whole question of rebirth with action here and now; your continuation is the ripples you create when you act in the world. He promotes a form of Buddhism that he calls Engaged Buddhism: one must not just sit in a cave or a monastery meditating; one must meditate while acting, not just by pumping metta (loving kindness), but by making a difference. Engaged Buddhism is affirmation. One responds to what is actually happening; one does not run away from it or ignore it; one reacts to it in the most appropriate and skillful way one can. However, to create his modern view of Buddhism, Thich Nhat Hanh has had to drop discourses on reincarnation as some continuation of a subtle self. In his words, "There is no birth and no death, only continuation,"[26] just as the ocean continues after the wave has ceased to be seen. Thich Nhat Hanh sees his own reincarnation, or more properly his continuation, in the monks, nuns and lay people he has taught and worked with over the eight decades of his life. Their lives continue his, and his ripples will continue to create new ripples through them. But the question can be asked, does Engaged Buddhism really express acceptance, or is it correction?

In the West we don't sit back and accept life on its own terms; we usually choose correction. This has worked wonders for us: Advances in science and medicines arise because we don't accept life the way it is, we try to change and improve it. Affirmative cultures don't seek or value change—what's the point? Many affirmative cultures don't believe things can change. Acceptance can lead to stagnation and perpetuation of things that do need changing, such as civil rights, universal suffrage, education for all, and universal health care. These things were won because people did not accept the status quo. There is something slippery about the affirmation of life offered by Vedanta, Tantra and Mahayana Buddhism; accepting life just as it is is not always the most skillful choice. Of course there is a downside to correction, too: The consequence of changing the world is that ... it changes! And sometimes in ways we don't like—species extinctions, global warming, war.

Every model, every philosophy, has its unanswered questions and unanswerable questions. Don't think that any of these maps are complete. Remember the questions the Buddha refused to answer because they were not conducive to study, to the challenge of living your life right here and right now? All traditions have these unanswerables; this is where faith arises. When the answers cannot be known, the disciple is urged to *believe*, because that is what the saints and sages believed. You may ask, "Why is my atman trapped in delusion created by Maya? Why would God want me to suffer? Why does he inflict ignorance upon me?" Ramakrishna would answer, "That is Maya's play."[27] Not a very helpful answer. Ramakrishna believes that without misery, there can be no happiness. But if the goal is to transcend these opposites, why produce them in the first place?

Chapter 20: Guru Yoga

Vande gurunam charanaravinde

Sandarshita svatmasukavabodhe

Nishreyase jangalikayamane

Samsara halahala mohashantyai [1]

— The Opening Ashtanga Yoga Chant

"I bow to the two lotus feet of the (plurality of) Gurus" [2]

The paths we follow in our lives and in our spiritual journeys are not always well marked, easy to discern, or cleared of obstructions. While King Arthur's knights chose to enter the forest where no one had gone before, that is a touch choice! A guide or guru who has been where we are trying to go, one who has gone through what we are facing, can be invaluable. A teacher or mentor is essential for success, if only, as in the Buddha's case, to show you where not to go and what doesn't work. A teacher need not have been to the top of the mountain to show you how to walk the next hundred yards; we can find teachers all around us, but a guru is a horse of a different color.

॥ ॐ ॥

Dad made a mistake.

A big mistake!

A fatal mistake.

The gods were lounging around Indra's palace, admiring the work of Vishvakarman and the lotus ponds he added last night, when the conversation turned to their favorite obsession: Dad's Mistake. It wasn't so much that Dad forgot to do something, he did it all—he created the whole universe, but he added something that did not need adding.

Indra, befitting his status as the alpha-male, decided it was time for them to pay Dad a visit and demand an explanation. Off they all went on their quest to find the creator and obtain the answer they were due. Dad wasn't hard to find; after all, he is everywhere! When his boys approached him, he was gardening, planting a few bulbs for the spring. Indra and the others bowed deeply, paid their father appropriate homage, arranged themselves in a circle around him and, when he finished with his digging and had laid his trowel down, asked the question.

"Dad," began Indra, "you know we love you and we love what you have done with the universe and all; great job there. I couldn't have done it, but we have one question that really puzzles us, and quite frankly disturbs us."

"What is your question, Indy?"

"With all you created, why did you have to create … him!" asked Indra, pointing over his shoulder to his quiet, brooding brother Yama. "He is always following us around, giving us the evil eye, waiting to pounce when we least expect it. Why did you have to create Death?"

"Hi, Yam!" said the father. Turning back to Indra, he said, "Well, Indy, as you know, I am not the man I used to be because, well … I am now all of you! I don't remember why I created Yama. It seemed like a good idea at the time, but I just don't remember anymore." Seeing the looks of concern on his sons' faces, he asked, "But why is it such a big deal? What's the problem with Yama?"

"What's the problem?" they all shouted at once.

"Dad," said Indra, "Yama is Death! Who wants to die? We sure don't. How can we get rid of him?"

"Beats me," said the father, "but maybe you should go ask Vishnu. He is a pretty smart guy—he'll be able to answer you."

⊰ ⊱

T.K.V. Desikachar (1938-) is a wonderful storyteller, a trained engineer, and a venerable teacher from one of the first families of yoga, son of the famed Krishnamacharya who was the teacher of Pattabhi Jois, B.K.S. Iyengar and many others. Desikachar's eyes twinkle as he spins tales of the gods, and along the way he intersperses his views on the meaning of the various symbols, helping Westerners to understand their import. In the current story, called "Churning the Cosmic Ocean," he explained that this is a story about the guru and the assistance rendered by the master to the disciple who seeks immortality.[3] The guru here is Vishnu, and the immortality sought is spiritual immortality—liberation—although to unopened ears it would seem to refer to physical immortality.

⊰ ⊱

Bowing at the edge of the Cosmic Ocean, the devas paid homage to the sleeping divinity. "Vishnu," began Indra, "is there any way that we can live forever? We seek a way to banish Yama from our presence and never have to face Death."

Vishnu answered, "Yes, there is a way to immortality, but it will take a lot of hard work. At the bottom of the Cosmic Ocean, there is a substance called amrita. Obtain it, and you obtain everlasting life."

In their excitement at hearing Vishnu's words, the gods lost their composure, forgot to thank Vishnu, and dove pell-mell into the ocean, heading straight to the bottom of the waters, each trying to outswim the others, and, as always, Indra was in the lead. Down and down they went, for weeks and weeks, but the Cosmic Ocean is infinitely deep, and they were not even close to the bottom. Finally even Indra had to give up and come back to the surface.

"Vishnu!" moaned the gods, "The ocean is too deep; we can't reach the amrita. How can we get it?"

⚛ ⚛

Intention is wonderful; without it, nothing gets started. But too much raw enthusiasm results in a lot of wasted splashing around. Settle down and wait for the teacher to teach.

⚛ ⚛

"Of course it is too deep for you. It is infinite! The only way to obtain amrita is to bring it to the surface. You must churn the Cosmic Ocean like a maid churning milk into butter. Churn, and the nectar will come to you."

Excitedly the gods dispersed, each seeking a paddle big enough to stir the waters to its depths, but none could be found that would make the slightest impact. Dejected, the gods returned to Vishnu and sought his counsel.

"You weren't listening. The ocean is infinite—to churn it, you require a paddle that is also infinite. You need to use Mount Meru."

Mount Meru, the Holy Mountain, home of the gods and center of the entire universe, is infinitely tall, wide and dense. It would not be easy for the entire company of gods to lift the mountain off its moorings, but they were inspired by their cause and managed to raise it up, invert it, and place it in the center of the ocean. In dismay they watched as the mountain plunged into the deep and disappeared. They returned, dejected, to Vishnu.

"Vishnu," moaned Indra, "Mount Meru—it sank! We need something to support it, to hold it up."

"All right," said Vishnu, "I will come and help you out."

Vishnu incarnated as the great tortoise, Kurma, and dove to the bottom of the Cosmic Ocean, as only Vishnu could. There, snuggling down into the roots of the world, he took Meru upon his back, lifting the mountain up above the water's surface. Finally the paddle was in place, and the churning could commence.

⚬ ⚬

There is a pose in Hatha Yoga called *kurmasana*; it is named after Vishnu's second incarnation, the tortoise. The pose involves sitting on the floor with legs apart, placing your arms underneath your outstretched legs, folding the arms behind your back, clasping hands, and bringing your feet together behind your neck; thus you appear as a turtle tucking its head in, its back rounded up to the sky.

Desikachar explained that the tortoise is symbolic of your pelvis: It is the base from which your erect spine rises. The spine is Mount Meru, the world axis. We find the Holy Mountain in many mythologies—it is called Olympus, Sumeru or Harney Peak in South Dakota (according to Black Elk, the Oglala Sioux shaman). It is equivalent to the Bodhi tree and the Tree of Life in the Garden of Eden, all symbolic of your center, your axis of being. The guru is the one who helps you get your alignment right so that the real work can begin.

⚬ ⚬

Now the gods realized they needed a rope so they could pull and turn the paddle. They needed something that could span the distance between the two shores of the Cosmic Ocean and wrap around Mount Meru. They looked in all the stores, bought all the twine, ribbons, cables, ropes and yoga straps they could find, bound them together, but it was nowhere near long enough. With a sigh they went back to their master.

"Vishnu!" they complained, "Our rope isn't long enough. Mount Meru is infinitely thick and the ocean infinitely wide; we need a rope that is really long. Where can we find something like that?"

440

Vishnu, asleep and dreaming the dream of the universe, has as his bed the snake named Endless. "You can borrow Ananta," he offered.

Ananta worked beautifully; he easily covered the distance and wrapped himself three times around the Holy Mountain. The devas positioned on both shores started to pull on that mighty rope with all their strength, but the rope didn't budge; the mountain stayed still, and no waves crested the ocean's water. Once more they flew back to Vishnu.

"It is not working! We don't have enough strength to move the mountain. What should we do now?"

Vishnu regarded the gods as children and out of compassion taught them. "You will need to team up with the *asuras*; only then will your combined strength suffice."

"Not the asuras!" complained the devas. "We hate them. They are pure evil. We don't want to share amrita with them; we like the fact that they are mortal and will die."

"It is your choice," said Vishnu. "Either work with the asuras, or forget any hope of obtaining immortality."

⊰ ⊱

The asuras are the anti-gods. To the Greeks they were the Titans, to us mortals they are the first three chakras, which need to be accommodated if we want to progress along the spiritual path.[4] If you want to progress along the spiritual path, you have to come to terms with your base nature.

⊰ ⊱

Grumbling, the gods agreed to strike a deal with the asuras, but they decided amongst themselves that at the first opportunity, they would cheat the asuras out of the spoils of their joint efforts. The two parties took up their positions: the devas on one side of the Cosmic Ocean and the asuras on the other. The churning began. Finally, after all this preparation, some real action!

The waters bubbled and boiled, and a black slick appeared that spread slowly outward. Everywhere this darkness went, life withered and died. The gods and anti-gods both stopped churning, for the poison was coming close to them. Its stench alone told them that it was powerful enough to kill them. The surface of the ocean was covered in death; while the churning had stopped, the poison had not. In fear the gods fled to Shiva for protection and assistance.

Shiva listened and decided. He came to the shore and sucked up the slick, taking it all in one big gulp and saving the universe. But there was a problem. Shiva could not swallow the poison, for it would kill even him, but neither could he spit it back out, for it would destroy the universe. Instead he held the poison in his throat, and eventually, it was absorbed by his body, turning his throat a dark blue. From this time on, Shiva has been called Nilakanta, the Blue-Throated One.

❧ ❧

When our spiritual practice begins, there are a lot of preliminaries. We have to prepare ourselves under our teacher's guidance, ensure we have the right tools (physical and mental), know the right techniques, find the right place and companions. This is also a very dangerous time, because poisons often arise from our depths that prevent us from going any further. In the chant cited at the beginning of this chapter, there is the phrase, *halahala*. Halahala is poison. In the chant it is equated with samsara, but metaphorically this poison can range from friends and family despising what we are trying to do and ostracizing us or preventing us from continuing, to physical discomfort that can occur in the earliest days of fasting or exercising. It is now our guru, *jangalikayamane*—the jungle physician—Shiva, who protects us, and through his wisdom and self-sacrifice we are able to continue. We grow increasingly indebted.

⊰ ⊱

Back to work: The halahala removed, the churning began anew. The next things that rose from the water were white cows, wish-fulfilling trees, precious gems and beautiful virgins.[5] The churning stopped.

The gods and anti-gods fought over the booty, took whatever they could grab, and headed back to their camps in the woods. There they enjoyed their virgin cows and wish-fulfilling women until finally Vishnu sauntered through the camp. Seeing Vishnu startled Indra, and he remembered. "Hey, this is great, but we were trying to become immortals. What are we doing here? Let's get back to work."

⊰ ⊱

A yoga practice will generate many gifts: good health, impressive levels of flexibility and strength, reduced stress. All these are wonderful physical benefits, but if your intention was spiritual growth, these gifts can be distractions.

⊰ ⊱

The churning commenced once more. This time the gods and anti-gods ignored the precious gifts and concentrated; they churned harder and harder and finally, after many long years—amrita! And calamity!

Before the devas could get organized and gather the amrita, the asuras stole it all. Off the asuras ran, cackling and giggling, back to their camp. And off the devas slunk, to Vishnu once more.

"Vishnu," they whined, "it's not fair! The asuras stole all the amrita! We were going to steal it from them first, but they took it all and … it's not fair!"

"All right! Don't worry. Return to your camp and wait for me there."

Vishnu knew this was going to happen and already had his plans set. He went to the asura camp, turned himself into an irresistibly beautiful woman, and walked seductively past the anti-gods, who were debating how best to serve amrita. Some thought it should be served chilled like white wine, while others thought a sauce would be nice, perhaps as a gravy over some pulled pork. Vishnu caught their eyes and slowly turned and walked back into the woods. The asuras, overcome by lust, raced after the vision. Vishnu led them on a merry goose chase, lost them, doubled back to their camp, and stole away the amrita. He brought it safely to the devas, who bowed deeply to their master.

ॐ ह्रीं

Even after all the work, after all the yoga, even when final liberation is within reach and enlightenment almost guaranteed, there is one last obstacle. Greed and desire can manifest even in the most advanced practitioner and steal away the benefits of decades of dedication. In the end, it is only by the grace of the guru that the final achievement is accomplished. This is known as *shaktipata*, the direct transmission from guru to disciple of spiritual power. This is tariki—the way of the kitten, the way of the bodhisattva, the way of Saint Paul and Saint Augustine. Without outside spiritual help, salvation, enlightenment, freedom and immortality cannot be achieved.

✳ ✳ ✳

"O Devi, there are many gurus ... but hard to find in all the worlds ... is the guru who reveals the Self. Many are the gurus who rob the disciple of his wealth, but rare is the guru who removes the disciple's afflictions ..."

—The Kula-Arnava-Tantra[6]

Vande Gurunam charanaravinde was translated earlier as "I bow to the two lotus feet of the (plurality of) Gurus." The plurality of gurus here refers to the fact that your guru had his guru, who had his guru, and so on back into the dim recesses of time, until we come to the *one*: the original guru, Shiva, who in the Tantric and Hatha Yoga traditions is the one who revealed all the secrets. In the story of "Churning the Cosmic Ocean," it is Shiva who saves the whole world and allows the yoga to continue. Since Shiva is such an important figure for Hatha yogis—for he really is the main guy—it is worthwhile to listen to the story of how he gave Hatha Yoga to the world.

ॐ ॐ

Matsya means "fish." *Indra* means "lord." *Nath*, which can also mean "lord," came to refer to a sect of yogis who followed the teachings of Matsyendranath. Matsyendra, as he is also known, was a fisherman: the lord of the fishes, although one time the fish won.

On this particular day, Matsyendra was dangling a line from his small boat in the Bay of Bengal, hoping to catch something to assuage his hunger, when he felt the bite. No nibble was this—the fish struck fast and hard and almost pulled the rod out of Matsyendra's hands. Matsyendra pulled back, and the battle was on. For hours the two struggled, until Matsyendra realized that he was tiring faster than the fish, so he decided to make one last heroic pull to heave the leviathan out of the water. But the fish pulled even harder, and Matsyendra flew into the sea, where he was swallowed whole.

Living inside the belly of a huge fish is not much of a life, but Matsyendranath did what he could to pass away the time. Mostly he just meditated and lived off the food being ingested by his fish. It was his mediation that saved him; Matsyendranath was able to keep at bay the digestive acids of the fish through his power of concentration, and thus he managed to survive for 12 uneventful years.

On the last day of his captivity, Matsyendranath's fish was resting on the bottom of a river. On the bank of the river, in an open meadow, Shiva was picnicking with his

445

lovely wife, Parvati. While she prepared their lunch, Shiva began to explain to her the practice of Hatha Yoga. Parvati was not attentive, distracted by her picnic basket's contents, and all the good teaching Shiva was pouring forth was being wasted. In annoyance he barked at her, "Are you listening?"

While Parvati was not listening, there in the belly of the fish on the bottom of the river, Matsyendra was listening and listening very intently. When he heard Shiva's question, he replied, "Yes!"

Shiva heard the answer with his super-hearing and, using his super-seeing, looked into the water and found his real student: This was the reason he decided to teach today. Shiva drew Matsyendra forth from the fish, dried him off, took away the fishy-guts smell, and set him down in the meadow so that he could learn Hatha Yoga. That day Shiva taught 84,000 asanas, one for each animal and plant on earth. Thus was Matsyendranath the first human to be given this great gift of knowledge, a gift he was directed to share with deserving seekers of true knowledge.

⁂

Why did Shiva feel the need to share this teaching, why now, and why 84,000 asanas? Four, as we have seen, symbolizes wholeness; eight, being twice as much as four, is doubly whole. (How a whole can become twice as whole we will leave as an exercise in higher mathematics.) And if eight is more complete than four, imagine how complete 84 is! Then picture the degree of wholeness exhibited by 84,000. Do not take the number literally, of course; this simply symbolizes that Shiva taught all there was to teach. In some versions of the story, he taught just 84 asanas. It is also common in Yoga to find the number eight on its own or added to the end of a higher number: 8, 18, 108, 1008. Some gurus require their students to perform 108 sun salutations every morning, facing the rising sun. All of these amounts symbolize a complete practice or ultimate wholeness.

Why now? Prior to 1000 B.C.E., the religious teachings of the proto-Indo-Europeans living in India were based on the Vedas. These were the perfect teachings for the golden ages of the earliest yugas. After that time, the Upanishads superseded the Vedas and provided guidance and understanding, but when the god-man Krishna (Arjuna's friend—remember him?) passed away, we entered the Kali Yuga, and the Vedas and the Upanishads were no longer enough. Shiva, in his compassion, provided new teachings to guide mankind through the time, when the older books were no longer useful. For Tantrikas, Shiva's gift was the Tantra itself and all its books. For the Nathas, a casteless sect of followers of Matsyendranath, Shiva's gift was Hatha Yoga.

The obligation of a guru is to pass along what was given. Matsyendranath now had to find others to share what he had learned, and so he began to travel the land. There is an unwritten rule for wandering mendicants: Never spend more than three nights in one place. This rule made it possible for the sadhus to receive alms, because the locals never had to worry about any one ascetic remaining at the door for months on end. Matsyendranath's wanderings brought him one day to a village where his fame had preceded him:

⤙ ⤚

The life of a peasant woman is hard in any culture, but what makes life even harder is bearing no sons. Every day she would pray to Shiva to grant her wish and let her bear a boy-child, but throughout her days she remained barren. One fine morning her village was buzzing with the arrival of a miracle worker, a yogi who was said to have mastered the highest teachings and had a healing touch. She dared not hope, but she gathered her courage and approached master Matsyendranath.

Matsyendra considered the woman's condition and position; he had gained many followers in the years since receiving Shiva's gift, and he made no distinction based on caste or gender. He agreed to help the pleasant peasant, so in kindness he took the sack of ash that all Natha yogis wore, ash from the cremation grounds that was applied liberally over the body after bathing, and handed it to her.

"Here," said Matsyendra, nodding his head from side to side, "Take this ash home and brew a tea from it. Drink the tea, and you will bear a son." With a flourish he opened his palm and waved the bag toward the woman.

The woman bowed deeply, took the bag, and returned home. While she walked, weighing the dusty bag in her hands, blowing away the fine power that was leaking onto her old worn-out clothing, she reflected, "I may just be an ignorant old peasant woman, but I know this is not the way babies are made." In resignation she tossed the bag of ash onto a nearby dung heap and went home.

Matsyendra's wanderings took him all over the northern lands of India; never staying in one place more than three days leads to lots of moving around, but 12 years after the above incident, his travels brought him back to the same village. And he remembered! He recalled the peasant woman and his gift—that boy should be about 12 years old by now. He resolved to check in on him.

Matsyendra found the woman and asked how her son was doing. She replied, "You are a cruel man; I have no son!"

"But, I gave you the ash—it would have given you a boy. What did you do with it?" asked Matsyendra.

"You didn't expect me to believe you, did you? I know that is not how babies are made. I threw the ash away, onto a dung heap."

"Where? Show me!"

The woman led Matsyendra to the pile of cow dung where she long ago tossed the ash: The pile was still there. Matsyendra looked closely at the mound and then shouted, "Come out of there!"

Out from the dung came a 12-year-old boy. Matsyendra named him Goraksha, cow protector. They traveled together for many years, and in time Goraksha became an even greater yogi than his guru and made the teachings of Hatha Yoga immortal.

⊰ ⊱

Matsyendra and Goraksha are legendary figures, larger than life, but they most likely were historical men.[7] They lived at a time when, in England, the legends of King Arthur were also growing. Legendary figures take on fantastic abilities, and so it was with Goraksha: He became a charismatic miracle worker who gathered a large following, supposedly wrote many books, and inspired a tradition that has lived and evolved for a millennia. However, the Hatha Yoga of Matsyendra and Goraksha was nothing like what passes today in the West for Hatha Yoga. The modern emphasis on asanas, the physical postures, was minimal in the earliest versions of Hatha Yoga. The earliest texts allocated more time to the Tantric tools of breath management (*pranayama*), energy seals (*mudras*) and energy valves (*bandhas*) than to postures, naming only 15 to 32 asanas. It wasn't until the late 18th century that the number of asanas described began to rise. In the 19th and 20th centuries, an exponential increase occurred, so that today there are many thousands of postures taught, and Hatha Yoga has become mostly a physical fitness practice.[8]

* * *

The word *guru* literally means "the heavy one"; this does not refer to the guru's girth or physical weight, but to his spiritual density. The disciple, the *laghu*, which means "the lightweight one," is in orbit around his master's spiritual

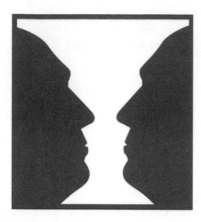

Figure 12: An Illusion: Do you see a vase or two faces?

center. The word can also be divided into its two component syllables: *gu* and *ru*, which mean "the remover of darkness." Your guru is the one who dispels your ignorance and brings you to the light. Your guru is your mother, your father, your god; whatever he says is Truth! and there is no debating or doubting him. Whatever he asks, you do.

The guru is said to have two feet: the red foot and the white foot.[9] The two feet symbolically refer to all the apparent opposites, the dualities of life: subject"object; you"me; life–death. The white foot is spiritual, the mystical teachings meant to be understood metaphorically; the red foot is material, the mundane reality of daily living. The disciple can look upon the guru's white foot and see God, the teachings about God, the teachings from God. But he can also look at the guru's red foot and see the human being, subject to frailties and error. Like an optical illusion which shows at first a vase and then two faces, these two aspects exist simultaneously in the single guru, and both aspects must be embraced as reality: The guru is transcendent of the seeming duality.

Joseph Campbell was fond of recounting a tale that displayed one guru's decidedly red foot, and perhaps there is a warning here for us in the West:[10]

༄ ༅

Laghu was late, but he was not to blame. He came running up to Guruji, breathlessly bowed down and kissed his feet, and waited for the reproach that was quick to come.

"You are late!" muttered the guru, barely acknowledging the prostrate man before him.

"I know, Guruji, please forgive me. I left home very early this morning and would have been on time, but when I came to the river, it was flooded. The bridge was washed away, all the boats had been torn from their moorings, and there was no way to cross. This is why I am late."

"Oh," replied the guru, softening his heart, "all right—but tell me, is the river still in flood?"

"Oh yes," came the reply. "The flood is very bad. All the bridges for dozens of mile have been washed away."

"So, how did you manage to get here? Did a boat finally arrive?"

"No, no boats."

"Then how did you cross the river?"

"Well," explained the student, "I remembered how you said once that my guru is truth and I was to think of you as God. So I began to meditate on you! I said to myself, 'guru, guru, guru,' closed my eyes, and began to walk ... and here I am!"

"Hmmmph" was all the guru could say. "Very well—let's proceed with the lessons for today."

The day was then like any other, but the guru could not get his student's story out of his mind. "My student meditated on me and was able to walk upon water! My power must be greater than I realized." All day long he was possessed by the story.

When he dismissed the student at the end of the day, the guru visited the swollen river, determined to test out his power. He composed himself, entered a deep meditative state, and, before attempting to walk upon the water, started to chant, "I, I, I ..."

The guru promptly sank and drowned.

⚜ ⚛

Remember the original Self who also thought "I" and became lost in the illusion of the world, became the world; and remember the Buddha who went backward past this point of identification with the self and regained the original state. A guru who confuses himself with his teaching will drown in the phenomenal world. The real guru is transcendent; he or she is beyond all dualities and beyond the ego associations that occur in the mind.

In the West we have a difficult time with the whole guru concept. We have our teachers, but in the West, independent thought is not only valued and encouraged, it is mandated. Students are expected to think for themselves, work out the answers, solve the problems, and challenge their teachers. Westerners find it very difficult to bow down before another human being and kiss his feet. This degree of submission strikes against our European heritage of independence; we may be able to submit to God (Mary Magdelena washed and kissed Jesus' feet), but in the West, God is not man and no man is God, save perhaps one. To bow down to another human being as if he were God is blasphemy. We just can't do it.

The degree of submissiveness of Eastern students to their teachers boggles the mind, and the challenging ways of Western students upset Eastern teachers.[11] The two cultures do not easily accommodate each other's ways. This is always a danger; when faced with maps that do not work for us, we may either reject all the good parts of the model, throwing the baby out with the bath water, or completely submit, surrendering too much to the new way and following paths that just don't take us where we need to go. Some Eastern gurus have been placed upon high pedestals by Western students, who failed to see the all-too-obvious-in-retrospect red foot. Some of the gurus fail their own high ideals, and their fall from grace is shocking. Their communities are blown apart when revelations of sexual misconduct, greed and secret amoral behaviors are revealed. Raising someone high above you is equivalent to bringing yourself down; a better strategy is to acknowledge the white foot, the teachings, while keeping in mind the red foot, the mundane teacher, who is simply the vehicle through which the teaching passes.

So which is it: Is a teacher invaluable, essential for walking the path, or does a teacher who shows you his path invalidate our sense of uniqueness? These are two very different maps, but, as always, one is not right and the other wrong. The question is always—which map is more useful for you? That depends upon your intention. A guru may be able to tell you the quickest, safest and easiest way to get from point A (here) to point B (there) because he has made the trip before and because he has made several other journeys that did not work out so well; he knows the pitfalls and the express routes from years of trial and error. This is probably what your own parents tried to teach you: "Learn from me, my child, and don't make the mistakes I made." However, the point of life is not to safely, easily and quickly get to the end of life! By following your guru's or your parent's path, all you have missed is *your* life. Life is not a destination; it is an experience—live it! The Western myths teach us to find our own path and not go where it is easy or safe, and who really cares how long it takes? What we need in the West from our teachers is not the path cleared for us, but training in how to walk the path. Teach us how to read a compass, how to wade through a swamp; teach us which animals are dangerous and which plants are safe to eat; teach us to survive when we are lost, but let us get lost!

Chapter 21: Living with the Mystical

In the beginning, God created the earth, and He looked upon it in His cosmic loneliness.

And God said, "Let Us make living creatures out of mud, so the mud can see what We have done." And God created every living creature that now moveth, and one was man. Mud as man alone could speak. God leaned close as mud as man sat, looked around, and spoke. Man blinked. "What is the purpose of all this?" he asked politely.

"Everything must have a purpose?" asked God.

"Certainly," said man.

"Then I leave it to you to think of one for all this," said God.

And He went away.

—*Cat's Cradle* by Kurt Vonnegut[1]

One of the functions of myth, the mystical function, is to answer the question, "What is the purpose of life, of my life?" We may as well ask, "What is the purpose of a sunset, a rainbow, a flower?"

⊰ ⊱

One day the Buddha's disciples had all gathered for a talk by the master, but when the Buddha arrived, settled in, regarded the monks and nuns before him, all he did was raise up a single flower. He did not talk. He held the flower and waited.

The monks grew restless. A few wondered to themselves, "What's up with the flower, Buddha?" but they dared not ask.

Finally, one monk looked up at the Buddha, saw the flower, and smiled. That monk was Maha Kashyapa. The Buddha smiled back to Maha Kashyapa and lowered the flower: Today's lesson had been received by at least one person.

⁂

Why are we here?

To be the eyes and ears and conscience of the Creator of the Universe, you fool.

—*Breakfast of Champions* by Kurt Vonnegut[2]

We can invest a lot of intellectual and spiritual energy in trying to answer "Why?" questions, but, as we saw long ago, not all questions have an answer. We can make up some plausible answers: Man is the moral agent of existence; the universe itself has brought us forth to be its own consciousness; we bring value and meaning to creation; without us, there is nothing—a deep, dreamless sleep. We are also thought, by some, to be here to fix the universe, a universe that is deeply flawed and filled with evil. We are here to _____: Fill in the blank with whatever the map you follow requires of you.

The search for meaning and purpose lends value and zest to life. Without a purpose we drift, without meaning we mope, become depressed, stop living. There are definite downsides to leading a meaningless life: no direction to follow, no reason to rise in the morning. However, there is also danger in a life filled with meaning; there is a judgment ahead to determine how well you have succeeded in fulfilling your mandate here on earth. In the Western religions, God is the judge. In the

East there is no personal judgment, but the laws of nature will determine what will become of you, based on your karma, the merits or demerits earned in this life. In modern secular life, man is the judge, both literally and figuratively.

The myths that require us to have and know our purpose, to know why we are here, are still only maps—and these are not the only possible maps we can choose to follow. Certainly, if these maps work for you and you are happy with life as it is, there is no need to look for a different map. But, as strange and counterintuitive as it may seem, there are models for living complete, fulfilled lives that do not require our lives to have meaning, that do not require us to have a purpose for simply being alive. To understand this, we need to look again with new eyes at the story from Genesis: the Garden of Eden.

✳ ✳ ✳

We have seen that God evicted man from Eden because he transgressed the conditions of his rental contract; he broke the law and paid the price. But that is only one way to look at this story, and it is a rather factually and historically implausible view whose obvious incongruity causes many to just dismiss the story as worthless. There is another way, a metaphorical way, to read the tale. Man *chose* to eat the fruit of the tree of knowledge; he *chose* to listen to his primitive instinct, in the form of the serpent (which the Bible does say was the wisest creature); he *chose* to exchange the fruit from the tree of immortal life for knowledge. This is a very telling point, for man is the conceptual animal. Watch as a baby acquires languages skills: One of the first and most frequent questions the toddler will ask is,

"What's that?"

That's a dog.

"What's that?"

That's a cat.

"What's that?"

That's your Aunt Linda.

We love to learn, we love to know, we love to put things into conceptual boxes so that we have a handle on them. Once we can define a thing, we think we know its essence. Names were kept secret in ancient times because to know a man's name was to have power over him. Yahweh kept his name secret, for to speak his name is to release his power, right here, where it cannot be properly contained or controlled. Naming things, creating concepts, is our nature.

A useful metaphor for our conceptualizing nature is that of a bowl. You can imagine a beautiful brass bowl used in a yoga class, one that is struck three times at the beginning and end of practices, or you can simply go get one of your breakfast cereal bowls—they both work equally well for this analogy. Now, place your finger on the rim of the bowl farthest away from you: This is "far." As soon as we create the concept "far," we automatically create the complementary concept "near"—place another finger on the rim closest to you. The rim of the bowl is the relative world, the world of concepts and duality. Touch now the right edge of the bowl; you have created a concept of "right," which automatically creates the concept "left." You cannot have "left" without "right," "near" without "far," "up" without "down," "good" without "evil," "beauty" without "ugliness," and so it goes. When the original Self first thought "I" it became afraid; as soon as you have the idea of existence, you bring into play the idea of nonexistence.

Whenever we create a concept, we are on the rim of the bowl; every concept, like yin and yang, begets its complement. This is one of the earliest teachings in the *Dao De Jing* by Lao Tzu:

Existence and nonexistence create each other.

Difficult and easy support each other.

Long and short contrast each other.

High and low attract each other.

Future and past follow each other.[3]

"Meaning" belongs here, too, as does "purpose"; once we create the need for meaning, once we create this concept and put it on the rim of the bowl, we instantly create the possibility that life will be "meaningless." If you seek meaning for life, for meaning in life, you create the reality that life can also be meaningless! If, however, you never seek meaning, if you never try to create a purpose for your life, then your life will never be meaningless, or purposeless. It is your longing for meaning that creates the suffering of having no meaning. People who do not seek the meaning of a flower are free to simply smile, like Maha Kashyapa; people who try to find the meaning of a flower struggle.

The Garden of Eden is the middle of the bowl: Put your finger there, in the empty place, the void of the middle space. This is where mankind was before we kicked ourselves out of the garden and headed out onto the rim of the relative world. The garden, the center of the bowl, is the absolute world that transcends concepts, transcends all dualities, transcends even a definition of itself, because to define this center in any way that is not a metaphor would be to put the center back on the rim of concepts.

꩜ ꩝

God did not kick man out of the Garden of Eden: We did it to ourselves!

꩜ ꩝

Life arrived on the earth long before meaning was sought. Life existed on our planet for billions of years before mud as man awoke, blinked, and asked, "What's it all about, Alfie?" Before man was even put in the Garden, there was life: plants and animals. It is only when we left the Garden that we felt the need for meaning; it was then that we became *rimsters*: people living on the rim of the bowl of concepts and dualities.

Just because my life lacks meaning does not make it meaningless. If you think that way, you are an old rimster, and you need to get back to the Garden, to the nameless center, to become a *centrist*, not a rimster. (Ah, but surely you see by now that if you call yourself a centrist, you just put yourself back on the rim again.) Rimsters have great difficulty with a-conceptual concepts. For example, the three poisons in Buddhism are greed, hatred and delusions; drop them, said the Buddha, and you are already in nirvana. But rimsters misunderstand. They think that the opposite of greed is not-greed or contentment, but not-greed is on the rim; it's another thing. The Buddha wants you to drop greed *and* not-greed, self *and* no-self, and go where no concepts exist: the middle ground. Many rimsters—and you may be one—have great difficulty with the instruction to drop all your attachments (another name for greed). You may feel deeply attached to your children; how can the Buddha tell us to become non-attached to our children? That is rimster thinking; that is not what he is saying. The Buddha is saying to go where there is neither attachment nor non-attachment.

"*Neti neti*," teach the Upanishads, "not this, not this!"[4] This negation is a common way to attempt to explain the center to rimsters: It can't be defined, so it is pointed to by saying what it is not. This negation often fails to enlighten or inspire, but this is the challenge in using concepts to teach the a-conceptual. When Joseph Campbell asked the Indian Guru Sri Atmananda and the saint Ananda Mayi whether one could live in the world or did one have to leave the world to find freedom, the answers were basically the same: For those living in the center of the bowl, it doesn't matter.

✳ ✳ ✳

Now we can understand the Catholic idea of original sin. Many people struggle with this concept: How can a brand-new baby, just arrived on this planet, so pure and innocent, already be a sinner? Seen literally, as a fact, this idea is impossible to accept; seen metaphorically, the idea makes sense. Every newborn baby is born with an innate urge to learn, to name, to conceptualize, to leave the Garden of the womb; it is hardwired into our DNA and we can't help ourselves. In the Catholic belief, every child bears the sin of Adam and must be absolved of this taint through Holy Baptism. The spiritual cleansing is meant to put us back into the emptiness of the bowl, but it doesn't take—soon the baby is learning to talk, and the sins begin.

The enlightened sage can see a stop sign, know that it is not really a stop sign, but stops anyway; he can live in both the absolute realm beyond concepts and duality and also in the relative world, playing the game just as well as anyone else. Just as an enlightened master knows the reality of the stop sign, he also knows that life has no inherent meaning, and yet he can choose to create meaning, realizing that it really doesn't matter.

You can do this, too, if you update your map. You can choose to set a direction for your life, make up a purpose, and work toward achieving this goal, but you can also know full well that in reality it doesn't matter if you achieve your goal or not. Life can have a meaning: Sure, go ahead and play that game, play as if your whole life depends upon it but also with the absolute knowledge that it is just a game.

This upgrade to the base map doesn't easily take. Many people intellectually agree with the philosophy espoused but can't incorporate the change at the visceral level. The software won't install. They may vocalize the appropriate noises when times are good, "Oh, it doesn't matter if I get the new job! What's important is the quality of life, not the quantity of money I have," but when they get fired from their current job, then the anxieties surface and the complaining begins. When the chips are down, the equanimity evaporates, and the real map is revealed.

"The problem with Yahweh is," said the Gnostics, "he thinks he is God!"[5] Yahweh is a name, an object which can be known, and thus lives on the rim; God is the unknowable, residing in the center. "The highest leave-taking," remembering what Meister Eckhart said, "is leaving god for God." Leave behind your *idea* of god for the *experience* of God—return to the center. The center of the bowl is the sacred space, and we have seen it called by many names: the Garden of Eden, the Grail Castle, Nirvana, Emptiness, Buddha Nature, the dance of Shiva, the dream of Vishnu, Turiya—the fourth syllable of Aum. The center of the bowl is not *saguna* Brahman, which is Brahman with qualities, but *nirguna* Brahman, which is Brahman without qualities; not Jesus, the historical man on the cross and on the rim, but Christ who rose again; not the wave, but the ocean. All of these terms risk putting us back on the rim, but read properly as symbols and not as concrete facts, they point beyond themselves to the transcendent: indescribable, ineffable ... and here we can say no more.

Man with his understanding cannot know what the rain is saying when it falls upon the leaves of the trees or when it taps at the window panes. He cannot know what the breeze is saying to the flowers in the fields.

But the Heart of Man can feel and grasp the meaning of these sounds that play upon his feelings. Eternal Wisdom often speaks to him in a mysterious language; Soul and Nature converse together while Man stands speechless and bewildered.

— Kahlil Gibran from *The Voice of the Master*[6]

* * *

Joseph Campbell felt that what most people were looking for was not a purpose for their life; they were not asking "Why?

Why am I here?" They were not looking for meaning. They were seeking a deep *experience* of life![7] This he named "bliss."

Bliss, in Campbell's definition, is not restricted to a pleasant feeling; it is a deep joy that comes from being fully alive, from following the map that leads you to what you most enjoy—that which you do with en-*joy*-ment. This goes beyond purpose or meaning to wholeness. This is not pleasure! It is much more fundamental than that, and to understand this point we need to look at the causations of pleasure and suffering once more, to see their conditional nature, to see how firmly they are planted on the rim of the bowl.

❧ ❧

There was something about Mary Jane. Sixto was borderline depressed, anxious and growing more antisocial each day, but that first time Mary Jane took his hand, sitting together silently in the park, Sixto really looked at her. He wanted to caress her face, but she was looking up into the sky. His heart exploded with love, and he vowed in that singular moment to dedicate his whole life to being with her, to studying her face so that he would see it every time he closed his eyes, to bring her presence with him wherever he went.

❧ ❧

The kneelers were hard and hurt, but she stayed kneeling despite the pain, probably, if truth be told, because of the pain—she at least felt something! Her arms were gathered protectively in front her, allowing her hands to remain in prayer. The church was dimly lit, and, even though it was almost noon, little light came through the high, stained-glass windows. The priest that passed by ignored her, obviously in a hurry to be somewhere else. She sighed and released her head into her hands, and she turned her gaze toward the crucifix suspended high above the altar. At that same moment, a light—a cloud must have been obscuring the sun but had now moved on—a brilliant beam of light, colored and enhanced by the rose quartz window, shattered the gloom and illuminated Christ's face. Immediately, joy exploded within her. She remained kneeling, transfixed by the experience; Jesus was looking directly at her, into her, and talking to her, although not in words. At that same moment, everything changed, and she knew she would come to church every day for the rest of her life, to this pew, to this very spot.

꿍 ꙡ

It was a hard climb, bitterly cold, and death was waiting for just a moment's carelessness. Finishing the sheer wall of granite, the slope was quite gentle now; he clambered up to the summit and for the first time allowed himself to soak in the view from the top. And it was amazing. He had trained for years, given up his career, lost his family; his only friends now were climbers. But it was worth it. The view was awesome, and he stood speechless in its presence. The rush was explosive; he would spend the rest of his days seeking the intense wonder of this moment over and over again. This would be his life, and his death.

꿍 ꙡ

The ineffable center of the bowl, the point with all the metaphoric names, can be experienced but only described in symbols. But even the experience defies conceptualization. Names have been applied with the hope of explaining what was perceived: joy, bliss, love, rapture, awe, wonder, ananda. These names help a little, for we have all had tastes of these strong emotions, but a name does not invoke the experience, for these peak experiences are not caused, they just are.

In the three vignettes above, the hero of the piece experienced something extra-ordinary: For a brief moment, they touched the center of the bowl, left their normal life; they experienced the transcendent and were blown away by it.

But in each case, they wanted to capture it, to hold onto it, to be able to find it again—they looked for the cause of it. This is where mistakes are made.

The center of the bowl is the place of no death. Only things that are born can die, and the center was never born; it has always been there. It existed long before man came along and created the rim of concepts that surround it. There is nothing there, so there is nothing to die, nothing to be born; nothing caused it, nothing can erase it. It is the deathless and the unborn; it is beyond time and beyond eternity; it is beyond causation. To look for the cause of bliss is to cast yourself into confusion.

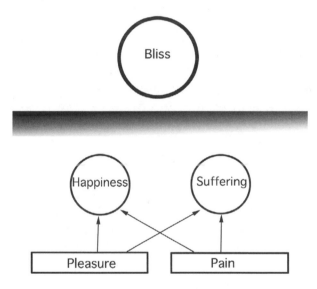

Figure 13: Happiness and suffering are conditional

We confuse pleasure with happiness, pain with suffering, the presence of pleasure and the absence of suffering with joy. Happiness and suffering have causes: pleasure and pain. Joy has no cause.

Pleasure is simply sensations that we like, that we want; pain is simply sensations that we do not like and do not want.

How we react to these sensations create either happiness or suffering, thus we see that both happiness and suffering are dependent conditions that arise by mental processes. It is possible to experience pleasure and choose to be happy about it, but it is also possible to experience these nice feelings and be unhappy or sorrowful. For example, tasting that second slice of cheesecake may be delicious, but you are not really enjoying it due to your guilt over succumbing to temptation once again. Pain may cause suffering, or it may also lead to happiness, like when the intensity of your workout has left you sore and aching, but you are happy in the knowledge that you are ready for the triathlon you will be running next week.

Beyond the conditioned arising of happiness and suffering is joy; we could again call it by many names, so let's use Joseph Campbell's famous term: bliss. Bliss has no cause; it is the experience of being in the center of the bowl. We can't explain this save by metaphors, so let's tell another story, the story of the blue sky.

> Sometimes it rains in Vancouver, sometimes it rains a lot. There are days in winter when the sun is not seen, the clouds are persistent, the rain just a drizzling mist hugging the ground. And yet, above the clouds there exists the blue sky. One day the clouds part briefly and a quick glimpse of sky is seen. It makes you joyful to see that blue space, but it is soon covered over again. Disappointed, you look around to see who created the gap in the clouds that provided that amazing experience of blue. You were with Mary Jane; she must have been the one who caused the clouds to part. Or you were kneeling in church when it happened, so going to church, you think, was the cause of the joy. Or you were by yourself in nature, and thus it was being in nature that allowed the glimpse. You look for a cause and latch on to the nearest plausible

explanation, and then you seek to replicate that cause, hoping to replicate the exact same experience.

≈ ≈

The clouds are metaphors for the stuff of life: The clouds are our thoughts and all the drama that comes and goes in any life. Behind the cloud is the sky, symbolic of the center wherein bliss is found. The reality is that the blue sky is always there, regardless of how many clouds appear in our lives. For a time we may be lucky and experience the blue sky, the joy of being, the bliss of doing what we love, but then the clouds come again, as they will, and we are back in the dullness of our daily lives. Nothing causes the blue sky, but it can be obscured and hidden from us. When we dispel the confusion that thinks bliss can be created, we no longer have to look for a cause or blame someone or something when it goes away, because it can't go away; the blue sky is always there, we just fail to see it sometimes. Faith is the skill that allows us to know that the blue sky is there even when dark storm clouds block the view, when lightning, thunder and hard rains make it impossible to experience happiness. Bliss is always available.

≈ ≈

Swami Satcitananda is in deep—there is no way to reach the yogi right now. He is gone; the outside world has been turned off. He sits, with eyes open but unseeing; ears listening only to the inner sound of Aum. In his deep samadhi, the yogi experiences exquisite joy: the deep reality, *sat*, of concentrated meditation; conscious only of consciousness, *cit*; and it is sheer bliss, ananda.[8]

≈ ≈

The Buddha mastered bliss, he reached the deep level of samadhi, but he found that this state of supreme consciousness was not the solution to old age, sickness and death he had been seeking, because at some point you have to come out of samadhi and rejoin the world again. He looked for a more permanent solution. The yogi Satcitananda reached the blue sky, but in so doing he left the world behind; the Buddha sought a way to have his cake and eat it, too. (And why not! If you go to the trouble of baking a cake, why not eat it, too?)

There is another level: samadhi without trance.[9] A bliss is available that doesn't require us to go anywhere different, a bliss that can be found right here in the every-day world, in living life as it is right now. The Buddha and many master yogis, like Yogananda and Ramakrishna, have found the path to this state of being.

The miracle is not to walk upon the water: the real miracle is to walk upon the earth.

— Lin Chi – ninth-century C.E. Chan master[10]

Thich Nhat Hanh, a modern living Buddha affectionately known as Thay, which is Vietnamese for "teacher," explains how being in the center, entering nirvana, does not require us to go anywhere:

We are entirely capable of touching the ultimate dimension. As I write this page, I am aware that my feet are on the ground in Plum Village, standing on French soil. I am also aware that France is linked to Germany, Spain, Czechoslovakia, and Russia, and even to India, China and Vietnam. Thinking globally, I see that I am standing on more than just a spot, because when I touch Plum Village, I touch all of Europe and Asia. China is just an extension of the small piece of land under my feet. Standing on one part of the Eurasian continent, I am standing on the whole continent.

This kind of awareness transforms the spot you are standing on to include the whole Earth. When you practice walking meditation and realize that you are making steps on the beautiful planet Earth, you will see yourself and your walking quite differently, and you will be liberated from narrow views or boundaries. Each step you take, you see that you are touching the whole Earth. When you touch with that awareness, you liberate yourself from many afflictions and wrong views.[11]

Following your bliss, in Joseph Campbell's view, is to joyfully engage in the sorrows of life, engaging in the world with all its challenges, dramas, dark clouds and storms. These clouds do not destroy joy, they simply hide it from us, but it is there if you know how to look. You don't have to go to the Promised Land; the promised land is within you right now. Look within, and you begin to become transparent to the transcendence that is immanent.

✳ ✳ ✳

Dance, when you're broken open.

Dance, if you've torn the bandage off.

Dance in the middle of the fighting.

Dance in your blood.

Dance when you're perfectly free.

—Rumi – 13th -century C.E. mystic and poet[12]

The visual artist, the performing artist, the poet, the musician: These are the people whose works transport us past the clouds to the blue sky beyond. If a mystic wants to communicate, she must become an artist, for only through symbols can the experience be transmitted. Proper art, in James Joyce's definition, is art that arrests us, that opens us to transcendence. If you ask an artist what his work means, and if the artist doesn't like you, warns Joseph Campbell, he may tell you![13] To create a meaning for art is to put it on the rim; it is to make the art improper—either pornographic or didactic. The intention of art is to render an experience upon the beholder. When you behold a work of art in any medium and become stopped, when the mind is stopped, when you gaze in wonder—you are there.

How to get there on your own, though, is the question myths can answer. This is the mystical function of myth—to render you transparent, to open you to the mystery, to provide the experience of bliss. At the mystical level, prayer becomes silent contemplation; prayer stops being a request. We go past requests of God, past praise *of* God, into silent stillness. No words suffice, no thoughts disturb; we simply experience what is arising and passing. We accept life, we affirm life, we experience life. We do all this with awe.

✳ ✳ ✳

We build awe through opening to life, to the experience that is in front of us right here, right now—and an effective way to do that is to cultivate doubt.

What is this?

—Zen kôan

Where there is great perplexity there is great awakening

Where there is little perplexity there is little awakening

Where there is no perplexity there is no awakening.

—Kusan Sunim – Korean Zen master[14]

Great doubt, explains Stephen Batchelor, is akin to misplacing your car keys and wondering where they have gotten to.[15] You don't know, and you wonder wordlessly; unhelpful thoughts come, but they don't bring an answer, so you return to simply not knowing. Although his teacher Kusan Sunim used the word *doubt*, Batchelor prefers the term *perplexity*. When you are wondering, perplexed, you are wide open; it is in this state that experience is most raw. Kôans were invented to create this sense of perplexity, of wondering. The point of a kôan is not to find an answer; their paradoxical nature is meant to take you off the rim of the bowl, beyond logic and rationality to where there are no answers, just an experience. There are several well-known kôans:

- Does a dog have Buddha Nature: no!
- What was your face before your parents were born?
- If you meet the Buddha, kill him!
- Why did the Bodhidharma come from the West?
- How many angels can dance on the head of a pin?
- What is the sound of one hand clapping?

These are not meant to yield logical answers (although Bart Simpson exploded the usefulness of the last one when he proceeded to clap with one hand by rapidly opening and closing it). These and other questions are meant only to create the mental state of openness, of wonder. Looking for a real answer is like asking the artist what her art means. Look for a "real" answer, and you'll miss the opportunity for transcendence. As Carl Jung observed, life itself can present us with kôans:

> The serious problems in life, however, are never fully solved. If it should for once appear that they are, this is the sign that something has been lost. The meaning and design of a problem seem not to lie in its solution, but in our working at it incessantly.[16]

The Buddha faced such a real life problem: His exposures to old age, sickness and death caused great personal puzzlement for him, which led to his dedication to find an answer. This is not a historical truth, but an archetypal truth, and one that each one of us goes through at some point: Why do *I* have to get sick, to grow old, to die? This is the great puzzle and used in the right way, can be very therapeutic.

We live with great kôans: Why am I here? Why do I have to die? What's it all about? Douglas Adams in his *The Hitchhiker's Guide to the Galaxy* provided an answer to his ultimate kôan of life, the universe and everything: the answer was 42, which did not seem very enlightening or helpful. In the story, it was realized that this mundane answer was given because the question was not articulated properly. A new question had to be formulated—this is the action of rimsters, the people who insist on logical answers and thus logical questions. The quest in the *Guide* was to find the ultimate question, which turned out to be, *What do you get if you multiply six by nine? Forty-two?* When faced with such inconsistencies, the rimster can come to only one conclusion: *... there [is] something fundamentally wrong with the universe.*[17] This is the fall in the Garden; this is Angra Mainyu pouring darkness into the world; this is the view that the universe is fundamentally flawed and needs correcting. But when we do not seek an answer to the question, there is no flaw, there is no fall, there is no answer—there is only the experience of life. For that, one has to leave the rim and listen.

Yoga begins with listening, said Richard Freeman, a well-respected Yoga teacher and scholar.[18] Richard pointed out that listening opens the student to space: When you really listen, you create space. For example, when you listen to a good friend who is going through stormy times, if you are really listening, you are giving her space to be who she needs to be in that moment. If you are not truly listening, if you are thinking about what you will say to her when she stops for breath, when you inject your opinions—"I told you not to go out with him! I told you, he was bad news right from the start!"—then you are closing down and taking away space. Listening is the highest, subtlest sense, and it is associated in Samkhya and Tantra with *akasha*: space. Listening is akin to wonder, to questioning it is an opening to what is, without analysis or judgment, an experiencing of life not a conceptualization of it.

✳ ✳ ✳

We have seen that religions have lost the mandate to describe cosmology to us. That has properly been taken over by scientists who render their stories for us based on proof and the ability for their models to be falsifiable, something no religion could ever tolerate. Religions have also lost their mandate to dictate the social order to us. That has properly been taken over by secular governing bodies, although many fundamentalists of various religious stripes are still trying to impose their ideas on how we should live, for example by trying to dictate what rights a woman has over her own body, or whether gays have the right to marry. Since religions no longer serve the first two functions of mythology, the cosmological and the sociological, they turn instead to the psychological function. It is not surprising to see ministers being trained in pastoral counseling. While this has always been a part of their job, today clergy are deliberately studying the sciences of psychology and psychotherapies to help their flocks with the inevitable dramas and crises of life. What else is left for them?

Is there a role still for religions in the final function of mythology, the mystical? Can religion still render the mystical experience today? This is not a role for scientists nor for politicians, so where do we turn if not to our spiritual teachers? Unfortunately, for many Westerners, the church and other organs of faith fail to render any sense of mystery, due mostly to their insistence on keeping to myths that don't work cosmologically or sociologically, and thus lose all credibility; the void is keenly felt. We grasp now at so-called "New Age" philosophies and beliefs or listen avidly to Eastern roshis and gurus with names ending in *ananda* or beginning with *swami*. We try to find new unknown territories where perhaps the mysterious can still be found—not within where they properly lie, but "out there" on planets circling distant stars with imaginary god-like inhabitants who can out-science our scientists. (There are no more geographies left to explore here on planet Earth; there are no places left where Shangri-La, the Garden of Eden, or El Dorado may lie hidden still; thus, many feel they have to look to the stars, where imagination is still free to be creative. If you believe that alpha-aliens from the Omega Omnicluster are coming to save you, and if this map is serving you well, allowing you to live your life more skillfully, then go ahead, follow that map and play that game, but don't insist that your map is the only map that works, and don't be surprised when others refuse to follow you.)

The problem with importing teachings from afar is that their symbols do not resonate within our psyches; their maps don't fit our landscape. There are certain aspects of the Eastern philosophies that do find some purchase, and there is much we can learn from them; but many rituals don't speak to us and indeed may distract some of us from the real value of what the East has to offer. Western followers of Eastern ways miss the point and try to imitate their Eastern gurus by copying their dress, adopting new spiritual names, or learning another language. This is entering the forest along someone else's path; it is not the Western way of seeking our own unique path through life.

Nonsecular Buddhism (mostly from the older Theravada tradition as opposed to the Mahayana or the Pure Land traditions) comes closest to speaking to us, for it does not require any change to our cosmological understanding or social structures, and it does offer many valuable psychological insights. What doesn't work for those of us raised in the West? The strong emphasis found in the East on the guru-student relationship (your guru is god and will set your spiritual life's course for you); the dismissal of the physical and phenomenological world; and the acceptance of dharma/karma/varna—that your secular life and role in society is predetermined for you and you must do what you are told. What can work for us in the West? The views of the oneness of everything, the nonduality of interbeing, and pragmatic psychological truths. We need to leave behind what doesn't work, take what does work, and integrate that into what we already have that works. As we have seen, not all Western maps are useless, but there are some places not marked on our maps, and these are areas we need to explore.

The Three Attitudes to Life: Reprised

In the middle of the bowl, there is no concept of wrong or right, thus affirmation is not the only way or the right way, rejection is not the wrong way, and neither is correction. Real life includes all of these strategies, some of the time; successful maps are not simple! There are times to affirm life, times to reject life and times to correct life, and wisdom, acquired through attention to experience, is required to know which action is most appropriate at which times. We affirm life, for example, when we accept the stages of aging, gracefully growing older. We reject life when it inflicts suffering too difficult to bear; we shut down and go away for a while to recover, take a holiday, go on retreat, or—the ultimate rejection—seek assisted suicide (which, of course, is not yet sanctioned in Western societies for religious and ethical reasons, even though secular compassion would permit it). We correct life when it gives us disease, disabilities or conditions that we won't accept and refuse to reject; we seek a cure through medicine, science and technologies, and social change.

To effect this integration of Eastern understanding with Western individualism requires a process, *bhavana*, as the Buddha recommended (a bringing forth or cultivation)—in other words, a ritual. There still could be a role for the clergy, for the church, if it allowed their rituals to be pathways to transcendence, to allow for the experience of the mystical rather than work to prevent such an experience, as Jung claims religions exist to do.[19] A ritual that is formalized, set in concrete, set up for everyone to follow, cannot render a unique experience that you alone attend. Let the ritual put the participant front and center so that the experience of the ritual is rendered upon the individual directly. The key is *your* action your dance your ritual your experience.

The ritual of the Catholic Mass, properly personalized, can render the mystery in either the Western view, dualistically, where God and his creation are not one, or in the Eastern way, nondualistically, where you are God. The important thing is that it is meant to be *your* experience, you *are* Jesus—through the miracle of bread and wine transformed into the body of Jesus, and of which you partake—and then you leave the rim of the bowl and leap with faith to the unnameable center. Recall that in the West, the religious path leads to a *relationship* with God, while in the East it leads to an *identification* with God. In the Catholic soteriology, we are human, as Jesus is, and we take him into ourselves through Holy Communion. But Jesus on the rim became Christ, once he was baptized by John the Baptist, and Christ is God: "Only God can know God" goes an old Tantric saying.[20] The knower is Christ; the known is God and the relating principle between Christ and God is the Holy Spirit. That is what we can partake of, if the Catholic ritual is *personally* experienced. Even if an Eastern philosophy applies, the ritual still works: You *become* God when you become Jesus who is Christ, who is God. The key is the *experience*: either the experience of beholding God, knowing God (living at the level of the sixth chakra); or the experience of being God (the seventh chakra). Satcitananda applies in both models: God is ultimate truth (*sat*); Jesus is the knower (*cit*); the Holy Spirit is the relationship between the knower and the known (*ananda*)—the bliss of the beatific vision.[21] Understood mythically, the ritual is powerful;

understood as a pantomime of some historical event, the ritual is sterile.

(Orthodox Catholics may have a great deal of difficulty with the idea that we can leave the rim and become Christ through Jesus, and thus God through Christ. That implies a nondualism foreign to the basic belief structure that man is not God; to claim you are is blasphemy, and yet, getting back to the Garden implies exactly that. Remember Genesis 3:22: "Elohim said, Behold, Man is become as one of us, to know good and evil. And now, lest he stretch out his hand, and take also of the tree of life, and eat, and live for ever ...!"[22] Elohim is a plural noun, and we find in all versions of this verse the pronoun *us* is used. The gods were quite worried that man would become like them: a god. If we jump back into the Garden, into the center, we in effect do become Him.)

* * *

The middle of the bowl is an empty space; that is what makes a bowl useful. A path is an empty space; again, that is what makes it useful. To build our rituals, we need to clear an empty area in our lives, a sacred area both in time and in space: the sacred space. A church, a temple, an altar, a rock on the seashore, a sunlit meadow, a seat under a tree, the bank of a river, a small room in your home or a corner of a room, a yoga studio: These are special places, set aside or outside the normal everyday experiences of life; these can become sacred spaces within which your ritual is enacted. As important as geography is, sacred space also includes a temporal dimension: You must set aside a repeatable time for the ritual to be conducted. Whatever space you choose, and Joseph Campbell noticed that in India some people simply paint a red line around a rock to render the space sacred, and whatever time you choose, these must begin with an emptiness and an emptying.[23] Now you are ready for the ritual to begin. You are ready to transcend the rim of the bowl, the everyday mundane aspect of life, and make the leap to the unknown: to listen, to dance.

A ritual is the enactment of a myth—either in a very literal way, or in an extremely abstract way.

—Joseph Campbell – *An Open Life*[24]

Of course, once you have made the leap and landed on the yonder shore, it is time to leave the ferryboat that took you across; the enlightened master can live in the relative and absolute worlds at the same time. Rimsters need specific sacred spaces, but from the center, every place is a sacred space and every moment is eternity. Eternal life is no more a question of time than the Promised Land is a place. As Black Elk said:

I was standing on the highest mountain of them all, and round about beneath me was the whole hoop of the world. [But anywhere is the center of the world.] And while I stood there I saw more than I can tell ... for I was seeing in a sacred manner ... And I saw that the sacred hoop of my people was one of many hoops that made one circle.[25]

He also observed:

The first peace, which is the most important, is that which comes within the souls of people when they realize their relationship, their oneness, with the universe and all its powers, and when they realize that at the center of the universe dwells Wakan-Tanka,[26] *and that this center is really everywhere, it is within each of us."*[27]

He is talking, of course, about the center of the bowl. Thich Nhat Hanh has also observed that we can create the sacred *without* having to go anywhere. This is an advanced practice, but one that is eminently achievable with intention and attention:

Mindfulness is the energy of being aware and awake to the present moment. It is the continuous practice of touching life deeply in every moment. To be mindful is to be truly alive and at one with those around us. Practicing mindfulness does not require that we go anywhere different.

We can practice mindfulness in our room and on our way from one place to another. We can do very much the same things we always do—walking, sitting, working, eating, talking—except we learn to do them with an awareness of what we are doing.[28]

In this advanced practice, everything becomes sacred: all places, all times, all people. There are no longer any boundaries, and there is no within and nothing without. This is the whole point of the teaching of the Tantrikas in the East and the Gnostics in the West. Sufis, the mystics of Islam, know that they wear two robes: the inner robe is the mystical garment, but the outer robe is cloth of culture.[29] When they meditate they take off the outer orthodox robe and dance, but when they walk among ordinary people, they don the outer robe once again.

The way to find your own myth is to determine those traditional symbols that speak to you and use them, you might say, as bases for meditation. Let them work on you. A ritual is nothing but the dramatic, visual, active representation of a myth. By participating in the rite, you are engaged in the myth, and the myth works on you—provided, of course, that you are caught by the image. But when you just go through the routine without real commitment, expecting it to work magically and get you to heaven ... you've turned away from the proper use of these rites and images.

— Joseph Campbell – *Pathways to Bliss*[30]

The Mystical Function of Mythology: Summary

The red face of the moon rose above the eastern horizon just as the sun sank beneath the western waters. A thin line of clouds above the setting sun was set aflame: a radiant pink fire reaching out and calling us by name. The sky deepened its hue, turning indigo from blue; while Venus, a moth with white wings, brightly shone; she followed her lover and soon she was gone. Appearing, as the evening faded to night, from north to south, a ribbon of light: a galaxy of whirling stars winked to us.

> We sat,
>> we saw,
>>> we wondered;
>>>> then we were blown asunder.

The mystical function of mythology is neither the last nor the least of the four functions; we saved its exploration to the end so that the full context of its importance could be appreciated. Joseph Campbell claimed that the mystical function is the first and primary function of mythology. The cosmological function exists to feed the mystical, to create awe. And so it goes throughout the cycle of the four functions of myths. The cosmological invokes the mystical through its stories and models; the sociological function mirrors the cosmos through its inflections of social structures—as in heaven, so one earth; the psychological function emerges from the social structures explaining our roles in life; and the mystical function expounds upon the personal, providing the purpose and meaning of life, and ultimately a deep experience of life.

While the four functions can be seen as a circle, there are definitely strong affinities between the social and personal, and between the cosmological and mystical. A good cosmological myth awakens the sense of wonder and awe that motivates us to experience the mystery of life. When we view the pictures from the Hubble space telescope or lie on our backs in a desert night watching meteors flash through the sky, we can feel our place in the universe; we are humbled and we are alive. The story of the Big Bang or the fantastic idea that all life has evolved from primal cells tenaciously clinging to the earliest rocks of our planet, while the heavens brought down sulfur rain and asteroids, fascinates and awakens the mystical sense of ananda.

The sociological function defines our role in the cosmos: to serve something greater than our individual self, to serve society or gods. In the East bowing down to "thou shalt" is the highest virtue: dharma. In the West "I want" is the prime motivator, and our unique path is the surest way to happiness; our secular laws guarantee us the right to pursue it. But extremes do not work, and having social rules imposed upon us by our myths is not always wrong, nor using myths to find our own personal road to bliss always right. There are times to allow our myths to dictate our social roles and times to allow a myth to guide us in our personal development. Taken to excess, any map, any model, any myth leads to dysfunction.

There are new times ahead never before experienced, and the old maps won't work there. Sure, there are some pieces of the old maps that will still prove useful, but a new synthesis is needed: We need new poet prophets, seers of science and mystic artists to illuminate the way before us. There is a dance that has been going on for a long time, and although the music and the steps are changing, the dance itself must continue— for the dance, like Shiva's lila, is life itself.

Epilogue: Transcending Boundaries — Going Beyond Your Map

⇥ ⇤

God summoned a council of His creation, and from the sky came the Great Eagle, from the river came the Sage Salmon, from the plains came the King of the Buffalo, and from Mother Earth came her heart, the Blind Mole. They gathered and listened to God's need:

"I have a problem and I am hoping you can help me. I have created a new creature, as you all have witnessed, and I have called him *man*. But man is never happy! He is always discontented, seeking happiness in temporary things, complaining about pain that comes with simply being alive. Man is always asking me to do something for him, but when I help one man, another complains. I can't continue like this—I need to hide somewhere so that man can learn to deal with his problems on his own. But I can't find a place to hide that will conceal me from his intelligence. Do you have any ideas for me?"

Eagle said, "Come with me. I know a spot on the far side of the moon. Man will never see you up there."

God replied, "Man's science will one day take him to the moon. I will be discovered if I go there."

Salmon said, "Come with me. I know a grotto at the bottom of the deepest trench in the ocean. Man will never find you there."

God replied, "Man's curiosity will take him deep inside the ocean, and he will see me. I can't hide there."

Buffalo said, "Come with me. I know an endless pit at the edge of the great plain. We can cover you and hide you there."

God said, "Man is exploring everywhere on this world, above it and within it. I can't hide in the earth, either."

Finally, Blind Mole spoke, "Then, hide yourself inside man. He will never look there for you."

God clapped excitedly: "Done!"

He hid within.

♨ ୫

Back home it was Christmas Eve, but we could no longer talk to the folks back home. We were in darkness: There was no sunlight here, there was not even the light of Earth to help us navigate. We were alone as no men had ever been before. It wouldn't last—we were moving fast, and we were busy, too busy to worry about what would happen if we made a mistake. But then ...

One hundred kilometers above the far side of the moon, out of sight of both the Earth and our sun, our capsule turned. We were finally facing in the direction we were travelling, but we weren't ready for what we were about to see. Rising just above the ugly, scarred face of the moon slipping quickly beneath us, we saw home and could only think of two words: "My God!" For the first time, humanity was witness to Earthrise.

We had no instructions about what to do; we had no sense that this would be a momentous occasion. But, my God, it was an awesome sight. There we saw our home shining six times brighter than the full moon on a cloudless night, hanging in a sea of stars, a blue-white candy holding such sweetness. When the wonder wore off, we did the only thing we could think to do: We took pictures.

♨ ୫

When the Apollo 8 astronauts, on December 24, 1968, rounded the backside of the moon and beheld for the first time what no human had ever seen, our own planet rising beautifully above the stark ugliness of a dead world, they were in awe. Bill Anders had the only color camera on board, and he took the most famous photo in NASA

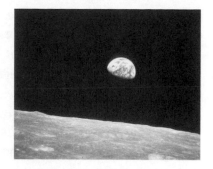

Figure 14: Earthrise - taken by the astronauts of Apollo 8

history: Earthrise.[1] As moving as this image and the visceral, heartfelt response was to the moment, even more important for all of us on planet Earth was the observation, noted by every single astronaut who has ever left this world, that our globe, when seen from space, has not a single borderline drawn upon it. There are no nations' names seen from space; there is just one solitary nest for humanity. There are no boundaries.

Ancient and current myths define us in relation to others: the group we live with, the tribe or the nation, defines who we are and how we are to act with respect to others, those who are not us. Love is reserved for those who are like us; contempt, suspicion and hatred are reserved for those who are not us. We are divided, not just from our fellow man; our myths also tell us that we are separate from nature herself! We are not animals—animals are here to serve and benefit us. Life is a contest, and you are either with us or against us. How else can we read our myths when they tell us that there is evil inherent in the world and we have to choose which side we are on. Those who choose not to stand with us—and our side is always the good side—stand for evil and must be conquered. When there are only two sides, there are no options: You can only take one path.

Joseph Campbell once attended a speech by Zen master D.T. Suzuki in which he characterized Western religion: *Nature against God. God against nature. Nature against man. Man against nature. Man against God. God against man. Very funny religion!*[2] Following this myth has led mankind to a precarious precipice: Mother Nature has taken all the abuse she can tolerate, and now we are poisoning our own wells and water, affecting the health of our own children. We can no longer afford war between developed nations; the results would be global disaster. We can no longer afford the belief that "my map is the right map" or "my god is the one true god" or "my way is the only way, and you are either with me or against me." We can no longer afford conflict between classes or races, and we can no longer afford the imaginary and artificial boundaries that our cultures and their stories have fostered since time out of mind. We have to move beyond boundaries—we *are* moving beyond boundaries—however, the stories needed to help us are but precious and few.

Some poets, some mystics, and some scientists are talking to us today: the poet Thich Nhat Hahn's definition of no-self— there is no separation and everything inter-is; the mystic Chief Dan Seattle's reputed wisdom—"We are part of the earth and it is part of us"; the scientist James Lovelock's vision of Gaia— *The Earth system behaves as a single, self-regulating system comprised of physical, chemical, biological and human components.*[3] They are all providing pieces for new artists to bring together in a grand new mythology of the oneness of life, which will lead toward a more sustainable model for society *and* individuals to follow. The only appropriate group today is the whole planet—just as the astronauts have seen it—without divisions.

The new mythologies can be no more predicted in detail than you can predict what you will dream tonight, but the trends and motifs have been foreshadowed. While technology changes, the basic structure of our psychic landscape does not. We can take from the older myths and maps the things that still work; we can deliberately transcend and leave out that which doesn't. Our new myths will sing of man who works with nature, and nature will continue to provide for man; man will continue to grow closer to his fellow beings, and secular laws will enshrine civil rights for every human being, as well as the rights of animals and plants; the primacy of nature will become first obvious, then supported; God will be found in his inward home as the source of spiritual energies that will support man's endeavors to achieve wholeness, both as individual persons and as a global society; and in this wholeness, God's nature will be revealed. Our new myths will be based on current cosmologies, the sciences of the 21st century, not the archaic sciences of thousands of years ago. We can pray that this will be so.

*   *   *

But how do we pray now? In the past, four ways were open to us, and these can still serve today at various levels. At the personal level, prayer is petition: "Please God, help me!" Here we are dealing with the function of mythology relating to our personal life. This is a valid form of prayer and useful at the personal, psychological level even when we modify our understanding of God from something "out there" to a great power ""in here." Prayer as petition is a form of individual psychotherapy.

At the social level, revealing our interactions with others, prayer moves beyond petition to the nobler intent of intercession: "Please God, help the people suffering in Haiti...." This form of prayer begins to dissolve boundaries and is the form we need to master today. It builds and is based upon compassion, not just for those we love but for all beings and for nature, as well.

At the cosmic level, prayer becomes devotion. Praise and gratitude are offered for everything we receive; we no longer ask anything *of* God, but we give thanks *for* what we already have. Gratitude for what this world has provided does not require that we stay with the old maps and the concept of a personal God, it can work through simply living graciously— that is, with grace and gratitude.

Finally, at the mystical level, prayer is silent. We go past petition and praise into stillness. No words suffice, no thoughts disturb … we simply experience what is arising and passing.

In the future our prayers may simply be the ritual of living our life to the fullest, the quest for wholeness and the tasting of what already is.

* * *

The Greek gods were right to worry about mankind climbing up toward them. We have already reached the heavens and destroyed the gods there. This is not meant to be taken literally: We did not build a real tower of Babel, but intellectually we have climbed so high that we have reached the plane of gods … and found them lacking. Remember! As Joseph Campbell often pointed out, the Virgin Birth is not a question of biology, and the Promised Land is not a question of geography. The answers we seek are not found "out there" but "in here." Where is Zeus today? Gone. Where is Odin or Jupiter, Enlil or Ra? Gone. Surpassed. Man *did* eat of the fruit of the tree of knowledge and became "like us" just as the God of Genesis feared. And what is left?

Joseph Campbell felt that the old myths were failing all around us, and what is left is the lifeless rubble of what was built before.[4] His metaphor is not apt because, as he himself knew very well, myths are living things. Like all living things, when they die—and they do—they decay not into rubble, lifeless inanimate stone, but into soil, into the humus from which the next wave of life arises. From the old myths, new shoots are coming up today.

The myths that guide us throughout our life are our life maps, and we cannot not have a map! We can choose to follow the maps that our culture has laid out before us, but many of these ancient maps no longer work: Their metaphors are worn out; their stories are laughable and unbelievable. They leave us adrift, uncertain and floundering in the waters too deep to swim safely through. So we grab on to any flotsam and jetsam that floats by—the myths of other cultures or other times that equally fail to support and succor us. There is another way: If we can recognize our myths as maps, we can draw better maps to help us navigate more skillfully through life. It is time for today's poets, scientists, artists, and mystics to come together and reveal the new maps, to lead us to an unbounded future.

Perhaps *you* will be the one to dream this new myth and sing its song.

> *I may not be changing the world, but I am changing people. That is what's necessary—it's got to be done.*

> — Joseph Campbell – from *Sukhavati*[5]

Acknowledgements

I owe a great debt to all the teachers who influenced me over the course of my life and who showed me their maps, and taught me how to find my own. I would like to acknowledge the influence of these great teachers, some of whom I have never met in person and others whom I had the great fortune and honor to have spent some time with. Joseph Campbell and Carl Jung are the two greatest influences and their wisdom shines throughout this book, for they taught me how to look at maps, both my own and those of the myths and stories that influenced our culture. My gratitude extends to the Joseph Campbell Foundation for the work they have done in keeping Campbell's wisdom alive, and for their permission to include several slices of Campbell's work in this book.

I would like to express my great appreciation for everyone who supported the creation of this book. To my publisher, Tom Doherty – thank you for believing in the project! To my friends who read the manuscript and offered valuable feedback and ideas: Nis Bojin, Reinhard Pekarek and Paul Grilley. Thanks also to Charleen Davis for her tireless efforts in editing the manuscript. I would like to give a special acknowledgement to Valérie Vasquez for sending me her wonderful photos of India. And, to Stephen Batchelor who encouraged me in this endeavor and provided so much wisdom through his own writings. To my partner, Nathalie Keiller – thanks for putting up with my mental absences while I was lost at my keyboard for so long. To all my students who listened to the early versions of this book while it was still incarnated as a series of power point slides. To Dan Clements and Gloria Latham – thank you for allowing me the opportunity to present these ideas to your yoga teachers in training. Finally, thanks to all those, too numerous to name, who inspired me, both in person and through their books and recordings: my deep debt to you can never be repaid.

Endnotes

A Note On Mythology

1. Vandiver, Elizabeth. "Introduction." *Classical Mythology*. DVD. Chantilly, Virginia, USA: The Teaching Company, 2000.

2. See Vandiver, Elizabeth. "What is Myth?" *Classical Mythology*. DVD. Chantilly, Virginia, USA: The Teaching Company, 2000.

3. "Mythology, which was the bane of the ancient world, is in truth a disease of language." *Lectures on the Science of Language delivered at the Royal Institute of Great Britain in April, May and June, 1861* by Max Müller, (Charles Scribner and Company), 1886, page 21.

4. See Vandiver, Elizabeth. "What is Myth?" *Classical Mythology*. DVD. Chantilly, Virginia, USA: The Teaching Company, 2000.

5. Ibid.

6. Ibid.

7. Ibid.

8. See Joseph Campbell, *Pathways to Bliss*. Novato, CA; New World Library, 2004, – page 104 – 107.

9. See Vandiver, Elizabeth. "Why is Myth?" *Classical Mythology*. DVD. Chantilly, Virginia, USA: The Teaching Company, 2000.

10. Vandiver, Elizabeth. "Why is Myth?" *Classical Mythology*. DVD. Chantilly, Virginia, USA: The Teaching Company, 2000.

11. Ibid.

An Introduction to Myths, Maps and Models

1. Quotation from Joseph Campbell, *Sukhavati*. San Anselmo, CA; The Joseph Campbell Foundation, 2005, 2:56 of video.

2. John 14:6

3. See *The Elegant Universe: Superstrings, Hidden Dimensions, and the Quest for the Ultimate Theory* by Brian Greene, (W.W. Norton & Company), 2003, pages 81–82.

4. See *Critique of Pure Reason*, by Immanuel Kant, Marcus Weigelt, editor, (Penguin Classics), 2008. See also background retrieved from *http://www.scaruffi.com/phi/kant.html*

5. In a dialogue between Heisenberg and Einstein, Einstein admitted, "but it is nonsense all the same ... In reality the very opposite happens. It is the theory which decides what we can observe." – See, Physics and Beyond: Encounters and Conversations, by Werner Heisenberg (translated by Arnold J. Pomerans) New York: Harper, 1971, p. 63.

6. See "To Be Quantum is to be Uncertain", *New Scientist* June 23, 2012. Despite Einstein's hope that it is simply our model of the universe that is insufficient, we know now that it is impossible to know everything about a particle because to do so would violate the Second Law of Thermodynamics.

7. See *An Incomplete Education* by Judy Jones and William Wilson, page 533, (Ballantine Books), 1995. Retrieved from *http://www.miskatonic.org/godel.html*

8. See *Joseph Campbell, The Hero's Journey*. Novato, CA; New World Library, 1990, page 134.

9. See Hróbjartsson A, Norup M (June 2003). "The use of placebo interventions in medical practice—a national questionnaire survey of Danish clinicians". *Evaluation & the Health Professions* 26 (2): 153–65

10. See Kaptchuk TJ, Friedlander E, Kelley JM, Sanchez MN, Kokkotou E, et al. (2010) "Placebos without Deception: A Randomized Controlled Trial in Irritable Bowel Syndrome". *PLoS ONE* 5(12): e15591. doi:10.1371/journal.pone.0015591. Retrieved from *http://www.plosone.org/article/info%3Adoi%2F10.1371%2Fjournal.pone.0015591*

11. Thanks to Georg Feuerstein for coining this term: while a cosmonaut is an explorer of the reaches of outer space, a psychonaut is an explorer of the psychic space within and its contents.

12. See *The Portable Jung* edited by Joseph Campbell, translated by RFC Hull, (Penguin Books), 1976, page xxi.

CHAPTER ONE: THE CREATION OF ALL THINGS

1. There is an ongoing debate over when the earliest Upanishads were compiled: the dates range from as early as 800 B.C.E. according to the 19th century scholar Max Müller, to whom most

people defer, to as late as 500 B.C.E. according to Dasgupta. See *The Shape of Ancient Thought* by Thomas McEvilley, (Allworth Press, an imprint of Skyhorse Publishing, Inc.), 2002 for a more detailed discussion of the various views.

2. The Vedas, which means *knowledge*, are the oldest texts of Hinduism and represent an early form of religion that emphasized rituals and sacrifice along with many tales of a pantheon of gods. The uncertainty in dating the Upanishads extends also to the dating of the earlier Vedas: some scholars believe these texts existed in some form as early as 3,000 B.C.E. while others feel they were created perhaps as late as 1,000 B.C.E. Again, see *The Shape of Ancient Thought* by Thomas (Allworth Press, an imprint of Skyhorse Publishing, Inc.), 2002 for a more detailed discussion.

3. John 10:30

4. Al-Hallaj said, "I am the Truth," which means I am God, because Truth is one of the ninety-nine names of God. See *From Primitives to Zen: A Thematic Sourcebook of the History of Religions* by Mircea Eliade, (Harper Collins), 1967, pages 523-524.

5. There is an awkwardness and misrepresentation arising whenever we use the term "the unconscious" to denote our deep psyche, for the deep is far from unconscious! It knows what is going on; it has first access to our sensory inputs; it is aware and very much conscious.

6. As with many ancient dates, there is controversy over when the Buddha was born. Some scholars hold to the year 563 B.C.E., while recently a later date of 480 B.C.E. has been proposed. There is no archeological evidence that proves when the Buddha lived or died. All we seem to know for sure is how long he lived; which was to the ripe old age of eighty. See *The Shape of Ancient Thought* by Thomas McEvilley, (Allworth Press, an imprint of Skyhorse Publishing, Inc.), 2002, page 426.

The Buddhist creation story cited was formed in part by the earliest Buddhist teachings, the Abhidharma, which is sometimes considered part of Theravada Buddhism (the Buddhism of the Elders; the oldest or original teachings of the Buddha), but for the most part this myth was compiled by a Buddhist scholar around the 4th Century C.E. named Vasubandhu in a commentary on the Abhidharma, called the *Abhidharmakośa*.

7. See *Joseph Campbell Audio Series: Volume 1 –The Individual in Oriental Mythology*; I.1.2 – 7, "God in the Levantine Orient", produced by the Joseph Campbell Foundation.

8. See *Understanding the Bible* by Stephen L. Harris, (McClelland & Stewart), 1985.

9. The Hebrew word for Eve is *Havva* or *Hawwa*. Havva eventually changed into the Latin form Eva, and then into Eve in English. Hawwa means *to live* or *the source of life*.

10. Plato believed that the power of the soul resided in the brain, which was connected to the penis through the spine: when stimulated the fluid of the soul flowed down the spine and out of the body with each ejaculation, which explains how new life and a new soul is generated through sexual congress. This is very similar to the Tantric and pre-Tantric philosophies of India where a man's vital energy, called *ojas*, found mostly in his semen, was meant to be preserved and enhanced through sexual control. See *The Shape of Ancient Thought* by Thomas McEvilley, (Allworth Press, an imprint of Skyhorse Publishing, Inc.), 2002, pages 208–211.

11. See the article by Lévi-Strauss: "The Structural Study of Myth". *The Journal of American Folklore* Vol. 68, No. 270, Oct. - Dec., 1955.

12. "It required tears and lamentations on her part to prevail upon Adam to take the baleful step." *The Legends of the Jews: Volume 1* by Louis Ginzberg [1909] page 42.

13. See Midrash, Rabbi Meir Zlotowitz, Bereishis, *Genesis/A New Translation with a Commentary Anthologized from Talmudic Midrashic and Rabbinic Sources* (Mesorah Publications Ltd.), 1977, p.72 on Genesis 1:27.

14. W. W. Malandra states: "Controversy over [Zoroaster's] date has been an embarrassment of long standing to Zoroastrian studies. If anything approaching a consensus exists, it is that he lived ca. 1000 B.C.E., give or take a century or so, though reputable scholars have proposed dates as widely apart as ca.1750 B.C.E. and 258 years before Alexander." ZOROASTER ii. GENERAL SURVEY in *Encyclopaedia Iranica Online*, originally published: July 20, 2009. Retrieved from *http://www.iranicaonline.org/articles/zoroaster-ii-general-survey*

15. Isaiah 44:28 and 45: 1- 3.

16. See Luke 23:13. The King James Version of the Bible reads: "Verily I say unto you, This generation shall not pass away, till all be fulfilled."

CHAPTER TWO: THE MAGIC OF MYTH

1. *Der Cherubinischer Wandersmann* by Angelus Silesius (1657) 2.102

2. Obviously, these priests had been watching too much *Lord of the Rings*!

3. To understand the current dating of the age of the universe see the article, "Best Map Ever Made of Universe's Oldest Light: Planck Mission Brings Universe into Sharp Focus" in *Science Daily* March 21, 2013.

4. See *The Cosmic Landscape: String Theory and the Illusion of Intelligent Design* by Leonard Susskind (Little, Brown and Company), 2006.

5. See the article, "Is String Theory in Trouble?" in *The New Scientist*, December 17, 2005.

6. Ibid.

7. See *A Universe from Nothing*, by Lawrence Kraus, (Free Press), 2013, page 175.

CHAPTER THREE: LIVING IN ACCORD WITH OUR NEIGHBORS

1. *The Power of Myth* by Joseph Campbell and Bill Moyers, (Doubleday), 1988, page 32.

2. See *The Historical Atlas of World Mythology: The Way of Animal Powers, volume 1* by Joseph Campbell, (Alfred Van der Marck), 1983, page 234.

3. See *Woman the Gatherer*, by Frances Dahlberg, (Yale University Press), 1975.

4. Yahweh was often mentioned with his aspects of thunder and lightning. For examples see Exodus 19: 16; Job 26:14; Psalms 29:3.

5. The question lingers in archeology and philology: who were the proto-Indo-Europeans? This is an important, fascinating and highly contentious question. The path to an answer weaves its way through accusations of racism, colonial thinking, new age wishes, as well as the more sedate sciences of archeology and philology. There are proponents emotionally invested in certain answers who would place the ancestors of the Aryan Indi-

ans and Europeans in the heart of India herself six thousand years ago or longer, and there are scholars who claim that India was culturally overrun by early Aryan invaders from another land.

Philology is the discipline of tracing the commonality between languages, a practice that is not new: the Greeks and Romans also noted that languages change and evolve. Sir William Jones, in 1786, speculated that there was a common source language pre-dating the Indian Sanskrit and many European languages such as Greek, Latin, Celtic and German (and thus English.) This observation started heads to scratching: could it be that India was the *source* of the great civilizations of antiquity? Arthur Schopenhauer [1788 - 1860] believed that India was the source of Christianity. For a time many believed that Sanskrit was not just cognate with the European languages (which means related to) but was the source. This European love affair for India did not last, and soon the newer discoveries in Egypt, and of its antiquities, overshadowed India; scholars began to believe Egypt was the font of all civilization: an idea too that did not last long.

There are two main possibilities for the earliest proto-Indo-Europeans, those people who gave birth to the cultures that arose in India and Europe as well as some parts of the Middle East. The most current and commonly accepted theory holds that these people arose somewhere above and between the Caspian and Black Sea; that they were a herding culture; and that they were the first to domesticate the horse, and were the inventors of the war chariot. The other theory, propounded mostly in India or by scholars sympathetic to the belief that British colonization of India had a negative effect on India's purported history, is that the early Aryans were native to India, have existed there since before antiquity and that their culture and language diffused to the West, and seeded the great civilizations of Egypt, Sumer and Greece. If this theory is true then there never was an Aryan invasion of India and all of Indian history is of domestic development. However, if the first theory is true, then at some point these early Indo-Europeans moved, whether by slow immigration or by waves of conquest, into the Indus valley and later onto the Gangetic plains.

Recent philological investigations are now indicating that the original homeland for the proto-Indo-Europeans was Anatolia, the region of modern day Turkey. It was from there that waves of

Indo-European people expanded East, South and West, taking their language and gods with them.

For the purposes of our investigations the theory we will follow is that the earliest proto-Indo-Europeans were nomadic, horse-master warriors, invading from another land (but from where and exactly when, we do not know); they expanded throughout Europe becoming known as the Celts, Germans and Greeks; through central Asia where they became known as the Persians; and into India where they became known as the Aryans.

For a more detailed review of the many possible theories of the proto-Indo-Europeans, the validity of the various claims, and the affect of these early Indo-Europeans upon both European and Indian history and philosophy, see *The Shape of Ancient Thought* by Thomas McEvilley published by Allworth Press, an imprint of Skyhorse Publishing, Inc., 2002. For the latest philological evidence that shows Anatolia as the ancient homeland for the proto-Indo-Europeans see *Mapping the Origins and Expansion of the Indo-European Language Family* by Remco Bouckaert et al in Science 24 August 2012, Volume 337 no. 6097 pages 957 – 960. To understand the Out of India theory see *In Search of the Cradle of Civilization* by Feuerstein, Frawley and Kak.

6. Deuteronomy 6: 10 -12

7. See *The Power of Myth* by Joseph Campbell and Bill Moyers, (Doubleday), 1988, page 104.

8. Ibid, page 104.

9. See *Transformations of Myth through Time* by Joseph Campbell, (Harper & Row), 1990, pages 81 – 84.

10. See *The Power of Myth* by Joseph Campbell and Bill Moyers, (Doubleday), 1988, page 106.

11. See "Uncovering Civilization's Roots." *Science* 17 February 2012: Vol. 335 no. 6070 pp. 790-793 DOI: 10.1126/science.335.6070.790.

12. See *Pathways to Bliss* by Joseph Campbell, (New World Library), 2004, page 57.

13. Numbers 15: 32-36

CHAPTER FOUR: THE GREAT CYCLES

1. See *The Power of Myth* by Joseph Campbell and Bill Moyers, (Doubleday), 1988, pages 62-64.

2. Ibid.

3. See *Joseph Campbell Audio Series: Volume 1 –The Individual in Oriental Mythology*; I.1.2 – 9, "The Humbling of Indra", produced by the Joseph Campbell Foundation.

4. "The Humbling of Indra" comes from the *Brahma Vaivarta Puranam*, which is one of the twenty or so most important Puranas, collectively known as the Mahapuranas. The exact date that it was written down is unknown, sometime in the first millennium of our common era, but it was likely recited orally long before it was captured on paper.

5. See *Joseph Campbell Audio Series: Volume 1– The Individual in Oriental Mythology*; I.1.2 – 7, *"God In the Levantine Orient"*, produced by the Joseph Campbell Foundation.

6. See *Myths and Symbols in India Art and Civilization* by Heinrich Zimmer, (Princeton University Press), 1972, pages 13-16.

7. See *The Indus script and the Zg-Veda* by Egbert Richter-Ushanas, (Shri Jainendra Press), 2001, page 16.

8. Assuming one human day and year is the same as God's day and year. This was worked out in 1658 C.E. by Archbishop James Ussher [1581 – 1656] who calculated that the world began in 4004 B.C.E.

9. See Genesis, Chapters 6 to 9, for the story of Noah and the flood.

10. Vandiver, Elizabeth. "Humans, Heroes and Half-Gods." *Classical Mythology*. DVD. Chantilly, Virginia, USA: The Teaching Company, 2000

11. Empedocles [490 – 430 B.C.E.] promoted a theory of cyclical time that also had four phases, the first and last being the Age of Love: this approach mirrored the Indian Jain view of six eras of degeneration followed by six era of regeneration, quite different than the cycles we looked at earlier. Some version of the cyclical nature of time can be found in the teachings of Pythagoras, Heraclitus and Plato, as well as within Hesiod himself. Aristotle [384 – 322 B.C.E.] said, "Time itself is thought to be a circle." With the rising influence of Zoroastrianism, the West abandoned

this concept in favor of linear time. For a comparison of the cosmic cycle within various Eastern and Western cultures, see *The Shape of Ancient Thought* by Thomas McEvilley, (Allworth Press, an imprint of Skyhorse Publishing, Inc.), 2002.

12. It was the emperor Constantine who in 321 C.E. made Sunday the day of rest from our labors. Country people, however, were allowed to freely attend to the cultivation of the fields. See Joseph Cullen Ayer, *A Source Book for Ancient Church History* (New York: Charles Scribner's sons, 1913), div. 2, per. 1, ch. 1, sec. 59, g, pp. 284, 285.

13. See *The Masks of God: Occidental Mythology* by Joseph Campbell, (Penguin Books), 1976, page 46.

14. See *The Golden Bough: A Study of Magic and Religion* by Sir James George Frazer – (Project Gutenberg), eBook Chapter 24, section 3.

CHAPTER 5: VARNA, DHARMA AND KARMA

1. *Brih* means to make great or to expand, and is related to our English word *breath*.

2. See *Joseph Campbell Audio Series One: Volume 1 – The Celebration of Life*; I.1.1 – 6, "The Third Function of Mythology", produced by the Joseph Campbell Foundation.

3. Interestingly, the Persian version of the word *Aryan* gave rise to the name of their country, Iran – the Persians and the Indians are believed to be descended from the same wave of proto-Indo-Europeans.

4. See *Autobiography of a Yogi* by Yogananda, (The Self-Realization Fellowship), 2002, page 380-381.

5. See *Philosophies of India* by Heinrich Zimmer, (Princeton University Press), 1989, page 59.

6. See *The Shape of Ancient Thought* by Thomas McEvilley, (Allworth Press, an imprint of Skyhorse Publishing, Inc.), 2002, specifically his chapter "The Problem of the One and the Many".

7. These edicts are from the Institutes of Vishnu. See *The Sacred Books of the East, Vol. 7*, edited by Max Müller, (The Clarendon Press), 1880.

8. "Institutes of Vishnu", *The Sacred Books of the East, Vol. 7*, edited by Max Müller, (The Clarendon Press), 1880.

9. Deuteronomy 25: 11-12 – the King James Version of the Bible reads: "When men strive together one with another, and the wife of the one draweth near for to deliver her husband out of the hand of him that smiteth him, and putteth forth her hand, and taketh him by the secrets: Then thou shalt cut off her hand, thine eye shall not pity her."

10. Deuteronomy 23:1 – the King James Version of the Bible reads: "He that is wounded in the stones, or hath his privy member cut off, shall not enter into the congregation of the Lord."

11. When new ideas did arise the orthodox Hindus subsumed them into the workings of society rather than let the new replace the old: the Buddhist threat was quite strong for many centuries. Like Jainism, it was a casteless worldview that could have stripped the Hindu concept of varna away, but eventually the attractive teachings of Buddhism were brought into an updated version of Vedanta, and the Buddha was cast as just one more incarnation of Vishnu: the threat was effectively neutralized. With this absorption of Buddhist teachings into Vedanta by the sage Shankara [788 – 820 C.E.], and with the Islamic conquest of India, by the 14th century Buddhism became virtually extinct in India.

12. See *Philosophies of India* by Heinrich Zimmer, (Princeton University Press), 1989, pages 160-162.

13. See *The Shape of Ancient Thought* by Thomas McEvilley, (Allworth Press, an imprint of Skyhorse Publishing, Inc.), 2002, Chapter 4, "The Doctrine of Reincarnation".

14. As we will see later, Shiva gave us eighty-four thousand Hatha yoga asanas: supposedly one for each plant and animal on earth. This may be an echo of the ancient Egyptian idea of passing through the rounds of plant and animal incarnations before becoming once again a human.

15. Herodotus, *The Histories* page 145-146 revised edition, April 29, 2003: translated by Aubrey de Sélincourt, revised with an introduction and notes by A.R. Burn (Penguin Books 1954, Revised edition 1972) Copyright © the Estate of Aubrey de Sélincourt, 1954. Copyright © A.R. Burn, 1972.

16. *The Shape of Ancient Thought* by Thomas McEvilley, (Allworth Press, an imprint of Skyhorse Publishing, Inc.), 2002, page 99.

17. Ibid.

18. The Buddha stated: "Not by birth is one an outcast; not by birth is one a brahmin. By deed one becomes an outcast, by deed one becomes a brahmin." See the SaCyutta Nikaya: Vasala Sutta, verse 21.

Chapter 6: Boundaries

1. See Deuteronomy 5 and Exodus 20, as well as Matthew 19-18 King James Version.

2. Numbers 25 and 31

3. As quoted in *The Jewish Paradox: A Personal Memoir*] by Nahum Goldmann, as translated by Steve Cox, (Grosset & Dunlap), 1978, page 99-100.

4. Isaiah 1: 15-17

5. In the Constitution of Medina, written by the Prophet Mohammed sometime around 622 C.E., Mohammed described the rights of the various ethnic communities within Medina, which included Christians, Jews and Muslims. He included all these people in the Ummah.

6. Alan Watts Podcast: "Following the Middle Way" #3, 2008-08-31. Retrieved from *www.alanwattspodcast.com*

7. For the full version of this speech see the film, *Home*. Selections of the speech are reprinted here with kind permission: *Home* [motion picture film] Southern Baptist Convention. Radio and Television Commission, 1972: Southern Baptist Historical Library and Archives, Nashville, Tennessee.

8. The text used was written by Ted Perry, inspired by a speech of Chief Seattle. The original speech was reported in the *Seattle Sunday Star* on Oct. 29, 1887, in a column by Dr. Henry A. Smith.

9. See *Thus Spoke Chief Seattle: The Story of An Undocumented Speech* by Jerry L. Clark in *Prologue Magazine of the US National Archives*, Spring 1985, Vol. 18, No. 1.

10. See *The Revenge of Gaia: Earth's Climate Crisis & The Fate of Humanity* by James Lovelock, (Penguin Books), 2007, copyright © James Lovelock, 2006, page 3.

11. *The Revenge of Gaia: Earth's Climate Crisis & The Fate of Humanity* by James Lovelock, (Penguin Books), 2007) copyright © James Lovelock, 2006, page 22

12. See *The Better Angels of our Nature: Why Violence Has Declined* by Steven Pinker, (Penguin Books), 2012, page 49.

CHAPTER 7: THE ARC OF AGING

1. See *The Power of Myth* by Joseph Campbell and Bill Moyers, (Doubleday), 1988, page 81, and *Joseph Campbell Audio Series One: Volume 1 – The Celebration of Life*; I.1.1 – 9, "An Australian Initiation", produced by the Joseph Campbell Foundation.

2. As stated in the Laws of Manu, Chapter 2, verse 36: "In the eighth year from the conception of a brahmin, in the eleventh from that of a kKshatriya, and in the twelfth from that of a vaisya, let the father invest the child with the mark of his class."

3. See the Kula-Anarva-Tantra XIII – 106.

4. This particular story was a favorite of Joseph Campbell, who relished relating it with several comic flourishes. See *The Gospel of Sri Ramakrishna: Abridged Edition*, 1996, (originally © 1942) translated by Swami Nikhilananda - page 258.

5. See *Joseph Campbell Audio Series One: Volume 1 –The Thresholds of Mythology*; I.2.1 – 15, "The Stages of Life – India", produced by the Joseph Campbell Foundation.

6. The psychologist Erik Erikson depicted eight stages of life by expanding the first stage of infancy into three separate stages.

7. See *Spontaneous Evolution* by Bruce Lipton and Steve Bhaerman, (Hay House), 2010, page 38.

8. See *Introduction to Quantitative EEG and Neurofeedback* by Budzinski, Budzinski, Evans and Arbarbanel, (Academic Press), 2008.

9. The average age for getting married in 1980 was 25.9 and 28.5 years old for women and men respectively; by 2000 the average age increased to 31.7 and 34.3 years old, at least in Canada, according to *Statistics Canada*. They also reported that the average age for a woman to become a mother for the first time was 29.7 years old in 2004, while it was below 27.0 years old in 1976. Retrieved from *http://www.statcan.gc.ca/help-aide/site-eng.htm*

10. See *Joseph Campbell Audio Series One: Volume 1 – The Celebration of Life*; I.1.1 – 8, "The Fourth Function of Mythology" produced by the Joseph Campbell Foundation.

11. See "The Proceedings of the Royal Society B," *Biological*, November, 2009 - vol 276, p 1674.

12. See "Middle age: A triumph of human evolution," *New Scientist* 08 March 2012 by David Bainbridge for a deeper investigation of this topic.

13. Ibid.

14. *Four Acts of Personal Power: How to Heal Your Past and Create a Positive Future* by Denise Linn, (Hay House), 2006. Also released as: *Sacred Legacies: Healing the Past and Creating a Positive Future*, (Random House), 1999.

15. The term "fury of democracy" is from a statement by Edmund Randolph – the 2nd Secretary of State of the USA and first Attorney General.

16. *The Complete Works of Benjamin Franklin*, (G. P. Putnam's Sons), 1887, page 219.

17. See *Sisters in Spirit: Iroquois Influence on Early American Feminists* by Sally R. Wagner, (Book Publishing Company), 2001.

18. "Middle age: A triumph of human evolution," *New Scientist*, 08 March 2012 by David Bainbridge.

19. See *Joseph Campbell Audio Series One: Volume 1 – Man and Myth*; I.4.1 – 5, "Traditional and Humanistic Orders" produced by the Joseph Campbell Foundation.

CHAPTER 8: THE GOALS OF LIFE

1. See *The Gospel of Sri Ramakrishna*, translated by Swami Nikhilananda, (Ramakrishna-Vivekananda Center), 2007, originally © 1942.

2. With three notable exceptions: Aphrodite's tricks and Eros' arrows have no effect on the three virgin goddesses – Athena, Artemis and Hestia.

3. There are several treatises on politics ascribed to the legendary Brihaspati and most of these were undoubtedly written by actual people, perhaps some even named Brihaspati, but we don't know what the legendary Brihaspati actually wrote or if he existed at all. Heinrich Zimmer states in his book *Philosophies of India* (published by Princeton University Press, 1989, pages 36-37) that the definitive book on artha is the *Kautiliya Arthashastra* written by a legendary figure, Kautiliya, an advisor to

Chandragupta Maurya, the founder of a great kingdom in the 4th century B.C.E.

4. Matthew 19: 23-24, Mark 10:24-25 and Luke 18: 24-25. Interestingly, for the past couple of hundred years there have been some people who claim that the "eye of the needle" is actually a very low gate in Israel. However, the term "eye of the needle" was used elsewhere in the Bible and in the Jewish Midrash, and the context shows it meant the eye of an actual sewing needle, signifying the difficulty of achieving some aim.

5. *The Shambhala Encyclopedia of Yoga*, by Georg Feuerstein, ©1997 by Georg Feuerstein, page 187. Reprinted by arrangement with Shambhala Publications Inc., Boston, MA., *www.shambhala.com*

6. *Philosophies of India* by Heinrich Zimmer, (Princeton University Press), 1989, page 41.

7. See *Baksheesh & Brahmin* by Joseph Campbell, (The Joseph Campbell Foundation, printed by New World Library), 2002, page 202.

8. See *The Gospel of Sri Ramakrishna*, translated by Swami Nikhilananda, (Ramakrishna-Vivekananda Center), 2007, originally © 1942, pages 410-411.

9. Ibid, page 238 and 411.

10. See *Dreams* by C.G. Jung, (Princeton University Press), 1974, page 29: "The question may be formulated simply as follows: What is the purpose of this dream? What effect is it meant to have?" See also page 67: "In psychological matters, the question 'Why does it happen?' is not necessarily more productive of results than the other question 'To what purpose does it happen?' "

11. Ibid, page 36: "I believe that it is true that all dreams are compensatory to the contents of consciousness."

12. Ibid, page 233.

13. See *Baksheesh & Brahmin* by Joseph Campbell, (The Joseph Campbell Foundation, printed by New World Library), 2002, page 131.

CHAPTER 9: THE SOUL QUESTION

1. See *Dante: The Divine Comedy 1 Hell* by Dorothy Sayers, (Penguin), 1949, pages 13-15.

2. Dante's *Il Convivio*(The Banquet), translated by Richard H. Lansing, (Garland Library of Medieval Literature), 1990, pages 40-41. Here we have substituted the word "story" for Lansing's original edit of "text" in the first line of the quote.

3. *Collected Ancient Greek Novels* by B.P. Reardon, (University of California Press), 2008, page 11.

4. Jung describes the missing fourth of the Trinity as the anima, the Holy Mother, which is often, being feminine, placed in darkness. For many, the dark feminine is the devil herself: the witch that scares the bejesus out of them. The fourth arm of the crucifix points downward and represents the devil: one cannot have evil without good, and Jesus' presence on earth was to balance the evil one's effect on the world; but you can't have a symbol of the Trinity without including Satan as well. Dante's descent to hell was a descent into his own darkness, where he would be provided the opportunity to round out his threes with a fourth. See *Dreams* by C.G. Jung, (Princeton University Press), 1974, pages 225-226

5. The original allegory involved chariots, not cars: "The Self (atman) is the owner of the chariot; the body is the chariot; awareness (buddhi) is the charioteer; the thinking function (manas) is the bridle; the senses (indriya) are the horses...the individual Self is called the enjoyer." From the Katha Upanishad 3.3-4.

6. *Philosophies of India* by Heinrich Zimmer, (Princeton University Press), 1989, page 79.

7. See a discussion on this topic in Georg Feuerstein's *The Yoga Tradition*, (Hohm Press), 2001, and *The Shambhala Encyclopedia of Yoga* by Georg Feuerstein, (Shambhala Publications), 1997, pages 236-237.

8. See *Yoga: Immortality and Freedom* by Mircea Eliade, (Princeton University Press), 2009, pages 8–10.

9. This quotation is from a private correspondence between Paul Grilley and the author: April 28, 2013.

10. There is some evidence that Mahavira reformed Jainism by taking many ideas from the equally ancient Ajivika religion, which was even stricter than Jainism. See *The Shape of Ancient Thought* by Thomas McEvilley, (Allworth Press, an imprint of Skyhorse Publishing, Inc.), 2002, page 278-280.

11. Ibid, page 279. In the Ajivika view, by contrast, it doesn't matter how much you clean your cup, you have to go through a predetermined number of incarnations, eighty-four thousand to be exact, before you are free. This view is even more pessimistic than Jainism, because the Ajivika teachers claim that there is no way to shorten your allotted time: there is no such thing as free will – everything is pre-determined. For the Ajivikas, the only benefit in practicing their yoga is to gain special, magical powers that make this particular incarnation more pleasant.

12. See *Philosophies of India* by Heinrich Zimmer, (Princeton University Press), 1989, page 182.

13. Ibid, page 181.

14. See *The Shambhala Encyclopedia of Yoga,* by Georg Feuerstein., (Shambhala Publications Inc.), ©1997 by Georg Feuerstein, page 132.

15. Ibid. Also see the "Yoga Sutra of Patanjali": 1-24 for the definition of Ishvara.

16. See *Philosophies of India* by Heinrich Zimmer, (Princeton University Press), 1989, pages 216–217, for the story of King Anandakumara, the second-to-last incarnation of Parsvanatha.

17. See *Yoga: Immortality and Freedom* by Mircea Eliade, (Princeton University Press), 2009, Chapter 8: "Yoga and Aboriginal India".

18. *Philosophies of India* by Heinrich Zimmer, (Princeton University Press), 1989, page 219.

19. Metis was a goddess and Zeus' first wife. There was a prophecy concerning their children: Metis would bear a son who would overthrow Zeus, just as he had overthrown his father. When Metis was pregnant with Athena, Zeus did not wait around for the prophecy to be fulfilled. He ate Metis! Swallowed her up whole. This is one of the few times that the Fates were foiled. It is interesting that *Metis* means *wisdom*: perhaps this story describes how Zeus acquired his wisdom: from a woman or from his inner woman. Notice also where wisdom is kept: in the gut! Perhaps this story is an aetiology of the final overthrow of the goddess culture by the patriarchal culture: the masculine consumed the feminine. In any case, eventually Zeus developed a splitting headache and to get some relief he asked Hephaestus to use an

axe and split open his head. Hephaestus did so and out popped Athena – she took over as the goddess of wisdom.

20. As in all these historical theories, there is no consensus. Some Vedic scholars would protest the claim that Vishnu was a Dravidian god: they feel he was clearly the solar deity described in the Rig Veda. He may have been, but it also may have been that the Indo-Europeans compiled the Rig Veda after they assimilated the Dravidian culture. Vishnu's skin color is blue like the sky, as is the color of his avatars Rama and Krishna: this may bespeak of his origins – as the Dravidian sky god. See Klaus K. Klostermaier's *A Survey of Hinduism*, (State University of New York), 1994, pages 145 and 297.

CHAPTER 10: MATTER VERSUS SPIRIT

1. There was an Oscar winning movie in 1990 called *Ghost*, in which a dead Patrick Swayze follows around his wife, played by Demi Moore. He is a ghost, and in one scene he is surprised to find that he can jump through a door and land on the other side. His spirit body is unaffected by a material door. But what is glossed over is the fact that he is standing on the equally material floor! Why doesn't he fall through the floor just as easily as he passed through the wall? This is an inconvenient realization best not thought about if you believe in the separation of spirit and matter.

2. Katha Upanishad: 6–17. See *The Sacred Books of the East: The Upanishads, Part 2* by Max Müller. While the Katha Upanishad describes the atman as thumb-sized and located at the heart, in the Svetashvatara Upanishad it is described as being both infinitesimally small, just one-hundredth the size of a hair, but also infinitely large; it is neither male nor female, nor neuter!

3. *The Dragons of Eden* by Carl Sagan, (Random House), 1977, page 7.

4. *Astounding Hypothesis: The Scientific Search for the Soul* by Francis Crick, (Touchstone), 1995, page 3.

5. *Neuronal Man* by Jean-Pierre Changeux, translated by Laurence Garey, (Princeton University Press), 1997, page 169.

6. Michael Lemonick, "Glimpses of the Mind", article in *Time Magazine* July 17, 1995.

7. See *The Spiritual Brain: A Neuroscientist's Case for the Existence of the Soul*, by Mario Beauregard and Denyse O'Leary, (Harper Collins), 2008, Chapter 5: "Are Mind and Brain Identical?"

8. *Taboo of Subjectivity: Towards a New Science of Consciousness* by B. Alan Wallace, (Oxford University Press), 2000, page 82.

9. Excerpt from *Quantum Reality: Beyond The New Physics* by Nick Herbert, ©1985 by Nick Herbert. Published by Doubleday, an imprint of the Knopf Doubleday Publishing Group, a division of Random House LLC. All rights reserved, page 249.

10. *The Spiritual Brain: A Neuroscientist's Case for the Existence of the Soul* by Mario Beauregard and Denyse O'Leary, (Harper Collins), 2008, page 107.

11. See *Sake & Satori: Asian Journals – Japan* by Joseph Campbell, (The Joseph Campbell Foundation, printed by New World Library), 2002, page 21.

12. We are referring here to Advaita Vedanta. Just as Christianity has many different schools and views that are dramatically different (such as the agnostic tradition and the orthodoxy of the Catholic tradition), Vedanta comes in a variety of flavors: Advaita Vedanta is the most common and holds to a strict non-duality, all is one; however, there are qualified dualistic views and even strictly dualistic views of Vedanta as well, such as the Dvaita Vedanta of Madhva. In the same vein there are multiple views of Maya: she can range from being a creative power of nature which is the ultimate energy of the universe, to the illusory nature of existence, to simply the relative versus absolute reality. See *The Yoga Tradition* by Georg Feuerstein, (Hohm Press), 2001, and *The Shambhala Encyclopedia of Yoga* by Georg Feuerstein, (Shambhala Publications), ©1997 by Georg Feuerstein.

13. Joseph Campbell offers this analogy of light bulbs and consciousness in many of his books and talks, such as *Myths to Live By* by Joseph Campbell, (Penguin Books), 1993; *Reflections on the Art of Living: A Joseph Campbell Companion* edited by Diane K. Osbon, (Penguin Books), 1993; and *Thou Art That: Transforming Religious Metaphor* by Joseph Campbell, (New World Library, 2001.

Chapter 11: The Individual in Society

1. Bob Dylan's song proposed that if you are not a servant of God, you are a servant of the devil. From Bob Dylan's Slow Train Coming album released in 1979 by Columbia Records.

2. John Lennon's song of reply to Bob Dylan, from the John Lennon Anthology, released in 1998 by Capitol Records.

3. "Job's Submission and Prometheus' Humanism"Joseph Campbell Audio Series One: Volume 1 – Symbolism and the Individual, I.1.3–08;" Job and Prometheus – Loyalty to God or to Man", Joseph Campbell Audio Series One: Volume 1 – Mythology East and West, II.1.2– 06, Joseph Campbell Foundation.

4. Walter Burkert, a German scholar of Greek mythology, believes that rituals become myths. First there is the ritual that serves some social function, and then a myth grows up around the ritual to explain why it is necessary.

5. *Myths to Live By*, by Joseph Campbell, (Viking Press), 1993, page 167.

6. This is a Shiite Muslim story of the fall of Lucifer. See *Transformations of Myth Through Time* by Joseph Campbell, (Harper and Row), 1990, page 247.

7. Peredur was the name of the Parzival character hundreds of years earlier, in a Welsh myth of the King Arthur and the Grail. It is fascinating to read the story of Peredur and see what parts von Eschenbach kept, left out or modified, but that is beyond our scope.

CHAPTER 12: MYTHS FOR WOMEN

1. *Philosophies of India* by Heinrich Zimmer, (Princeton University Press), 1989, 166.

2. Vishnu Smriti 25-14.

3. Artharva Veda 18-3-1.

4. Elizabeth Vandiver, "Monstrous Females and Female Monsters," Classical Mythology. DVD. (Chantilly, Virginia: The Teaching Company, 2000).

5. Hippolytus was not gay; he just didn't want anything to do with sexuality. As Elizabeth Vandiver points out, "In a society with high infant mortality and many enemies, it was the absolute, unambiguous, unarguable duty of every male citizen to marry and beget children whether he wanted to or not." See Elizabeth Vandiver, "Monstrous Females and Female Monsters."

6. Genesis 19.

7. Judges 19: 20–29.

8. This version of the sacrifice of Iphigenia is taken mostly from Aeschylus' Oresteia, but there are milder versions where at the last minute Artemis allows a deer to be substituted for the girl. It is in Euripides' version of the story that Iphigenia goes willingly to the sacrifice.

9. Genesis 12: 11–16.

10. Genesis 20.

11. Genesis 22.

12. Judges 11: 30–40.

13. In the Oresteia, Apollo defends Orestes from the charge of murdering his mother by pointing out, in the proper scientific models of the day, that Orestes' mother was not a blood relative, because she was merely the host of the fetus. See Elizabeth Vandiver, "Blood Vengeance, Justice, and the Furies," Classical Mythology. DVD. (Chantilly, Virginia: The Teaching Company, 2000).

14. "Vishnu, Padma, and Brahma—Dreaming Creation,"Joseph Campbell Audio Series One: Volume 1 – The World Soul, I.2.5–7, Joseph Campbell Foundation.

15. Here we are making a distinction: shakti without the capital letter represents the impersonal energy of creativity; with the capital letter, Shakti represents a goddess who personifies that energy.

16. *The Shambhala Encyclopedia of Yoga* by Georg Feuerstein, (Shambhala Publications), 1997, page 269.

17. Indeed, Mohammed had many wives! He had 12 or 13: the stories vary.

18. Dr. Francesca Stavrakopoulou makes this statement in the BBC documentary "The Bible's Buried Secrets, Episode 2: Did God Have a Wife? 24, February 2009. Retrieved from *http://www.bbc.co.uk/programmes/b00zw3fl.*

19. In 598 B.C.E. Nebuchadnezzar conquered Israel, deported the population in three waves to Babylon, and in 587 B.C.E. destroyed God's temple. How could this happen? How could God have allowed his own house to be destroyed and his people defeated? Someone must have screwed up big time. As the rab-

bis contemplated this mystery, the idea arose that the conquest and destruction the Jewish people experienced was a punishment for their failure to abide by the agreement they had with God. The very first commandment was to have no other gods: the priestly scribes in exile decided to write down the definitive version of the five books of the Torah, and in creating these works they removed any references to Asherah, although a few faint allusions still remain. It was in this period that the Jewish religion became truly monotheistic. For further evidence of Asherah's role in early Jewish worship, and the links between the Canaanite and Jewish cultures, see the work of Dr. Francesca Stavrakopoulou, "The Bible's Buried Secrets, Episode 2: Did God Have a Wife?"

20. We can say re-creation here because Durga was originally widely worshipped in India before the arrival of the proto-Indo-Europeans. See *Yoga: Immortality and Freedom*, by Mircea Eliade, (Princeton University Press), 2009, page 343.

21. There are only three important virgin goddesses in Classical mythology: Athena, Artemis and Hestia, a sister of Zeus. Hestia means hearth: she was the goddess that looked after the home life, and there are very few myths about her.

22. See *Joseph Campbell Audio Series One: Volume 2 – The Function of Mythology*; II.1.11, "Our Rapidly Changing Social Orders", produced by the Joseph Campbell Foundation.

23. See *Baksheesh & Brahmin* by Joseph Campbell, (published by The Joseph Campbell Foundation, printed by New World Library), 2002, page 155.

24. See *Buddha* by Karen Armstrong,(Phoenix/Orion Books), 2002, pages 138-142

25. Ibid.

26. *Buddhist Cosmology: Philosophy and Origins* by Akira Sadakata, (Kosei Publishing Co), 2009, page 117.

27. Gospel of Saint Thomas: 114

28. See the *The Global Gender Gap Report 2011* by the World Economic Forum.

29. Ibid. These rankings are for 2011.

30. There are many versions of the story of the Handless Maiden. Its roots go back to medieval Europe. Jacob and Wilhelm Grimm

wrote the two most popular versions in their anthologies of myths and folk tales, but its theme can be found woven into many myths. The version we are using is mostly based on the story as told by Robert A. Johnson in his book *The Fisher King and the Handless Maiden*, (Harper Collins), 1995.

31. See "Sounds True: Insights at the Edge"Podcast with author: Dr. Clarissa Pinkola Estés on her book *The Dangerous Old Woman: Myths and Stories of the Wise Woman Archetype*, (Sounds True, Incorporated), 2010.

32. Marlo Thomas. (1972). Free to be you and me [Recorded by Alan Alda and Marlo Thomas]. On *Atalanta* [audio]. n.d.: Arista Records. This was a project created by Marlo Thomas to provide her niece with a more wholesome mythology to grow up with. It has since been used by many mothers to teach their young daughters what a woman can do.

33. See the Charles Perrault (1628-1703) version of "Red Riding Hood"in *Perrault's Fairy Tales* which predates the Brothers Grimm's version and is available from Wordsworth Editions in a 2004 volume of their Children's Classics.

34. Alix Olsen. (2001). Eve's Mouth. On *Built Like That* [cd]. n.d: Subtle Sister Productions. Retrieved from *www.alixolson.com*

35. See Vandiver, Elizabeth. "Culture, Prehistory, and the Great Goddess."*Classical Mythology*. DVD. Chantilly, Virginia, USA: The Teaching Company, 2000.

Chapter 13: Myths of Love

1. *We: Understanding The Psychology of Romantic Love* by Robert A. Johnson, (Harper Collins), 1983, page xi.

2. See *The Fisher King and the Handless Maiden* by Robert A. Johnson, (Harper Collins), 1995, page 6.

3. Ibid.

4. Matthew 22: 39

5. Ovid's *Metamorphoses*, Book 4 translated by A. S. Kline, (Borders Classics), 2004, pages 55–92.

6. These statistics are from the UNICEF, Human Rights Council. See the website Statistic Brain.com. Retrieved from *http://www.statisticbrain.com/arranged-marriage-statistics/*

7. See Vandiver, Elizabeth. "Gods are Useful."*Classical Mythology*. DVD. Chantilly, Virginia, USA: The Teaching Company, 2000.

8. See *Myths to Live By* by Joseph Campbell, (Viking Press), 1993, page 151.

9. The word used in the earliest Greek versions of the Bible was *doulos*, which means a slave, bondsman or a man of servile condition.

10. Ephesians 6:5. Also see Colossians 3:22 22: "Servants, obey in all things your masters … fearing God:"

11. Mark 10:9

12. Mark 10:8

13. See *Joseph Campbell Audio Series One: Volume 1 – Man and Myth*; I.4.1– 10, "The Moth and the Flame", produced by the Joseph Campbell Foundation, 2002.

14. In his book, *We: Understanding The Psychology of Romantic Love*, Robert Johnson bases his retelling of the story of Tristan mostly on a version written by Béroul (see *The Romance of Tristan and Tristan's Madness*, published by Penguin Books, in 1970.) The version summarized in our story has some elements from Johnson's version, but is based mostly on the tale written by Gottfried von Strassburg [See *Tristan with the Tristan of Thomas* by Penguin Classics and translated by Professor A.T. Hatto, (Penguin Books), 2004.

15. *We: Understanding The Psychology of Romantic Love* by Robert A. Johnson, (Harper Collins), 1983, page 70.

16. Recall that the number three represents incompleteness, while four represents wholeness. The number three occurs many times in Tristan's story, and we can see over and over again how incomplete his life is: Morold shouts three times before he is killed; the love potion lasts only three years; there are the three Isoldes; and there is the three-sided triangle between Mark, Isolde and Tristan that could be healed by the fourth, by Isolde of the White Hands, but unfortunately Tristan rejects her.

17. See *Joseph Campbell Audio Series One: Volume 1– Confrontation of East and West in Religion*; I.2.3–10, "The West – Relationship to the Divine", produced by the Joseph Campbell Foundation.

18. Jayadeva's poem dates from around 1175 C.E. This was one of the early versions of the love affair between Krishna and Radha, but in the 14th century C.E. the Brahmavaivarta Purana expanded upon the theme. It is in this latter story that thousands of gopis get to share in Radha's bliss. See *The Masks of God: Oriental Mythology* by Joseph Campbell, (Penguin Books), 1976, page 352–364.

19. *The Gospel of Sri Ramakrishna, Abridged Version* by Swami Nikhilananda, Ramakrishna-Vivehananda Center, 1996, reissued, (© 1942) page 42.

20. See *Joseph Campbell: The Hero's Journey – Joseph Campbell on His Life and Work* edited by Phil Cousineau, (published by The Joseph Campbell Foundation, printed by New World Library), 1990, page 104.

Chapter 14: The Horror of Life

1. See *Myths to Live By* by Joseph Campbell, (Viking Press), 1993, pages 103-104.

2. Oppenheimer was referring to a line from the Bhagavad Gita: Chapter 11, verse 32. In Georg Feuerstein's translation of the Gita, the line reads: "I am time, mighty wreaker of the world's destruction, engage here in the annihilation the worlds." (See The Bhagavad-Gîtâ, by Georg Feuerstein, with Brenda Feuerstein, ©2011 by Georg Feuerstein and Brenda Feuerstein. Reprinted by arrangement with Shambhala Publications Inc., Boston, MA. *www.shambhala.com*, page 233).

3. See Plato's *Timaeus*

4. See *Joseph Campbell Audio Series One: Volume 1 – The Celebration of Life*; I.1.1 – 14, "Out of Death Comes Life - the Plant World as Inspiration", produced by the Joseph Campbell Foundation, 2008.

5. See *Philosophies of India* by Heinrich Zimmer, (Princeton University Press), 1989, page 565.

6. Joseph Campbell describes two attitudes of Shiva: first, the path of fire and of the sun, of quitting the world forever and never coming back; and second, the path of smoke and of the moon, of returning. In this second attitude, Shiva would be depicted with his eyes open gazing up at Kali. See *Joseph Campbell Audio Series One: Volume 1 – The World Soul*; I.2.5 – 6, "Shiva and Shava –

Two Attitudes of Yoga", produced by the Joseph Campbell Foundation.

7. The Brihadaranyaka Upanishad

8. See *The Masks of God: Oriental Mythology* by Joseph Campbell, (Penguin Books), 1976; and *Yoga: Immortality and Freedom* by Mircea Eliade, (Princeton University Press), 2009; and *Philosophies of India* by Heinrich Zimmer, (Princeton University Press), 1989.

9. See *The Golden Bough* by James Frazer, (Simon & Brown), 2013, Chapter 47 – Lityerses, section 3 – Human Sacrifices for the Crops. Compare this to 1 Corinthians 6: 19 -20: "You are not your own, for you were bought with a price."

10. See *The Masks of God: Oriental Mythology* by Joseph Campbell, (Penguin Books), 1976, page 5.

11. See *Philosophies of India* by Heinrich Zimmer, (Princeton University Press), 1989, page 566

12. Ibid.

13. See *CNN News: Pat Robertson says Haiti paying for 'Pact with the devil'*, January 13, 2010 broadcast. Retrieved from *http:// articles.cnn.com/2010-01-13/us/haiti.pat.robertson_1_pat-robertson-disasters-and-terrorist-attacks-devil?_s=PM:US*

14. See *Christian Broadcasting Network: The 700 Club*, September 12, 2005 broadcast. Retrieved from *http://mediamatters.org/research/2005/09/13/religious-conservatives-claim-katrina-was-gods/133804*

CHAPTER 15: THE CHARACTERISTICS OF LIFE

1. See the Vinaya Pitaka: Book IV – Mahavagga (The Book of The Discipline)

2. Often the tree is called the *bodhi tree*, and this is translated frequently as the tree of illumination, but *bodhi* means awakening, not illumination as is often believed. However, either interpretation works.

3. *The Middle Length Discourses of the Buddha, A Translation of the Majjhima Nikaya* translated by Bhikkhu Nanamoli & Bhikkhu Bodhi, (Wisdom Publications), 1995, page 655.

4. See Stephen Batchelor podcasts of a series of talks he gave at Gaia House in July, 2006: "Going Against the Stream". Retrieved from *http://www.stephenbatchelor.org/index.php/en/audio-archive*

5. See *The Questions of King Milinda* by Thomas William Rhys Davies, Book II, Chapter 1,"The Distinguishing Characteristics of Ethical Qualities," (Forgotten Books), 2007.

6. See Stephen Batchelor podcasts of a series of talks he gave in Beatenburg, Switzerland, March, 2008: "A Middle Way." Retrieved from *http://www.stephenbatchelor.org/index,.php/en/audio-archive*

7. See Stephen Batchelor podcasts of a series of talks he gave at Gaia House in July, 2006: "Contingency and Emptiness". Retrieved from *http://www.stephenbatchelor.org/index.php/en/audio-archive*

8. See Hardy, Grant. "Nagarjuna and Vasubandhu – Buddhist Theories."Great Minds of the Eastern Intellectual Tradition. DVD. Chantilly, Virginia, USA: The Teaching Company, 2011

9. *Verses from the Centre: A Buddhist Vision of the Sublime* by Stephen Batchelor, (Riverhead Books), 2001, page 22

10. This refers to the famous Zen kôan where master Joshu was asked if a dog had Buddha Nature, and he replied, "mu!"Now the student, who knows that all things possess Buddha Nature, has to figure out why this dog doesn't.

11. See *The God Delusion* by Richard Dawkins, (Mariner Books), 2008, specifically his chapter "The Roots of Morality: Why Are We Good,"for a discussion of this point.

12. This translation from the Dhammapada is by Stephen Batchelor. Most renditions of this text translate the word *atta* as a reflexive pronoun *himself,* but truly it means *self.* The discomfort of translators to leave the word as a noun and instead use a pronoun is due to their belief that Buddha never admitted to the existence of a self. [See *The Pali Canon: Source Texts for Secular Buddhism* from Stephen Batchelor, found at his web site *www.stephenbatchelor.org/index.php/en/stephen/study-tools*

13. *Confession of a Buddhist Atheist* by Stephen Batchelor, (Spiegel & Grau), 2010, page 152.

14. Ibid.

15. See *The Analects of Confucius,* Book 17, Chapter 2 in "The Chinese Classics" Translated into English with Preliminary Essays and Explanatory Notes by James Legge. *Vol. 1. The Life and Teachings of Confucius. Second Edition* (N. Trübner), 1869.

16. *Confession of a Buddhist Atheist* by Stephen Batchelor, (Spiegel & Grau), 2010, page 152.

CHAPTER 16: THREE ATTITUDES TOWARD LIFE

1. Mundaka Upanishad, III.i.1

2. For a detailed description of this early form of yoga practiced by chariot warriors see *Sinister Yogis* by David Gordon White (The University of Chicago Press), 2009, pages 59 – 72).

3. See *The Masks of God: Oriental Mythology* by Joseph Campbell, (Penguin Books), 1976, page 132.

4. Ibid, page 255-257.

5. Sutta Nipata translated by K.R. Norman in *The Group of Discourses, Second Edition*, (Pali Text Society), 2001, page 50.

6. Stephen Batchelor from a podcasts of a series of talks he gave at Gaia House in July, 2006: "Democracy of the Imagination". Retrieved from *http://www.stephenbatchelor.org/index.php/en/audio-archive*

7. Ibid.

8. See the Encyclopedia Britannica entry on Ananda: Retrieved from *http://www.britannica.com/EBchecked/topic/22668/Ananda#ref828218*

9. See *Confession of a Buddhist Atheist* by Stephen Batchelor, (Spiegel & Grau), 2010, page 231 – 236.

10. See the Kalama Sutta

11. Luke 9:60

12. *The Messianic Idea in Israel* by Joseph Klausner, translated by W.F. Stinespring, (George Allen and Unwin, Ltd.,), 1956, page 59.

13. Well, at least the orthodox Jewish God won't show up, but some versions of Judaism do allow adult women to make up the minimum required number.

14. *The Power of Myth* by Joseph Campbell and Bill Moyers, (Doubleday), 1988, page 218.

15. See *Zen Flesh, Zen Bones* by Paul Reps, (Tuttle Publishing), 1998, page 38.

16. See *Joseph Campbell Audio Series One: Volume 1 – The Fourth Function of Mythology*; I.4.4 – 2, "Rejection, Affirmation, and Amelioration,"produced by the Joseph Campbell Foundation.

17. See *Philosophies of India* by Heinrich Zimmer, (Princeton University Press), 1989, pages 345-347.

18. Thanks to Erich Schiffmann for this specific flavor of the story: see his audio recording of *"The Wave and The Ocean"*, 2006, at his web site. Retrieved from *http://erichschiffmann.com*

CHAPTER 17: AUM IN FOUR SYLLABLES

1. *Joseph Campbell Audio Series One: Volume 1– The Mystical Traditions of India*; I.3.2– 4, "The Symbolism of AUM", produced by the Joseph Campbell Foundation.

2. John 1:1

3. Saul, in this case, is Saul David Raye who shared this story during a yoga class early on the morning of December 13, 2003, which was the last day of his advanced Thai Yoga Therapy training. The author was one of the students waiting in Down Dog.

4. *Pra* from *prakriti* means "nature" and *nava*, cognate with our English word navy, means "boat." See *The Shambhala Encyclopedia of Yoga*, by Georg Shamba., ©1997 by Georg Feuerstein. (Shambhala Publications Inc.), 1997, page 225.

CHAPTER 18: MAHAYANA BUDDHISM

1. See *The Masks of God: Oriental Mythology* by Joseph Campbell, (Penguin Books), 1976, pages 298–299.

2. From Stephen Batchelor's talk at Spirit Rock Meditation Center in California – "The Life and Death of Siddhatta Gotama: Awakening", October 23, 2005.

3. See "Wisdom of the Mountain"talk by Alan Alan Watts Podcast August 31, 2008: "Following the Middle Way #3."Retrieved from *alanwattspodcast.com*

4. See *Buddhist Cosmology: Philosophy and Origins* by Akira Sadakata, (Kosei Publishing Co), 2009, page 118.

5. See *Buddhism; The Religion of No-Religion* by Alan Watts, (Tuttle Publishing), 1999, pages 68–69 .

6. See The Epistle of Paul the Apostle to the Romans, Chapters 7 and 8.

7. See *Philosophies of India* by Heinrich Zimmer, (Princeton University Press), 1989, pages 478–481.

8. See *Buddhist Cosmology: Philosophy and Origins* by Akira Sadakata, (Kosei Publishing Co,) 2009, page 116.

9. See *Joseph Campbell Audio Series One: Volume 1 – The Mystical Traditions of India*; I.3.2– 6, "The Reincarnating Principle", produced by the Joseph Campbell Foundation.

10. The Gospel of Saint Thomas: 113

11. *Touching Peace: Practicing the Art of Mindful Living* by Thich Nhat Hanh, (Parallax Press), 1992, page 121.

12. See *Buddha* by Karen Armstrong, (Phoenix/Orion Books), 2002, page 89.

13. Recall earlier that we defined dukkha, not as suffering, but as unsatisfactoriness or even sorrow. Here is where these terms get more confusing. The Four Noble Truths do imply *suffering*, more than the basal condition of the world, which is unreliability, because suffering is what the Buddha is trying to cure. He is not trying to stop dukkha, defined earlier as unsatisfactoriness or sorrow and inherently a part of existence: he is trying to stop us from turning dukkha into to suffering.

14. *Confession of a Buddhist Atheist* by Stephen Batchclor, (Spiegel & Grau), 2010, pages 153, 253-254.

15. See Chapter Seven: The Arc of Aging for this story

16. *Confession of a Buddhist Atheist* by Stephen Batchelor, (Spiegel & Grau, 2010, page 153.

17. Ibid, page 161.

CHAPTER 19: TANTRA YOGA

1. See *The Yoga Tradition* by Georg Feuerstein, (Hohm Press), 2001, page 342.

2. See *Philosophies of India* by Heinrich Zimmer, (Princeton University Press), 1989, page 62, footnote 26.

3. See *Tantra: The Path of Ecstasy* by Georg Feuerstein, (Shambhala Publications), 1998, page 68; and again note the comment by Heinrich Zimmer about the 'so-called nondualism' of Vedanta cited earlier: *Philosophies of India* by Heinrich Zimmer, (Princeton University Press), 1989, page 219.

4. The five veils of Maya are more properly called *jackets*, from the Sanskrit *kancuka*. The five jackets are *kalaa*, limited action; *vidya*, limited knowledge; *raga*, desire and attachments; *kala*, time; *niyati*, causality or fate. See *The Yoga Tradition* by Georg Feuerstein, (Hohm Press), 2001, page 269.

5. The Upanishads by Sri Aurobindo, (Lotus Press), 2001, page 32.

6. Often this is called a diamond body because most people have no idea what adamantine is. However, fans of Wolverine know: adamantine is the hardest substance in the universe.

7. There are various views of the siddhis offered by various schools. Eight *mahasiddhis* are often referred to: the ability to become very small; or very tall; to levitate; to travel anywhere instantly; to fulfill all desires; to have an irresistible will; to command the material universe; and to command the spiritual universe just as God can. See *The Yoga Tradition* by Georg Feuerstein, (Hohm Press), 2001, pages 367–368.

8. From a libation cup of King Gudea: this is a drawing of a vase of green steatite found at Telloh (Lagash), now at the Louvre. Originally published as figure 368c in *The Seal Cylinders of Western Asia*, by William Hayes Ward [1835 - 1916], Washington, 1910.

9. These five Dhyani Buddhas are: Vairochana, Akshobhya, Ratnasambhava, Amitabha, and Amoghasiddhi. See *Joseph Campbell Audio Series One: Volume 1* – Imagery of Rebirth Yoga; I.2.4 – 13, "Bardo Thodol - Descent through the Cakras", produced by the Joseph Campbell Foundation.

10. See *Transformations of Myth Through Time* by Joseph Campbell, (Harper and Row), 1990.

11. Ibid, page 144.

12. See *Joseph Campbell Audio Series Two: Volume 1 – The Sound AUM and Kundalini Yoga*; II.1.3 – 6,"Hearing AUM - Cakra 4", produced by the Joseph Campbell Foundation.

13. See *Tantra: The Path of Ecstasy* by Georg Feuerstein, (Shambhala Publications), 1998, page 155.

14. The analogy of the chakras to floors of a building comes from Joseph Campbell (See *Reflections on the Art of Living: A Joseph Campbell Companion* edited by Diane Osborn, (Harper Collins), 1991, page113).

15. See *Tantra: The Path of Ecstasy* by Georg Feuerstein, (Shambhala Publications), 1998, page 154.

16. See *Joseph Campbell Audio Series One: Volume 1 – Creativity in Oriental Mythology*; I.3.5 – 5, "Cakra of Purification", produced by the Joseph Campbell Foundation.

17. See *Joseph Campbell Audio Series One: Volume 1– Hinduism*; I.3.3– 6, "Learning the Lesson of Life", produced by the Joseph Campbell Foundation.

18. By contrast improper art is didactic: it teaches something, or tries to invoke some feeling or action from the observer. Improper art, in James Joyce's mind, includes all forms of advertising and commercial art. He called this form of art pornographical. See his novel *A Portrait of the Artist As a Young Man* by James Joyce, (Penguin Classics), 2003.

19. See *A Meister Eckhart* edited by Franz Pfeiffer, translated by C. De B. Evans (London: John M. Watkins, 1924 – 1931), No. XCVI ("Riddance"), I, 239.

20. Pope John XXII did eventually excommunicate Eckhart, but it was two years after Eckhart's death.

21. From the Heart Sutra of Mahayana Buddhism: "Gone, gone, gone beyond to the yonder shore".

22. See *Philosophies of India* by Heinrich Zimmer, (Princeton University Press), 1989, page 530.

23. See *The Gospel of Sri Ramakrishna, Abridged Version* by Swami Nikhilananda, 1996, (originally © 1942) pages 400 – 401.

24. The Gospel of Saint Thomas, verse 77.

25. See Stephen Batchelor's comments on rebirth in *Buddhism Without Beliefs*, (Riverhead Books), 1998, page 34 – 38.

26. *Understanding Our Mind* by Thich Nhat Hanh, (Parallax Press), 2006, page 242.

27. See *The Gospel of Sri Ramakrishna, Abridged Version* by Swami Nikhilananda, 1996, (originally © 1942) page 252

CHAPTER 20: GURU YOGA

1. This is a prayer from the *Yoga Taravalli* by Shankara circa ~ 800 C.E. It is translated by Pattabhi Jois [1915 - 2009 C.E.] as, "I worship the guru's lotus feet; Awakening the happiness of the Self

revealed; Beyond comparison, acting like the jungle physician; To pacify delusion from the poison of existence."*Yoga Mala* by Pattabhi Jois, (Eddie Stern/Patanjali Yoga Shala), 2000, page 15.

2. From *The Mirror of Yoga*, by Richard Freeman, © 2010 by Richard Freeman. Reprinted by arrangement with Shambhala Publications Inc., Boston, MA. *www.shambhala.com* pages 183.

3. Desikachar provided this interpretation of the story during a weeklong retreat, attended by the author, entitled *The Symbols of Yoga*. The version of the story related here is the author's rendition, not Desikachar's.

4. Curiously, for the Persians whose top god was named Ahura Mazda, their anti-gods were called *devils*. We obtain the word *devil* from the Sanskrit word *deva*. To the Persians, the Indian devas were devils, and to the Indians, the Persian god Ahura became their asuras. As a final quirk of language, even though the English word *devil* comes down to us via Persia, the English word *divine* stems from the same source: the Indian devas: these devils are divine.

5. As one might surmise, this story was written by men for men.

6. *The Yoga Tradition* by Georg Feuerstein, (Hohm Press), 2001, pages 11-12.

7. Versions of the myths of Goraksha and Matsyendra, along with what historical facts we have, can be found in *The Yoga Tradition* by Georg Feuerstein, (Hohm Press), 2001, pages 385–386.

8. The 14th-century Hatha Yoga Pradipika lists only 15 asanas and allocates only 38 stanzas out of 383 to postures, however, it does state that Shiva taught 84 asanas originally. The Gheranda Samhita, written perhaps late in the 17th century (the dates are disputed), listed 32 asanas. (See *The Yoga Tradition* by Georg Feuerstein, (Hohm Press), 2001, page 423.) For a more thorough review of the growth of Hatha Yoga as practiced today in the West, and how this Eastern practice was actually shaped by Western gymnastics and fitness regimes, see *Yoga Body* by Mark Singleton, (Oxford University Press), 2010.

9. See *The Mirror of Yoga*, by Richard Freeman, © 2010 by Richard Freeman, (Shambhala Publications Inc.), 2010, pages 185-186.

10. See Joseph Campbell, *Pathways to Bliss*. (New World Library), 2004, pages 58-59.

11. See *Joseph Campbell Audio Series One: Volume 1 – The Individual in Oriental Mythology*; I.1.2 – 2, "Individual Identity In the Occident and Orient", produced by the Joseph Campbell Foundation.dent and Orient", produced by the Joseph Campbell Foundation.

CHAPTER 21: LIVING WITH THE MYSTICAL

1. *Cat's Cradle* by Kurt Vonnegut, (Dial Press, an imprint of The Random House Publishing Group), 1998, page 265.

2. *Breakfast of Champions* by Kurt Vonnegut, (Dial Press, an imprint of The Random House Publishing Group), 1999, page 68.

3. Dao De Jing, Chapter 2. The text is attributed to the earliest Daoist sage, Lao Tzu, who supposedly lived in the sixth century B.C.E., however, scholars feel this legendary figure is more myth than man.

4. This is cited many times in the Brihadaranyaka Upanishad and other Indian sacred texts.

5. See *The Power of Myth* by Joseph Campbell and Bill Moyers, (Doubleday), 1988, page 62.

6. Kahlil Gibran from *The Voice of the Master*, translated by Anthony R Ferris, (Citadel), 2003, pages 58-59.

7. See *The Power of Myth* by Joseph Campbell and Bill Moyers, (Doubleday), 1988, page 1.

8. This particular form of trance is called *savikalpa Samadhi*: samadhi with trance: Higher than this state is *nirvikalpa Samadhi*, samadhi that doesn't require a trance. It is the ability to remain "in the center" and work on the "rim" simultaneously.

9. This is called *nirvikalpa Samadhi*.

10. *Touching Peace: Practicing the Art of Mindful Living* by Thich Nhat Hanh, (Parallax Press), 1992, page 1.

11. Ibid, page 122-123.

12. *The Essential Rumi* translation by Coleman Barks with John Moyne, (Harper Collins), 1995, page 281.

13. See *Joseph Campbell Audio Series One: Volume 1 – Personal Myth*; I.4.5 – 5, "Symbols of Childhood and Maturity", produced by the Joseph Campbell Foundation.

14. *Confession of a Buddhist Atheist* by Stephen Batchelor, (Spiegel & Grau), 2010, pages 62-65.

15. Stephen Batchelor - There is only one kôan and that is "you" – (~22:40 mark) Dharma Podcast #14 from Upaya.org, Recorded at Upaya Zen Center, Saturday Afternoon Sessions from "A Retreat on the Secular Buddha." Broadcast June 3, 2006 Retrieved from *http://www.upaya.org/dharma/dp-14-stephen-batchelor-there-is-only-one-koan-and-that-is-you*

16. *Modern Man in Search of a Soul* by Carl Jung, (Harcourt Harvest), 1965, Originally published in 1933, page 103.

17. *The Restaurant at the End of the Universe*, Episode 6 of the TV series *The Hitchhiker's Guide to the Galaxy* produced by the BBC and written by Douglas Adams: Copyright 1981.

18. From *The Mirror of Yoga*, by Richard Freeman, © 2010 by Richard Freeman. Reprinted by arrangement with Shambhala Publications Inc., Boston, MA. *www.shambhala.com*, page ix.

19. Jung wrote: "One feels much safer under the shadow of the Church, which serves as a fortress to protect us against God and his Spirit. It is very comforting to be assured by the Catholic Church that it "possesses" the Spirit, who assists regularly at its rites. Then one knows that he is well chained up. Protestantism is no less reassuring in that it represents the Spirit to us as something to be sought for, to be easily "drunk," even to be possessed." [From a 1954 letter from Carl Jung to Pere Lachat reproduced in *The Symbolic Life*, Volume 18 of *The Collected Works of C.G. Jung* translated by Gerhard Adler and R.F.C. Hull, (Princeton University Press), 1977, page 680.]

20. The Tantric saying *"nadevo devam arcayet"* means only a god can worship a god. See *Yoga: Immortality and Freedom* by Mircea Eliade, (Princeton University Press), 2009, page 208.

21. See *An Open Life: Joseph Campbell in Conversation with Michael Toms*, edited by Maher and Briggs, (Harper Collins), 1990, page 78.

22. This translation comes from the Darby Bible: many other translations omit Elohim and just say God, which minimizes the distinction noted here.

23. See *Joseph Campbell Audio Series One: Volume 1 – History of the Gods*; I.5.4 – 4, "Final Mystery of Being", produced by the Joseph Campbell Foundation.

24. *An Open Life: Joseph Campbell in Conversation with Michael Toms*, edited by Maher and Briggs, (Harper Collins), 1990, page 68.

25. Reprinted by permission from *Black Elk Speaks: Being the Life Story of a Holy Man of the Oglala Sioux, The Premier Edition* by John G. Neihardt, (State University of New York Press), © 2008, State University of New York, page 33. All rights reserved.

26. To the Sioux *Wakan-Tanka* is the name of the "Great Mystery"— all that is sacred or divine.

27. *The Sacred Pipe: Black Elk's Account of the Seven Rites of the Oglala Sioux* as told to Joseph Epes Brown, (University of Oklahoma Press), 1953, page 115.

28. *Happiness: Essential Mindfulness Practices* by Thich Nhat Hanh, (Parallax Press), 2009, page ix.

29. See *Joseph Campbell: The Hero's Journey – Joseph Campbell on His Life and Work*, edited by Phil Cousineau, (The Joseph Campbell Foundation, printed by New World Library), 1990, page 232.

30. *Pathways to Bliss* by Joseph Campbell, (New World Library), 2004, page 97, copyright © 2004; reprinted by permission of Joseph Campbell Foundation, *jcf.org*

EPILOGUE: TRANSCENDING BOUNDARIES

1. See "Apollo Astronaut Shares Story of NASA's Earthrise Photo": *http://www.nasa.gov/centers/johnson/home/earthrise.html*

2. *The Power of Myth* by Joseph Campbell and Bill Moyers, (Doubleday), 1988, page 56.

3. *The Revenge of Gaia: Earth's Climate Crisis and the Fate of Humanity* by James Lovelock, (Penguin Books), 2007, page xvi.

4. See *Joseph Campbell: The Hero's Journey – Joseph Campbell on His Life and Work*, edited by Phil Cousineau, (published by The Joseph Campbell Foundation, printed by New World Library), 1990, page 133.

5. Joseph Campbell, *Sukhavati*. San Anselmo, CA; The Joseph Campbell Foundation, 2005, 1:14:50, video.

Index

Page numbers followed by "n" indicate notes. Numbers in *italics* indicate photos or illustrations.

A